The Epilepsies 2

Blue Books of Practical Neurology
(Volumes 1–14 published as BIMR Neurology)

The Epilepsies 2

Edited by

Roger J. Porter, MD
Vice President, Clinical Pharmacology, Wyeth-Ayerst Research, Radnor,
Pennsylvania; Adjunct Professor of Neurology, University of Pennsylvania,
Philadelphia; Adjunct Professor of Pharmacology, Uniformed Services
University of the Health Sciences, F. Edward Hébert School of Medicine,
Bethesda, Maryland

and

David Chadwick, DM, FRCP
Professor of Neurology, Walton Centre for Neurology and Neurosurgery,
University of Liverpool, United Kingdom

Butterworth–Heinemann
Boston   Oxford   Johannesburg   Melbourne   New Delhi   Singapore

Library of Congress Cataloging-in-Publication Data

The epilepsies 2 / edited by Roger J. Porter, David Chadwick.
        p.   cm. -- (Blue books of practical neurology ; 18)
   Includes bibliographical references and index.
   ISBN 0-7506-9824-1
   1. Epilepsy.   I. Porter, Roger J., 1942- . II. Chadwick,
David. III. Series.
   [DNLM: 1. Epilepsy. W1 BU9749 v.18 1997 / WL 385 E6015 1997]
RC372.E653   1997
616.8'53--dc21
DNLM/DLC
for Library of Congress   96-50470
                                          CIP

British Library Cataloguing-in-Publication Data
A catalogue record for this book is available from the British Library.

The publisher offers special discounts on bulk orders of this book.
For more information, please contact:
Manager of Special Sales
Butterworth–Heinemann
313 Washington Street
Newton, MA 02158–1626
Tel: 617-928-2500
Fax: 617-928-2620

For information on all Butterworth–Heinemann medical publications available, contact our World Wide Web home page at: http://www.bh.com/med

10 9 8 7 6 5 4 3 2 1

Printed in the United States of America

Contents

Contributing Authors

Massimo Avoli, MD, PhD
Professor of Neurology, Neurosurgery, and Physiology, McGill University Faculty of Medicine, Montreal

Colin D. Binnie, MD, MA, BChir, FRCP
Professor of Clinical Neurophysiology, Department of Clinical Neurosciences, Kings College School of Medicine and Dentistry, London; Clinical Director of Clinical Neurophysiology, Kings College Hospital, London

David Chadwick, DM, FRCP
Professor of Neurology, Walton Centre for Neurology and Neurosurgery, University of Liverpool, United Kingdom

Robert J. DeLorenzo, MD, PhD, MPH
Professor and Chairman of Neurology, Virginia Commonwealth University, Richmond; Neurologist-in-Chief, Medical College of Virginia, Richmond

John DeToledo, MD
Clinical Associate Professor of Neurology, University of Miami School of Medicine

Orrin Devinsky, MD
Professor of Neurology, New York University School of Medicine; Chief of Neurology and Director, New York University-Hospital for Joint Diseases Epilepsy Center

Fritz E. Dreifuss, MB, FRCP, FRACP
Professor of Neurology, University of Virginia Health Sciences Center, Charlottesville

Olivier Dulac
Professor of Pediatrics, University René Descartes and Hospital St. Vincent de Paul, Paris

Frances Elmslie, MRCP
Clinical Research Fellow in Paediatrics, University College of London Medical School; Honorary Senior Registrar in Neurology, Great Ormond Street Hospital for Sick Children, London

R. M. Gardiner, MD, FRCP
Professor of Paediatrics, University College of London Medical School, London; Honorary Consultant Paediatrician, Paediatric Directorate, University College London Hospitals

Robert J. Gumnit, MD
President, Minnesota Comprehensive Epilepsy Program Epilepsy Care, Minneapolis; Clinical Professor of Neurology, Neurosurgery, and Pharmacy, University of Minnesota Medical School, Minneapolis

Martha J. Morrell, MD
Associate Professor of Neurology and Neurological Sciences, Stanford University School of Medicine, Stanford, California; Director, Stanford Comprehensive Epilepsy Center, Stanford University Medical Center, Stanford

John M. Pellock, MD
Professor of Neurology, Pediatrics, Pharmacy, and Pharmaceutics and Chairman of Child Neurology, Medical College of Virginia and Virginia Commonwealth University, Richmond; Director, Comprehensive Epilepsy Institute, Medical College of Virginia Hospitals, Richmond

Roger J. Porter, MD
Vice President, Clinical Pharmacology, Wyeth-Ayerst Research, Radnor, Pennsylvania; Adjunct Professor of Neurology, University of Pennsylvania, Philadelphia; Adjunct Professor of Pharmacology, Uniformed Services University of the Health Sciences, F. Edward Hébert School of Medicine, Bethesda, Maryland

R. Eugene Ramsay, MD
Professor of Neurology and Psychiatry, University of Miami School of Medicine

Alan Richens, MD, PhD, FRCP
Emeritus Professor of Pharmacology and Therapeutics, University of Wales College of Medicine, Cardiff, United Kingdom

A. James Rowan, MD
Professor and Vice-Chairman of Neurology, Mount Sinai School of Medicine, New York; Chief, Neurology Service, Bronx VA Medical Center, Bronx, New York

Simon Shorvon
Professor of Neurology, Institute of Neurology, University College, London University; Consultant Neurologist, The National Hospital for Neurology and Neurosurgery, London

Dennis D. Spencer, MD
Harvey and Kate Cushing Professor of Neurosurgery and Chief of Neurosurgery, Yale University School of Medicine and Yale-New Haven Hospital, New Haven, Connecticut

Susan S. Spencer, MD
Professor of Neurology, Yale University School of Medicine, New Haven, Connecticut; Attending Neurologist, Yale-New Haven Hospital, New Haven

Michael R. Sperling, MD
Clinical Professor of Neurology, Temple University School of Medicine, Philadelphia; Director, Comprehensive Epilepsy Center, Graduate Hospital, Philadelphia

William H. Theodore, MD
Chief, Clinical Epilepsy Section, National Institutes of Health, Bethesda, Maryland

Christopher M. Verity, MA, FRCP, BCh
Associate Lecturer, Clinical School, University of Cambridge, Cambridge, United Kingdom; Consultant Paediatric Neurologist, Addenbrooke's Hospital, Cambridge

Matthew Walker, MA, MRCP
Research Fellow, Department of Clinical Neurology, Institute of Neurology, University College, London University

H. Steve White, PhD
Associate Professor and Principal Scientist, Anticonvulsant Screening Project, Departments of Pharmacology and Toxicology, University of Utah, Salt Lake City

Series Preface

The *Blue Books of Practical Neurology* series is the new name for the *BIMR Neurology* series, which was itself the successor to the *Modern Trends in Neurology* series. As before, the volumes are intended for use by physicians who grapple with the problems of neurologic disorders on a daily basis, be they neurologists, neurologists in training, or those in related fields such as neurosurgery, internal medicine, psychiatry, and rehabilitation medicine.

Our purpose is to produce monographs on topics in clinical neurology in which progress through research has brought about new concepts of patient management. The subject of each monograph is selected by the Series Editors using two criteria: first, that there has been significant advance in knowledge in that area and, second, that such advances have been incorporated into new ways of managing patients with the disorders in question. This has been the guiding spirit behind each volume, and we expect it to continue. In effect, we emphasize research, both in the clinic and in the experimental laboratory, but principally to the extent that it changes our collective attitudes and practices in caring for those who are neurologically afflicted.

C. David Marsden
Arthur K. Asbury
Series Editors

Preface

Although a mere decade has passed since the first publication of *The Epilepsies* in this Butterworth–Heinemann series, striking advances in epilepsy research during these years have resulted in marked changes in the way we diagnose and treat our patients with epilepsy. In the past decade we have added, for example, magnetic resonance imaging as a near-routine diagnostic evaluation of difficult cases. Treatment regimens have likewise changed considerably, influenced by the addition to our armamentarium of a series of new antiepileptic drugs. Underlying these practical advances is a continuing expansion of our knowledge of the basic mechanisms of the epilepsies.

The Epilepsies 2 is a completely new volume. It fully reflects the excitement of new research in epilepsy and its application to the patient. The first three chapters are devoted to the science of antiepileptic drugs, neurophysiology, and genetics. The following three chapters provide the most recent understanding of the role of imaging and electroencephalographic techniques in the laboratory diagnosis of seizure disorders. Chapters 7 through 10 emphasize the latest clinical approach—the syndromic approach—to the diagnosis of epilepsy, in which we are now able to classify the patient and not just the seizure type. Chapters 11 through 13 address four of the latest antiepileptic drugs and their therapeutic role and are followed by four special chapters on difficult topics, such as status epilepticus and the pregnant patient with epilepsy. The last two chapters remind us that appropriate treatment is more than the prescription of antiseizure medications; as advocates for our patients we need to understand not only their internal psychological issues but how the external social system provides—or fails to provide—the needed support for a full and meaningful life.

We express our appreciation to the series editors and to Butterworth–Heinemann for their expertise and assistance in the creation of this volume. The book could not exist, of course, but for the collective sagacity and diligence of our chapter authors; we are very grateful for their efforts.

RJP
DC

xiii

The Epilepsies 2

1
Mechanisms of Antiepileptic Drugs

H. Steve White

There are more than 50 million epileptics worldwide. For some, seizures can be controlled with the standard antiepileptic drugs (AEDs), including phenytoin (PHT), carbamazepine (CBZ), the barbiturates and primidone, the benzodiazepines (BZDs), valproate (VPA), and ethosuximide (ESM). However, seizures in 25% of epilepsy patients remain resistant to these AEDs. Of these patients with refractory seizures, only a small percentage will become candidates for surgery and will have their seizures controlled by surgical intervention. Another category of epilepsy patients includes those whose seizures may be controlled, yet who experience chronic toxicity associated with their medications. Thus, there is a recognized need for more efficacious AEDs and AEDs with more favorable side-effect profiles.

Until 1993, physicians and neurologists had a relatively limited pharmacologic armamentarium at their disposal for managing patients with seizure disorders. The new era of AED therapy in the United States began in 1993 with the introduction of felbamate (FBM). Between July 1993, when FBM was approved, and December 1995, two new AEDs received market approval from the U.S. Food and Drug Administration (FDA): gabapentin (GBP) and lamotrigine (LTG). The newest AED to reach the U.S. marketplace is topiramate (TPM), which received final FDA approval on December 24, 1996. Four additional drugs, vigabatrin (VGB), tiagabine (TGB), oxcarbazepine (OCBZ), and zonisamide (ZNS), are registered in other countries and are under clinical investigation in the United States. A fifth drug undergoing clinical evaluation in the United States is remacemide (RCM). Potentially, all of these drugs represent new therapeutic options for patients suffering from epilepsy. More important, they provide renewed hope for patients with seizure disorders resistant to pharmacotherapy and patients whose seizures may be controlled but only at the expense of serious adverse effects associated with the taking of their medication.

Many of the new drugs differ from the standard AEDs in their proposed mechanism or mechanisms of action. This may explain their apparent efficacy in clinical trials in which they are added to therapeutic regimens that often include one

1

or more of the established AEDs. After a brief review of the preclinical models used in the search for novel AEDs and some mention of the mechanisms underlying burst firing, the remaining discussion focuses on the proposed mechanisms of action of currently available AEDs and those investigational AEDs that may soon become available.

PRECLINICAL IDENTIFICATION OF NOVEL ANTIEPILEPTIC DRUGS

Screening for Efficacy in Animal Seizure Models

For the most part, the new AEDs currently available or under clinical development resulted from the routine screening of thousands of chemically divergent structures. Indeed, most of these drugs were ushered into the present arena in part by the efforts of the Antiepileptic Drug Development Program sponsored by the National Institute of Neurological Disorders and Stroke (NINDS), which began screening candidate AEDs in 1974. This program, which represents a collaborative agreement between government, the pharmaceutical industry, and academia, has screened almost 19,000 chemical entities in the maximal electroshock (MES) and subcutaneous pentylenetetrazol (scPTZ) tests.[1]

A number of widely different animal seizure models have been used in the search for new and novel anticonvulsant drugs to be used in the treatment of human epilepsy. At present, no single laboratory test will in itself establish the presence or absence of anticonvulsant activity or fully predict the clinical potential of a test substance. Of the many available animal models, the MES and scPTZ tests still represent the most commonly used models for the routine screening and identification of new anticonvulsant drugs. When conducted properly, these two tests are probably the best validated of all the in vivo seizure models (for a review and discussion see reference 2). Both tests have been validated in human studies and have, in essence, withstood the test of time. The electroencephalographic (EEG) record and resultant behavioral seizure after electroconvulsive shock therapy and PTZ administration in humans were found to be remarkably similar to those observed in animals. Furthermore, it was recognized early on that these tests display distinctly different pharmacologic profiles. For example, MES seizures could be blocked by PHT and phenobarbital (PB) but not trimethadione,[3] whereas PTZ seizures could be blocked by trimethadione and PB but not by PHT.[4] These observations, coupled with the finding that trimethadione was effective against petit mal attacks and ineffective in or worsened grand mal attacks,[5] provided the clinical correlation between anticonvulsant efficacy against human seizures and maximal and threshold seizures in animal models (Table 1.1).

These findings led to the suggestion that the MES test would identify drugs that may be active clinically against generalized tonic-clonic seizures, whereas the scPTZ test predicted clinical efficacy against generalized absence epilepsy (see Table 1.1). With one exception (i.e., PB), there does appear to be a reasonable correlation between the preclinical and clinical profiles of the established AEDs, such as PHT, CBZ, VPA, ESM, the BZDs, and PB. In the case of PB, it is effective in rodents against clonic seizures induced by the scPTZ test but is ineffec-

Table 1.1   Correlation between experimental animal models and clinical utility of established antiepileptic drugs

Experimental model	Generalized seizures		Partial seizures	Drugs
	Tonic and/or clonic	Absence		
MES (tonic extension)	+	—	—	CBZ, PHT, VPA, PB
scPTZ (clonic seizures)	—	+	—	VPA, ESM, PB, BZD
Electrical kindling (focal seizures)	—	—	+	CBZ, PHT, VPA, PB, BZD

MES = maximal electroshock; scPTZ = subcutaneous pentylenetetrazol; CBZ = carbamazepine; PHT = phenytoin; VPA = valproate; PB = phenobarbital; ESM = ethosuximide; BZD = benzodiazepine.

tive in humans for the treatment of generalized absence seizures. For this reason, the scPTZ test may be more useful for identifying drugs effective against myoclonic seizures.

In addition to the MES and scPTZ tests, the preclinical profile of most investigational AEDs is differentiated further on the basis of additional in vivo seizure models. Of the numerous animal seizure models available, the kindling model provides useful information regarding the potential ability of an investigational drug to limit focal seizures originating from discrete limbic brain regions (e.g., amygdala, hippocampus) and is thought to represent a model of complex partial seizures.[6, 7] This conclusion is supported in part by the pharmacologic profile of the kindling model. As summarized in Table 1.1, drugs effective against human partial seizures are also effective against fully kindled seizures in animals. Furthermore, the kindling model probably represents the most suitable model available for evaluating the ability of an investigational substance to prevent the acquisition of a seizure focus (i.e., antiepileptic versus anticonvulsant potential).

The MES test is thought to identify drugs that prevent seizure spread and the scPTZ test is thought to identify compounds that elevate seizure threshold. Beyond this limited description, very little can be said about the molecular mechanism of action of drugs active in these two animal models. Nonetheless, attempts to correlate the anticonvulsant profile of the standard AEDs with their proposed mechanisms of action reveals certain interesting trends (Table 1.2). For example, MES-induced tonic extension seizures can be blocked by drugs that act primarily by inhibiting voltage-sensitive Na^+ channels (PHT and CBZ) and in some instances by drugs that enhance gamma-aminobutyric acid (GABA)-mediated inhibitory neurotransmission at the $GABA_A$ receptor (i.e., PB and perhaps VPA). In contrast, clonic seizures induced by scPTZ are not blocked by Na^+ channel blockers but are blocked by drugs that reduce T-type calcium currents (ESM) and drugs that enhance inhibitory neurotransmission mediated by $GABA_A$ receptors (BZDs, PB, and perhaps VPA). Drugs with multiple mechanisms of action, such as VPA and perhaps PB, are active in both seizure tests. Fully kindled seizures are blocked by all of the drugs except ESM. Thus, ESM displays the narrowest and VPA the broadest preclinical profile of the standard AEDs, which is a finding that correlates with their clinical utility.

Table 1.2 Correlation between experimental animal models and proposed mechanisms of action of antiepileptic drugs (AEDs)

Experimental model	Established AEDs	Proposed mechanism of action
MES (tonic extension)	PHT, CBZ, VPA	Limit sustained repetitive firing by inhibiting voltage-sensitive Na^+ channels
scPTZ (clonus)	BZDs, PB, ESM, VPA	Enhance GABA Reduce T-type Ca^{2+} currents
Electrical kindling (expression)	PHT, CBZ, VPA, BZDs, PB	Multiple

MES = maximal electroshock; scPTZ = subcutaneous pentylenetetrazol; PHT = phenytoin; CBZ = carbamazepine; VPA = valproate; BZDs = benzodiazepines; PB = phenobarbital; GABA = gamma-aminobutyric acid.

It is important to note that a number of the newer AEDs, some of which appear to possess novel mechanisms of action, have been demonstrated to be active in one or more of these models. In this respect, as long as both tests are used in the routine screening for efficacy, it is not likely that novel anticonvulsant drugs will be missed. This is not meant to imply that such an approach should limit additional in vivo testing to differentiate further the anticonvulsant profile of new AEDs.

Mechanism-Based Antiepileptic Drug Development

The current era of AED development is driven largely by a greater understanding of the molecular mechanisms underlying seizure disorders. The mechanistic approach has, for the most part, been directed at development of drugs that enhance inhibition or reduce excitation. Within the central nervous system (CNS), inhibitory neurotransmission is mediated primarily by GABA. Evidence implicating a role for GABA in the epileptic process is provided by the observation that drugs that reduce GABAergic tone by inhibiting $GABA_A$ receptors (e.g., bicuculline) or block the chloride ionophore coupled to $GABA_A$ receptors (e.g., picrotoxin) induce seizures in laboratory animals. Furthermore, experimental seizures in animals and seizures in certain human epileptic syndromes can be reduced by drugs that potentiate GABAergic neurotransmission (e.g., BZDs and barbiturates). In addition to directly modulating the GABA receptor, drugs can enhance inhibition by preventing reuptake of neuronally released GABA and by blocking GABA metabolism. As discussed below, these two strategic approaches have led to the development of two clinically effective anticonvulsants (i.e., TGB and VGB).

Conversely, ongoing research efforts have led to a greater understanding of the processes underlying fast excitatory neurotransmission in the brain that is mediated primarily by glutamate and other excitatory amino acids.[8] Once released from presynaptic nerve terminals, glutamate activates three ionotropic receptor types: the α-amino-2,3-dihydro-5-methyl-3-oxo-4-isoxazolepropanoic acid (AMPA), kainate, and *N*-methyl-D-aspartate (NMDA) receptors.[9, 10] Each of these receptors is composed of families of subtypes that combine to form functional receptors with distinct biophysical and pharmacologic properties. There are four AMPA receptor subunits ($GluR_1$–$GluR_4$) that are differentially distributed

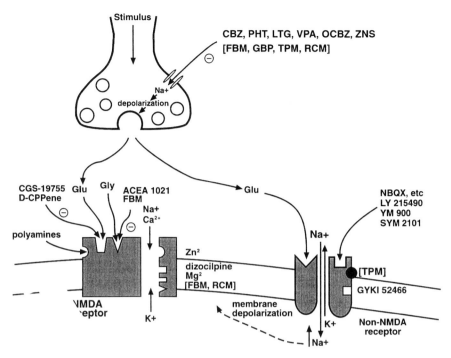

Figure 1.1   Proposed mechanisms of action of established and new antiepileptic drugs (AEDs) at the excitatory synapse mediated by glutamate. Several of the established and newer AEDs may act by blocking neuronal release of glutamate through an inhibitory effect on voltage-sensitive Na^+ channels. Once released from the presynaptic terminal, glutamate can bind to *N*-methyl-D-aspartate (NMDA) and non-NMDA receptors. Glycine is required as a coagonist at the NMDA receptor, which is coupled to an associated ion channel permeable to Na^+, K^+, and Ca^{2+}. The NMDA receptor complex possesses multiple modulatory sites that are targeted by several new generation AEDs. Drugs can decrease NMDA function competitively by binding to the NMDA receptor (e.g., D-CPPene or CGS-19755) or the strychnine-insensitive glycine receptor (e.g., ACEA 1021 and felbamate [FBM]) or noncompetitively by binding to a site within the open channel (e.g., dizocilpine, FBM, and remacemide [RCM]). Glutamate can also activate an ion channel coupled to the non-NMDA α-amino-2,3-dihydro-5-methyl-3-oxo-4-isoxazolepropanoic acid (AMPA)/kainate receptor that is permeable to Na^+ and K^+. Activation of the non-NMDA receptor by glutamate provides sufficient depolarization to relieve the Mg^{2+}-dependent block of the NMDA receptor. Drugs can block non-NMDA responses competitively (e.g., 6-nitro-7-sulphamoylbenzo[f]quinoxaline-2,3-dione [NBQX], etc.) or noncompetitively (GYKI 52466). Kainate-evoked currents can also be blocked by the new generation AED topiramate (TPM) (see text for further discussion). (CBZ = carbamazepine; PHT = phenytoin; LTG = lamotrigine; VPA = valproate; OCBZ = oxcarbazepine; ZNS = zonisamide; GBP = gabapentin.)

throughout the CNS. AMPA receptors expressing $GluR_2$ are permeable to Na^+ and K^+ (Figure 1.1) and are probably involved in mediating fast glutamatergic neuro-transmission. AMPA receptors lacking $GluR_2$ subunits display increased Ca^{2+} permeability and may be involved in certain pathologic states, such as ischemia[11] and epilepsy.[12] In addition, ongoing investigations suggest that direct activation of the $GluR_3$ subunit by $GluR_3$ antibodies contributes to drug-resistant seizures associated with Rasmussen's encephalitis.[13, 14] These two findings represent the first evidence linking an experimental disorder to the abnormal expression or altered regulation of a particular receptor subunit. Furthermore, they suggest that abnormal glutamatergic activity, abnormal subunit regulation, or both may contribute to synaptic reorganization in chronic epileptic foci that results in a pharmaco-resistant state.[15] The day will likely come when we see the introduction of drugs for epilepsy and other CNS disorders that target specific receptor subunits and the processes controlling their regulation.

The NMDA receptor is also composed of two major subunit families, i.e., $NMDAR_1$ and $NMDAR_2$ (see references 9, 16, and 17 for reviews). Thus far, eight splice variants have been identified for the $NMDAR_1$ subfamily. The $NMDAR_2$ subfamily is composed of four subunits ($NMDAR_{2A}$–$NMDAR_{2D}$). The NMDA receptor is coupled to high-conductance cationic channels permeable to Na^+, K^+, and Ca^{2+} and is activated by the combined presence of glutamate and glycine, which binds to a strychnine-insensitive site and serves as a coagonist (see reference 18). At resting membrane potentials, the NMDA receptor is blocked by physiologic concentrations of Mg^{2+}. Even in the presence of sufficient agonists, depolarization of the postsynaptic membrane by AMPA receptor activation is required to relieve the voltage-dependent Mg^{2+} block and render the channel ion-permeable. The NMDA receptor complex, which expresses a number of pharmacologically distinct modulatory sites (see Figure 1.1), has been implicated in a variety of normal and pathologic processes, including long-term potentiation, learning and memory, chronic neurodegenerative disorders, ischemia/hypoxia-induced neurotoxicity, and seizure disorders (see reference 9 for a review).

The evidence supporting a role for glutamate in the initiation and propagation of seizure activity is extensive. Antagonists aimed at NMDA and non-NMDA receptors and associated modulatory sites (see Figure 1.1 for specific examples) have been demonstrated to possess anticonvulsant activity in several different animal models of generalized seizures. However, in the kindled rat model of partial seizures, NMDA antagonists are not only ineffective in blocking expression of focal seizures, they also produce psychotomimetic-like behavioral side effects.[19] Similar disappointing results have been obtained in the clinic. For example, limited add-on clinical trials conducted on patients with drug-resistant complex partial seizures with one competitive NMDA antagonist and two noncompetitive antagonists had to be discontinued because of lack of efficacy and intolerable neurologic side effects (see reference 20 for a review and references). Thus, in this particular example, the mechanistic approach has not always led to a viable, clinically effective AED.

Molecular biology has provided new insight into the molecular conformation of glutamate receptors and will undoubtedly lead to the development of more efficacious and less toxic pure glutamate antagonists. It is still too early to assess whether drugs directed at the strychnine-insensitive glycine site or competitive and noncompetitive antagonists directed at the non-NMDA receptor will possess a more favorable efficacy and side-effect profile. As discussed below, it appears that three of the newer AEDs (i.e., FBM, TPM, and RCM) act in part by modulating glutamate receptor function (see Figure 1.1). In contrast to pure antagonists, these three drugs appear to function as low-affinity antagonists at the NMDA (FBM and RCM) and non-NMDA (TPM) receptor.

MECHANISMS UNDERLYING BURST FIRING

The exact cellular mechanisms underlying interictal and ictal events are not known; however, there are certain essential elements that are subject to regulation by anticonvulsant drugs. Although it is not the purpose of this chapter to provide an exhaustive description of the cellular and anatomic substrates of burst firing, a brief review of the key features will provide a framework for the discussion that follows (for more in-depth reviews see references 15, 21, and 22).

On a surface EEG tracing, the interictal event may be manifested as a spike, poly-spike, or spike and wave and occurs when a population of neurons is activated synchronously as a result of an imbalance in local inhibitory and excitatory processes. The intracellular correlate of the interictal spike is the paroxysmal depolarization shift (PDS), which is characterized by membrane depolarization that is sufficient to evoke a train of action potentials that is terminated by membrane hyperpolarization. A number of different inhibitory processes can contribute to the hyperpolarizing potential that ultimately limits the PDS. These may include activation of $GABA_A$ and $GABA_B$ receptors, voltage-activated K^+ channels, and Ca^{2+}-dependent K^+ currents (see reference 21 for a review and references). Thus, an ictal event can result when there is a sustained burst of spikes and depolarization that is not limited by sufficient "inhibitory" events. Inhibitory processes can be reduced as a result of an increase in extracellular K^+, which reduces the hyperpolarization resulting from an activation of K^+ channels or by reducing GABAergic neurotransmission. Because GABA-mediated inhibition is frequency dependent, it is reduced by repetitive stimulation. In contrast, excitatory pathways are often enhanced by repetitive stimulation. Thus, excessive stimulation of normal synaptic pathways, if not interrupted, can lead to reduced inhibition and enhanced excitation. If sufficient, these processes may contribute to a transition between the interictal event and a seizure and ultimately the spread of epileptiform activity from a seizure focus.

The ionic and cellular events underlying interictal and ictal firing have been studied most extensively in slice preparations in vitro. Within the hippocampus, spontaneous interictal spikes can be elicited by the application of a convulsant drug. A typical burst may consist of a calcium-dependent depolarizing potential underlying a series of sodium-dependent action potentials. Sustained depolarization can lead to activation of high-threshold voltage-dependent calcium channels that may result in a series of calcium-dependent action potentials followed by hyperpolarization.

To propagate burst discharges to other brain regions, additional mechanisms are required. In the hippocampus, bursts generated in the CA3 and CA2 pyramidal cells are propagated via the Schaffer collaterals to produce synchronous burst firing of CA1 cells. Within the thalamus, thalamic relay neurons are believed to rhythmically drive cortical neurons. The firing pattern of the thalamic relay neurons is determined in part by a balance between voltage-activated calcium currents and GABAergic inhibition. The low-threshold calcium current (T-type) plays a critical role in generating the characteristic 3-Hz spike and wave EEG pattern seen in generalized absence seizures.

Ultimately, there are numerous molecular mechanisms through which drugs can alter neuronal excitability and thereby limit or control seizure activity. However, three primary mechanisms appear to be targeted by most of the established anti-convulsants.[23] For example, drugs that block sustained high-frequency firing through an effect on voltage-sensitive Na^+ channels can disrupt burst firing, drugs that enhance GABA-mediated neurotransmission can elevate seizure threshold, and drugs that reduce voltage-dependent low-threshold (T-type) Ca^{2+} currents in thala-mocortical neurons can interrupt the thalamic oscillatory firing patterns associated with absence seizures. Likewise, drugs that reduce glutamatergic-mediated excita-tion can be expected to reduce burst firing elicited by synaptic stimulation. Although not a target of standard AEDs, this mechanism does appear to be targeted by some of the newer AEDs, including FBM, TPM, and RCM.

MECHANISMS OF ACTION OF STANDARD ANTIEPILEPTIC DRUGS

The remaining discussion focuses primarily on the proposed mechanisms of action of the standard AEDs (PHT, CBZ, VPA, and ESM, and the BZDs and bar-biturates) and the newer AEDs (FBM, GBP, LTG, TPM, VGB, TGB, OCBZ, RCM, and ZNS). Depending on the concentration used, multiple effects have been reported for most of these drugs; however, this discussion will be limited to those effects that are thought to result at therapeutic concentrations and thereby are presumed to represent their primary mechanism of action. Excellent reviews have been published in recent years and should be consulted for more in-depth discussion and references.[22–25]

Phenytoin and Carbamazepine

In animal seizure models, PHT and CBZ possess relatively narrow anticonvul-sant profiles. They are effective against tonic extension seizures induced by a number of stimuli, including electroshock, and several different chemoconvul-sants.[1, 26] Both AEDs are also effective in a number of electrical kindling mod-els.[24] These effects correlate quite well with their clinical effectiveness against generalized tonic-clonic and complex partial seizures, respectively. PHT and CBZ are ineffective against clonic seizures induced by PTZ and bicuculline. CBZ differs from PHT in that it is effective against clonic seizures induced by picrotoxin. Whether this effect contributes to a greater efficacy of CBZ over PHT in some epilepsy patients is not known.

PHT and CBZ have been shown to block post-tetanic potentiation (PTP), a process in which high-frequency stimulation results in transiently enhanced responsiveness to a subsequent single stimulation (for a review and references see reference 24). PTP has been suggested to contribute to facilitation of local exci-tatory discharges and enhanced spread from a seizure focus. In this respect, inhi-bition of PTP by PHT and CBZ may underlie their ability to limit seizure spread.

Table 1.3   Comparative mechanistic profile between established and newer antiepileptic drugs (AEDs)[a]

Site of action	Established	Newer
Limit sustained repetitive firing (Na$^+$ channel)	PHT, CBZ, VPA	FBM, GBP,[b] LTG, TPM, OCBZ, RCM, ZNS
Enhance GABA	BZDs, PB, [VPA]	VGB,[c] TGB,[d] FBM, GBP, TPM, [ZNS]
Reduce T-type Ca^{2+} channels	ESM, [VPA]	ZNS
Reduce glutamate-mediated excitation	[PB]	FBM, TPM, RCM

PHT = phenytoin; CBZ = carbamazepine; VPA = valproate; GABA = gamma-aminobutyric acid; BZDs = benzodi-azepines; PB = phenobarbital; ESM = ethosuximide; GBP = gabapentin; LTG = lamotrigine; TPM = topiramate; OCBZ = oxcarbazepine; RCM = remacemide; ZNS = zonisamide; TGB = tiagabine; FBM = felbamate; VGB = vigabatrin.
[a]For drugs enclosed in brackets, the reported effect requires verification; relevance to AED effect not fully understood.
[b]Mechanism not clearly established; binds to unique site; requires prolonged exposure.
[c]Inhibits GABA metabolism.
[d]Blocks neuronal and glial uptake of synaptically released GABA.

The cellular mechanisms by which these two drugs attenuate PTP and ulti-mately block seizure spread are not clearly understood. Many mechanisms of action have been ascribed to PHT since its identification by Putnam and Merritt in 1937.[27] The most appealing one is related to their ability to limit sustained repetitive firing of action potentials in neurons in culture (Figure 1.1, Tables 1.2 and 1.3).[28, 29] This effect, which occurs at free concentrations found in plasma of epilepsy patients being treated with PHT and CBZ, correlates with their ability to block MES-induced seizures in animals and tonic-clonic seizures in humans.

It is generally believed that the voltage-sensitive Na$^+$ channel underlies the ability of neurons to fire repetitively. As such, anticonvulsants that inhibit repeti-tive firing are likely to exert an effect on voltage-sensitive Na$^+$ channels. Indeed, in a number of studies, PHT and CBZ have been found to exert an inhibitory effect on voltage-gated Na$^+$ channels that is use- and voltage-dependent.[30–33] Thus, their effect on Na$^+$ currents is enhanced by sustained depolarization and high-frequen-cy firing. These latter properties account for the unique ability of PHT, CBZ, and other voltage-dependent Na$^+$ channel blockers to limit high-frequency firing characteristic of epileptic discharges without significantly altering normal patterns of neuronal firing.

In mammalian myelinated nerve fibers, PHT and CBZ have been demonstrat-ed to produce a shift in the steady-state inactivation curve to more negative volt-ages,[34] effectively reducing the degree of depolarization required to inactivate Na$^+$ channels. In addition, both drugs delayed the rate of Na$^+$ channel recovery from inactivation. Slight differences between PHT and CBZ in time dependence for the frequency-dependent block have been noted; it has been suggested that these subtle differences may account for differences in anticonvulsant efficacy between these drugs.

Voltage-, frequency-, and time-dependent inactivation of Na$^+$ channels by PHT has also been confirmed in isolated rat hippocampal neurons and *Xenopus* oocytes injected with human brain messenger ribonucleic acid (mRNA).[35, 36] All of these studies provide strong experimental evidence supporting an interaction of PHT and CBZ with the voltage-dependent Na^+ channel. By stabilizing the Na^+ channel in its inactive form and slowing its rate of recovery from inactivation, both drugs can prevent sustained repetitive firing evoked by prolonged depolarization, such as that found in an epileptic focus.

Ethosuximide

The preclinical and clinical profile of ESM differs markedly from that of PHT and CBZ. In experimental seizure models, ESM is primarily effective against clonic seizures induced by the chemoconvulsants PTZ, bicuculline, and picrotoxin. It is ineffective against tonic seizures induced by MES.[1, 26] Thus, in contrast to PHT, ESM is primarily effective in raising seizure threshold. In human epilepsy, ESM is effective against generalized absence and lacks efficacy in patients with generalized tonic-clonic and partial epilepsy. In this respect, it would not be too surprising to find that ESM possesses a different mechanism of action than PHT or CBZ.

Despite extensive investigation by numerous investigators, the mechanism of action of ESM remained somewhat elusive until 1989, when it was shown to reduce low-threshold, T-type, Ca^{2+} currents (see Tables 1.2 and 1.3) in thalamic neurons.[37, 38] This effect of ESM, which is produced at clinically relevant concentrations, is thought to represent the primary mechanism by which it controls absence epilepsy. Activation of T-channels in thalamic relay neurons generates low threshold Ca^{2+} spikes that are thought to contribute to the abnormal thalamocortical rhythmicity that underlies the 3-Hz spike and wave EEG discharge of absence epilepsy. ESM and dimethadione, the active metabolite of the antiabsence drug trimethadione, block positive currents in a voltage-dependent manner.[39]

Valproic Acid

Among the standard AEDs, VPA has perhaps the broadest preclinical and clinical profile. It is effective in a wide variety of animal seizure models, including tonic extension seizures induced by MES, clonic seizures induced by PTZ, bicuculline and picrotoxin, and electrically kindled focal seizures.[1] VPA is effective in humans against partial and generalized seizures. This broad profile of VPA can probably be accounted for by multiple mechanisms of action.

VPA, like PHT and CBZ, blocks sustained repetitive firing (see Figure 1.1, Tables 1.2 and 1.3) of mouse central neurons in culture[40] and rat hippocampal slices.[41] Results from considerable in vitro investigations support an effect of VPA on voltage-sensitive Na^+ channels. For example, VPA has been found in isolated *Xenopus laevis* myelinated nerves to inhibit Na^+ currents.[42] Furthermore, a reduction in Na^+ current was observed with VPA in neocortical neurons in vitro.[43] In rat hippocampal neurons, VPA decreased peak Na^+ currents in a voltage-dependent manner and produced a 10-mV leftward shift in the Na^+ inactivation curve.[44] Taken together, these results support an action for VPA at the voltage-sensitive Na^+ channel and provide a mechanistic basis for its ability to inhibit MES seizures in animal models and generalized tonic-clonic seizures in humans.

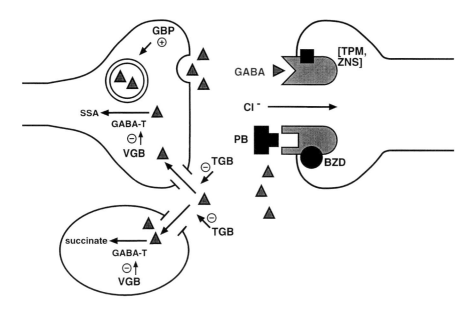

Figure 1.2   Interaction of established and newer antiepileptic drugs (AEDs) at the gamma-aminobutyric acid A (GABA$_A$) inhibitory synapse. Once released, GABA binds to the GABA$_A$ or GABA$_B$ (not shown) receptors. The GABA$_A$ receptor and its associated allosteric binding sites are coupled to a chloride-permeable ion channel. AEDs can enhance GABA at the postsynaptic receptor by increasing channel opening and burst frequency (e.g., benzodiazepines [BZDs] and topiramate [TPM]) or by increasing channel open and burst duration (e.g., phenobarbital [PB]). AEDs can also enhance GABA-mediated neurotransmission by blocking neuronal and glial reuptake of synaptically released GABA (e.g., tiagabine [TGB]). Vigabatrin (VGB) increases GABA levels within neuronal terminals and surrounding glial cells by irreversibly inhibiting GABA aminotransferase (GABA-T), which metabolizes GABA to succinic acid semialdehyde (SSA). Gabapentin (GBP) has also been observed to increase brain GABA levels through a yet to be defined mechanism. (ZNS = zonisamide.)

However, this effect alone is not sufficient to explain the broad preclinical and clinical profile of VPA. VPA has been observed to produce a modest reduction of T-type Ca^{2+} currents in primary afferent neurons,[45] to elevate whole brain GABA levels, and to potentiate GABA responses at high concentrations (see reference 24). These latter effects may contribute, either singly or in concert, to the anticonvulsant efficacy of VPA.

Benzodiazepines and Barbiturates

Once released from GABAergic nerve terminals, the inhibitory neurotransmitter GABA binds to GABA$_A$ and GABA$_B$ receptors. The GABA$_A$ receptor complex is a multimeric macromolecular protein that forms a chloride-selective ion pore (Figure 1.2). Thus far, multiple binding sites for GABA, anticonvulsant BZDs, barbiturates, neurosteroids, convulsant beta-carbolines, and the chemoconvulsant picrotoxin have been identified (for a review see reference 46). The $GABA_B$ receptor is coupled via a GTP-binding protein to Ca^{2+} or K^+ channels but does not form an ionophore and does not appear to contribute to the anticonvulsant action of BZDs or barbiturates. Thus, the principal anticonvulsant action of the BZDs and barbiturates is thought to be related to their ability to enhance inhibitory neurotransmission by allosterically modulating the $GABA_A$ receptor complex.

Although it is beyond the scope of this chapter to provide a complete review of the molecular biology of the $GABA_A$ receptor, some discussion is appropriate (for a more detailed description see reference 46). The $GABA_A$ receptor is thought to be a heteropentameric glycoprotein. Rapidly evolving molecular biology studies have thus far identified at least five distinctly different subunits (α, β, γ, δ, and ρ), most of which have multiple subtypes ($\alpha1–\alpha6$, $\beta1–\beta4$, $\gamma1–\gamma3$, and $\rho1–\rho2$) that can combine to form functional $GABA_A$ receptors. Although the exact conformation, stoichiometry, and number of GABA receptor isoforms is not known, the differential expression and distribution of various subunits within the neurons of the CNS is thought to confer pharmacologic specificity to drugs acting on the $GABA_A$ receptor.

GABA receptor current can be enhanced by increasing channel conductance, open and burst frequency, open and burst duration, or combinations of these variables. The BZDs and barbiturates enhance GABA-evoked current by binding to allosteric regulatory sites on the $GABA_A$ receptor.[47] Results from several studies have demonstrated that the principal effect of the barbiturates is to increase the mean channel open duration without affecting channel conductance or opening frequency.[48, 49] In contrast, the binding of a BZD to its allosterically coupled binding site enhances GABA receptor current by increasing opening frequency without affecting open or burst duration.[49–52]

Results from reconstitution experiments wherein specific GABA receptor subunits were transiently expressed in *Xenopus* oocytes, Chinese hamster ovary cells, or human embryonic kidney cells have provided a molecular basis for the differential regulation of GABA receptor current by these two classes of drugs. These studies, which were conducted in a variety of laboratories, have suggested that the allosteric regulatory site conferring barbiturate sensitivity appears to be contained in the α and β subunits.[53, 54] Whereas GABA receptors formed from α-1 and β-1 subunits are barbiturate-sensitive, they are BZD-insensitive.[53, 55] BZD sensitivity is restored when the γ-2 subunit is coexpressed with α-1 and β-1 subunits.[55] Thus, transient coexpression of the γ-2, α-1, and β-1 subunits in human embryonic kidney cells results in fully functional GABA receptors that are sensitive to the BZDs, barbiturates, beta-carbolines, and picrotoxin.

In addition to the γ subunit, the α subunit also plays an important role in determining BZD receptor pharmacologic properties. For example, sensitivity to the prototypical BZDs, diazepam and flunitrazepam, the beta-carbolines, the inverse agonist Ro 15-4513, and the antagonist flumazenil is influenced by the specific α subunit expressed. The original classification, which included type I and type II BZD receptor subtypes, has been further subdivided into type I, IIA, IIB, and III on the basis of whether α-1 (type I), α-2 and α-3 (type IIA), α-5 (type IIB), or α-4 and α-6 (type III) subunits are expressed (for reviews see references 55–57).

MECHANISMS OF ACTION OF NEW ANTIEPILEPTIC DRUGS

Felbamate

FBM (2-phenyl-1,3-propanediol dicarbamate) received FDA approval in mid-1993 and was the first new AED approved in the United States since 1978. Results from preclinical studies conducted by the NINDS Anticonvulsant Drug Development Program demonstrated that FBM possessed a broad anticonvulsant profile in animal seizure models.[58, 59] It is effective against tonic extension seizures induced by MES and the glutamate agonists NMDA and quisqualic acid. FBM is also active against clonic seizures induced by a number of chemoconvulsants. In syndrome-specific animal models of partial seizures, FBM has been found to reduce the seizure severity in corneal-kindled rats and PTZ-kindled rats and to raise the seizure threshold in amygdala-kindled rats.[60] Seizure frequency was reduced in monkeys made epileptic with focal injections of aluminum hydroxide. Additional studies have found it to be effective against pilocarpine-induced status. These results suggest a broad anticonvulsant profile in the clinic. In addition to its anticonvulsant properties, FBM has also been demonstrated to possess neuroprotectant properties in vitro and in vivo. For example, it has been demonstrated to inhibit hypoxia-induced injury in hippocampal slice preparations[61] and to produce marked neuroprotectant effects in neonatal rats in a rat model of hypoxia-ischemia when administered before[62] or after[63] the hypoxic-ischemic insult. FBM has also been demonstrated to possess neuroprotectant properties after kainic acid–induced status epilepticus.[64] In clinical trials, FBM demonstrated efficacy in patients with partial seizures and seizures secondarily generalized, including Lennox-Gastaut syndrome.[65] However, the current clinical utility of FBM is limited because of a high risk for hematologic and hepatic toxicity. Currently, the risk of aplastic anemia and liver disease has to be weighed against the potential benefit in seizure control.

From a mechanistic point of view, FBM remains a scientifically interesting AED. Like VPA, FBM is likely to possess multiple mechanisms of action that work in concert to support its broad preclinical and clinical anticonvulsant profile as well as its neuroprotectant action. The precise mechanism of action of FBM has not been clearly elucidated; however, it has been found to produce several effects that support its anticonvulsant and neuroprotectant actions (see Figure 1.1, Table 1.3). FBM reduces sustained repetitive firing in mouse spinal cord neurons in a concentration-dependent manner.[59] This effect of FBM is consistent with its ability to block tonic extension seizures in the MES test and occurs at concentrations ($IC_{50} \approx 300$ μmol/liter) that are achieved in the brains of animals receiving anticonvulsant and neuroprotectant doses of FBM[66, 67] and the brains of epilepsy patients treated with FBM.[68] Although suggestive of an interaction with voltage-dependent Na^+ channels, it remains to be determined whether FBM directly inhibits Na^+ currents in a voltage- and use-dependent manner like PHT and CBZ.

An effect on sustained repetitive firing in and of itself cannot totally explain FBM's broad preclinical profile. Investigations from several independent laboratories do not support a direct interaction between FBM and the NMDA-receptor ionophore. For example, FBM does not bind to the MK-801 binding site of the NMDA receptor-ionophore in mouse cortex and hippocampal membranes,[59] nor does it interact with the dextromethorphan binding site in guinea pig brain.[69] FBM can be further differentiated from competitive and noncompetitive NMDA antagonists by its inability to inhibit NMDA-induced lethality.[70]

Subsequent investigations have examined the possible interaction between FBM and two modulatory sites on the NMDA-receptor ionophore—i.e., the polyamine recognition site and the strychnine-insensitive glycine recognition site. The polyamine binding site is not affected by FBM as evidenced by the inability of FBM to modulate spermine-enhanced MK-801 binding.[67] On the contrary, therapeutic concentrations (≈300 µmol/liter) of FBM have been demonstrated to displace [^{3}H] 5,7-dichlorokyurenic acid binding, a competitive antagonist at the strychnine-insensitive glycine binding site of the NMDA receptor, to rat brain membranes[67] and to sections of human postmortem brain.[71] The standard AEDs—PHT, CBZ, PB, and VPA—were without effect at concentrations that far exceeded their therapeutic levels. This effect of FBM appears to correlate with its ability to reduce glycine-enhanced NMDA-evoked calcium transients in cerebellar granule cells.[72]

Results from additional in vitro and in vivo studies provide the best experimental evidence supporting an action of FBM at the strychnine-insensitive glycine receptor. For example, the neuroprotective effect of FBM in rat hippocampal slices is totally reversed by glycine[73] and the glycine uptake inhibitor histidine[74] but not by glutamate. The anticonvulsant effects of FBM have also been shown to be reversed by agonists acting at the strychnine-insensitive glycine receptor. For example, d-serine reverses the anticonvulsant effect of FBM in Frings audiogenic seizure-susceptible mice.[72, 75] Conversely, this effect of d-serine could be reversed by increasing the dose of FBM. Prior intraperitoneal administration of glycine has also been reported to reverse the ability of FBM to block MES- and NMDA-induced seizures[76] and audiogenic seizures in DBA mice.[77] Collectively, these results support an interaction of FBM with the strychnine-insensitive glycine receptor on the NMDA receptor-ionophore complex that may play an important role in mediating its anticonvulsant and neuroprotectant effects.[60]

FBM has been reported to enhance GABA-evoked chloride currents and inhibit NMDA-evoked currents[78] at concentrations (1 and 3 mmol/liter) higher than those required to block seizures in vivo and to inhibit sustained repetitive firing and displace 5,7-dichlorokyurenic acid from the strychnine-insensitive glycine receptor in vitro. The mechanism by which FBM enhances GABA-evoked currents is unknown. For example, FBM in concentrations up to 1 mmol/liter does not appear to affect ligand binding to the GABA, BZD, or picrotoxin binding sites on the $GABA_A$ receptor ionophore, nor does it enhance GABA-stimulated Cl⁻ flux into cultured mouse spinal cord neurons.[79] The ability of FBM to block NMDA-evoked currents is unique among the standard and newer AEDs. Despite its interaction with this receptor complex, FBM does not appear to produce the behavioral or pathologic impairment of the CNS associated with competitive or noncompetitive NMDA antagonists.[60]

In summary, FBM represents the first of the newer AEDs approved in the United States. It possesses a broad anticonvulsant profile in laboratory animals and human studies that appears to be related in part to multiple mechanisms of action thus far ascribed to this unique drug.

Gabapentin

The second of the newer generation AEDs to be marketed in the United States is GBP. GBP, 1-(aminomethyl)cyclohexaneacetic acid, was originally designed and synthesized as a drug to enhance GABA-mediated inhibition by mimicking the steric conformation of the endogenous neurotransmitter GABA.[80] In animal seizure models, it displays a broad anticonvulsant profile.[81, 82] It is effective against tonic extension seizures induced by a number of stimuli, including electrical and chemical. GBP is also active against clonic seizures induced by PTZ but not bicuculline, picrotoxin, or strychnine. In other seizure models, GBP blocks audiogenic seizures in DBA/2J mice, blocks tonic and clonic seizures in genetically susceptible gerbils, and reduces the behavioral seizure score in hippocampal-kindled rats. GBP is apparently ineffective against absence-like spike-wave discharges in Wistar rats. In human studies, GBP has demonstrated efficacy against partial seizures and secondarily generalized seizures.

The anticonvulsant profile of GBP is somewhat unique among the standard and newer AEDs, indirectly suggesting a novel mechanism of action (see Figure 1.1, Table 1.3). However, despite demonstrated efficacy in animal and human studies and numerous in vitro studies, which have described several potential mechanisms of action, the precise mode of action of GBP remains unknown. Although originally designed to function as a GABA-mimetic, results from studies have essentially excluded this as a possible mechanism of action. Unlike those AEDs that directly modulate voltage- and receptor-gated ion channels, there is a substantial time lag between the appearance of peak plasma and brain concentrations and GBP's time to peak anticonvulsant effect after intravenous administration.[83] This delay in anticonvulsant effect suggests that prolonged synaptic or cytosolic exposure to GBP is important and supports an indirect mechanism of action for GBP. This hypothesis is supported by in vivo and in vitro studies. For example, only after prolonged application of GBP was a reduction in sustained repetitive action potential firing observed.[84] The ability of GBP to limit sodium-dependent sustained-action potential firing in cultured mouse spinal cord neurons was observed at clinically relevant concentrations and was voltage- and frequency-dependent but developed slowly with prolonged exposure. The precise mechanism of this effect is not known; however, it is unlikely that GBP inhibits Na^+ currents in a manner similar to that of the established Na^+ channel blockers PHT and CBZ.

GBP has also been reported to increase GABA concentrations in discrete brain regions; this effect parallels its anticonvulsant time course.[85] Similarly, GBP has been reported to increase the cytosolic concentration of GABA in isolated neonatal rat optic nerves.[86] Since this preparation contains mostly axons from retinal ganglion cells and glial cells and lacks neuronal cell bodies and synapses, the majority of GABA is presumed to be localized in the glial compartment. The significance of this finding is that GABA can be released from glial cells in a calcium-independent manner by the GABA uptake inhibitor nipecotic acid.[87] For example, by acting as a substrate for the GABA transporter, nipecotic acid can release GABA by reversing the GABA transporter. Once released, GABA produces a $GABA_A$-dependent depolarization that is blocked by bicuculline. GBP pretreatment enhances nipecotic acid–induced depolarization presumably by increasing the amount of GABA that is released by reversal of the GABA transporter.[86] GBP has also been demonstrated to enhance nipecotic acid–induced inward currents in isolated CA1 hippocampal pyramidal neurons in culture.[88] Thus, it would appear that GBP possesses a unique ability to increase the concentration of releasable GABA in the glial and neuronal compartment. More recently, GBP has been reported to increase in vivo occipital lobe GABA levels in epilepsy patients.[89] This effect, determined using ^{1}H nuclear magnetic resonance spectroscopy, was significantly higher in controls than in those patients receiving GBP at 40 mg/kg per day.

GBP may increase brain GABA turnover by interacting with different metabolic processes. It has been demonstrated to enhance glutamate dehydrogenase and glutamic acid decarboxylase and inhibit branched-chain amino acid aminotransferase and GABA aminotransferase. Although any one of these effects could singly, or in concert with the others, contribute to the anticonvulsant action of GBP, it is not clear at this point which effects are important.[82]

Finally, GBP has been reported to bind to a novel site in rat brain preparations.[90] Specific [^{3}H]-GBP binding is not affected by any of the standard AEDs, including PHT, CBZ, VPA, PB, diazepam, or ESM. Furthermore, GBP binding is not displaced to any significant extent by NMDA or AMPA receptor ligands. On the contrary, [^{3}H]-GBP binding is displaced by unlabelled GBP and several structural GBP analogues, including 3-isobutyl GABA. It is also displaced stereospecifically by L-amino acids, including L-leucine, L-isoleucine, L-methionine, and L-phenylalanine, suggesting an association between the [^{3}H]-GBP binding site and the system L transporter of neuronal cell membranes.[91] However, the precise relationship between the GBP binding site and system L transporter is unclear, and any conclusions regarding the potential role of either site will require additional investigations.

In summary, GBP displays a unique anticonvulsant profile in animal studies and has demonstrated efficacy in human trials. Furthermore, results from in vitro and in vivo studies would also suggest that the mechanism of action of GBP is unique among the existing AEDs. Among the many possible hypotheses being tested, the two that appear most closely associated with its anticonvulsant action are related to the ability of GBP to enhance GABA turnover and release, and to interact with a unique binding site.

Lamotrigine

LTG (3,5-diamino-6-[2,3-dichlorphenyo]-1,2,4-triazine) represents the third new-generation AED to be marketed in the United States since 1993. LTG emerged from an antifolate drug development program that was based on the observation that chronic use of PB, primidone, and PHT reduced folate levels[92] and that folates induce seizures in laboratory animals.[93] However, LTG, despite its structural similarity to other antifolate drugs, displays only weak antifolate activity. Furthermore, results from structure-activity studies suggest that there is little correlation between antifolate activity and anticonvulsant potency.[24]

In experimental animal models, LTG possesses an anticonvulsant profile that most closely approximates that of PHT and CBZ. For example, it is effective against tonic extension seizures induced by MES and ineffective against clonic seizures induced by PTZ.[94] LTG has also been reported to be effective in reducing the after-discharge duration in anesthetized rats, dogs, and marmosets.[95]

Surprisingly, LTG appears to possess a broader clinical profile than would be predicted from its preclinical profile. LTG is useful for the treatment of partial and secondarily generalized seizures.[96] In addition, anecdotal reports from open label studies support the clinical evaluation of LTG in typical and atypical absence, atonic, and myoclonic seizures.[96] The results from preclinical studies suggest that LTG, PHT, and CBZ share a similar mechanism of action. However, anecdotal reports suggesting efficacy in patients with absence seizures argue that LTG possesses a broader mechanistic profile than PHT and CBZ.

LTG selectively blocks veratrine-evoked glutamate release and is without effect against KCl-evoked release.[97] Thus, it appeared from these studies that LTG, much like PHT and CBZ, acted at a voltage-dependent Na^+ channel, thereby decreasing presynaptic glutamate release (see Figure 1.1, Table 1.3). Subsequent studies demonstrated an ability of LTG to inhibit sustained repetitive firing in a voltage-dependent manner in cultured spinal cord neurons.[98] LTG was also found to inhibit sustained burst firing induced by ionophoresis of L-glutamate or high K^+, but it did not affect the first action potential of the burst.[99] These results, like those of the release experiments, were highly supportive of an interaction between LTG and voltage-sensitive sodium channels. Consistent with this hypothesis is the observation that LTG inhibits [^{3}H]batrachotoxin binding and veratrine-stimulated [^{14}C]quanidinium transport into synaptosomes.[98, 100] Confirmation was provided when LTG, in side-by-side studies with PHT and CBZ, was demonstrated to inhibit sodium currents of N4TG1 mouse neuroblastoma cells in a concentration-dependent manner.[31] This effect, like that of PHT and CBZ, was use and voltage dependent. In this study, all three AEDs slowed recovery from inactivation.

Based on these studies, it is likely that the anticonvulsant effect of LTG, like that of PHT and CBZ, is primarily caused by a direct interaction of LTG with the voltage-dependent Na^+ channel. This single mechanism of action is not sufficient to explain the apparent broad clinical profile of LTG. Thus, if the results from ongoing clinical trials continue to support the use of LTG in the management of generalized absence, it is highly likely that LTG will be found to possess one or more additional mechanisms of action.

Topiramate

TPM [2,3:4,5-Bis-O-(1-methylethylidene)-b-D-fructopyranose sulfamate] is a chemically novel AED available in the United Kingdom, Sweden, and South America and is the latest new AED to receive FDA approval in the United States. TPM displays an anticonvulsant profile in the MES and chemoconvulsant tests that most closely resembles that of PHT and LTG. It is effective against tonic extension seizures induced by MES and ineffective against clonic seizures induced by PTZ, picrotoxin, or bicuculline.[101] In amygdala-kindled rats, TPM is effective in reducing the seizure score and the after-discharge duration.[102] In spontaneously epileptic rats, TPM blocks tonic extension seizures in a time- and dose-dependent manner.[103] In this model, it is as efficacious as PHT and ZNS in reducing the duration of tonic extension. These mutant rats also display absence-like spike-wave discharges that are blocked by the antiabsence drugs trimethadione and ESM. In this model, TPM decreased the duration of spike-wave discharges in a time- and dose-dependent manner, whereas PHT and ZNS were without effect.[103] The ability of TPM to block tonic extension, amygdala kindling, and spike-wave discharges suggests a broad clinical profile that may include generalized tonic-clonic, partial, and absence epilepsy, respectively.

Results from three double-blind add-on trials with TPM have demonstrated efficacy against partial and secondarily generalized seizures in highly refractory patients. Based on anecdotal reports and limited clinical trials, TPM appears to be effective in reducing seizure frequency in patients with primary generalized epilepsy, including absence, and may provide some benefit to pediatric patients with Lennox-Gastaut syndrome.[104] As discussed below, a number of different mechanisms of action have been identified that may account for the broad anticonvulsant profile of TPM. At therapeutic concentrations (3–30 μmol/liter), TPM blocks voltage-sensitive Na^+ channels and kainate-evoked currents and enhances GABA-evoked chloride currents. In this respect, TPM appears to possess a unique ability to decrease excitation and enhance inhibition.

Although the mechanism of action of TPM has not been clearly elucidated, results from in vitro studies conducted thus far have revealed some similarities as well as some interesting and unexpected differences between TPM and PHT. Because TPM, like PHT, blocks MES-induced tonic extension, it might be anticipated that it would also limit depolarization-induced sustained repetitive firing. Indeed, TPM has been found to inhibit sustained repetitive firing in cultured hippocampal neurons in a use- and concentration-dependent manner.[105] Qualitatively similar results have been observed in cortical neurons (M. McLean, personal communication, 1996). In addition, McLean and colleagues have demonstrated that the ability of TPM to inhibit sustained repetitive firing is voltage dependent. The ability of TPM to limit sustained repetitive firing is suggestive of an interaction between TPM and the voltage-sensitive Na^+ channel. Preliminary results obtained from cultured neocortical neurons are consistent with this conclusion. In these studies, TPM was demonstrated to reduce voltage-activated Na^+ currents.[106] Ongoing investigations are attempting to characterize the mechanism of the interaction between TPM and voltage-activated Na^+ currents. In additional electrophysiologic studies conducted on cultured hippocampal neurons, TPM, at a therapeutic concentration of 10 μmol/liter, was reported to reduce the duration and frequency of action potentials within spontaneous epileptiform bursts.[105] These effects on sustained repetitive firing, Na^+ currents, and spontaneous burst firing are consistent with its apparent ability to reduce seizure spread and block MES-induced seizures in rodents.

TPM has also been reported to reduce kainate-evoked whole-cell currents in hippocampal neurons.[105, 107] This effect was evident at 10 μmol/liter and was concentration dependent from 10 to 100 μmol/liter. At 100 μmol/liter, TPM had no effect on NMDA-evoked inward currents. When compared with other AEDs, this effect of TPM on kainate-evoked currents is unique to TPM and is consistent with a decrease in neuronal excitability.

Inhibition of kainate-evoked currents, reduction of spontaneous burst firing, and depolarization-induced sustained repetitive firing may contribute to the ability of TPM to block MES-induced tonic extension in laboratory animals and partial and secondarily generalized seizures in humans. However, such effects do not necessarily support the ability of TPM to block absence-like spike-wave discharges in spontaneously epileptic rats and anecdotal reports suggesting efficacy against generalized absence epilepsy. TPM has been reported to enhance GABA-evoked chloride single-channel currents in cultured neocortical neurons.[108, 109] Kinetic analysis of single-channel recordings from excised outside-out patches demonstrated that TPM increased the frequency of channel opening and the burst frequency but was without effect on open channel duration or burst duration. In this respect, the effect of TPM on $GABA_A$ channel activity was similar to that observed with BZDs. However, in contrast to the BZDs, the ability of TPM to enhance $GABA_A$-evoked current was not reversed by the BZD antagonist flumazenil. This effect is consistent with the ability of TPM to block spike-wave discharges and its apparent efficacy against absence epilepsy. However, this effect would not be predicted from previous in vitro studies wherein TPM did not displace radiolabeled ligand binding to known binding sites on $GABA_A$ receptors.[101] Ongoing investigations are addressing the possibility that TPM modulates GABA currents through a novel interaction with a specific $GABA_A$ receptor subunit.

The studies conducted thus far suggest that TPM possesses multiple actions that contribute to its broad anticonvulsant profile. Effects on sustained repetitive firing, voltage-sensitive Na^+ channels, and non-NMDA receptors may account for its ability to prevent seizure spread and its efficacy against partial seizures secondarily generalized. Enhancement of GABA-mediated inhibition may contribute to its ability to elevate seizure threshold and its possible efficacy against absence epilepsy.

Vigabatrin

VGB [4-amino-5-hexanoic acid; (γ-vinyl GABA)] is widely available in Europe for the treatment of partial seizures and is in late-stage clinical development in the United States. Numerous preclinical studies have demonstrated VGB to be effective in a variety of experimental seizure models.[110] For example, it is active against strychnine- and sound-induced seizures[111, 112] and is effective in reducing the seizure severity in photosensitive baboons.[113] VGB has also been reported to inhibit the acquisition of amygdala kindling[114, 115] and the expression of fully kindled generalized seizures.[116] In a rodent model of absence epilepsy, direct injection of VGB into the median part of the lateral thalamus significantly increased the cumulative duration of spike and wave discharges.[117, 118]

VGB, a close structural analogue of the inhibitory neurotransmitter GABA, evolved from a mechanistically oriented drug discovery program that targeted GABA alpha-oxoglutarate transaminase (GABA-T; EC 2.6.1.19), which is the enzyme responsible for GABA metabolism (see Figure 1.2, Table 1.3). The presence of a vinyl function on the carbon next to the amine group transforms the substrate of GABA-T into an irreversible enzyme inhibitor. VGB was developed on the premise that inhibition of GABA-T would result in increased brain GABA levels and ultimately enhanced GABAergic neurotransmission. Subsequent studies demonstrated that VGB administration to laboratory animals produces a prolonged, dose-related inhibition of GABA-T and corresponding elevation of whole-brain GABA levels.[112, 119] An increase in all brain regions examined was observed; however, quantitative differences between brain regions were noted.[120] Likewise in human studies, VGB produces a dose-dependent increase in cerebrospinal fluid GABA levels.[121–123] In animal studies, there does appear to be a preferential increase in the GABA concentration in the synapto-somal-versus-nonsynaptosomal pool.[124] Thus, VGB treatment leads to an increased amount of presynaptic GABA available for release, which indirectly leads to increased GABAergic activity at postsynaptic GABA receptors. Presumably, this effect accounts for the primary anticonvulsant and antiepilep-tic mechanism of action of VGB.

Tiagabine

TGB [(R)-N-(4,4-di-(3-methyl-thien-2-yl)but-3-enyl)] nipecotic acid hydrochlo-ride] is a selective GABA uptake inhibitor (see Figure 1.2, Table 1.3) that emerged from a mechanistic-based drug discovery program designed to identify lipophilic GABA uptake inhibitors for the treatment of epilepsy (see reference 125 for a review). TGB is a potent anticonvulsant for a number of chemoconvulsant-induced seizures, including dimethoxyethyl-carboline carboxylate (DMCM)-induced clonus and PTZ-induced tonic and clonic seizures. It is effective against MES-induced tonic extension, but only at doses two- to threefold greater than the dose that produces motor impairment. In genetic epilepsy models, TGB is effective against sound-induced seizures in DBA/2 mice and GEPR rats. TGB produces par-tial protection against photically induced myoclonus in the photosensitive baboon, *Papio papio* (see reference 125). In the amygdala-kindled rat model of partial epilepsy, TGB has been reported to decrease after-discharge duration and seizure score of fully kindled rats at doses that do not produce motor impairment (see reference 125). Results from completed clinical trials suggest that TGB is effec-tive in patients with highly refractory partial and secondarily generalized tonic-clonic seizures.[126–128]

The principal mechanism of action of TGB appears to be related to its ability to inhibit neuronal and glial GABA uptake (see Figure 1.2). TGB is a potent inhibitor of GABA uptake in various brain regions.[129] It selectively binds to the GABA uptake carrier of neurons and glia in a reversible manner. TGB does display a slight-ly higher affinity for the glial GABA carrier; however, it is without effect at other neurotransmitter receptor binding or uptake sites. It is important to note that TGB is not a substrate for the carrier, nor does it stimulate GABA release. Treatment with TGB has been demonstrated to increase extracellular fluid GABA levels in vivo in animal[130] and human brains.[131] TGB, by inhibiting GABA uptake, increases the synaptic concentration of GABA, which leads to enhanced inhibitory neurotrans-mission. Electrophysiologically, TGB has been shown to prolong the pharmaco-logic effects of GABA. For example, in the hippocampal slice preparation, TGB prolongs the inhibitory postsynaptic potential and inhibitory postsynaptic current in CA1 and CA3 cells produced by exogenously applied GABA.[132–134] Collectively, these studies suggest that inhibition of GABA uptake is the primary mechanism through which TGB exerts an anticonvulsant effect.

Oxcarbazepine

OCBZ (10,11-dihydro-10-oxo-CBZ) is a derivative from the dibenzazepine series and is structurally related to CBZ (see reference 135 for a review). The keto substitution at the 10,11 position of the dibenzazepine nucleus does not affect the therapeutic profile of CBZ but does contribute to better tolerability in humans.[136–139] In vivo, OCBZ is rapidly and completely reduced to its active metabolite (10,11-dihydro-10-hydroxy-CBZ; HCBZ), which is thought to be responsible for OCBZ's anticonvulsant action.[140] HCBZ is a racemate that can be separated into two enantiomers, both of which appear to contribute to the anti-convulsant activity of HCBZ.[141]

The anticonvulsant profile of OCBZ and HCBZ is virtually identical to that of CBZ. They are both active at nontoxic doses against tonic-extension seizures induced by MES and essentially inactive against clonic seizures induced by PTZ, picrotoxin, and strychnine.[141, 142] Both compounds were found to possess activity against focal seizures in monkeys with chronic aluminum foci.[140] In developing rats, OCBZ and HCBZ also share a similar profile with CBZ. In this model they all displayed a dose-dependent ability to block PTZ-induced tonic extension seizures.[143] In comparative clinical trials, OCBZ was demonstrated to be as efficacious as and better tolerated than CBZ.[136, 138, 139]

OCBZ, HCBZ, and CBZ, as might be expected from the marked similarities in their preclinical profiles, appear to share a similar mechanistic profile (see Figure 1.1, Table 1.3) (see reference 144 for a review). OCBZ and HCBZ, like other drugs that block MES seizures (e.g., CBZ, PHT, VPA, FBM, LTG, and TPM) block sustained repetitive firing in cultured spinal cord neurons.[145] This effect, which is evident at therapeutic concentrations, is voltage- and frequency-dependent and suggests an interaction with voltage-sensitive Na^+ channels (see Figure 1.1). However, support for this conclusion must await direct confirmation by appropriate voltage-clamp studies.

Additional results from electrophysiologic studies with HCBZ and its two enantiomers in rat hippocampal slices suggest an effect on K^+ channels.[141] In these investigations, the ability of all three compounds to inhibit penicillin (1.2 mmol/liter)-evoked epileptic-like discharges was attenuated by the K^+ channel blocker 4-aminopyridine. Although not conclusive, these results suggest that the anticonvulsant action of OCBZ, HCBZ, and its enantiomers is mediated in part through an interaction with K^+ channels. Overall, OCBZ appears to represent a less toxic and equally efficacious alternative to CBZ that appears to exert its anti-convulsant effect through a similar mechanism of action.

Remacemide

RCM [($\pm$)-2-amino-N-(1-methyl-1,2,-diphenethyl)-acetamide] is a novel anti-convulsant substance undergoing clinical trials for the treatment of epilepsy and stroke (see reference 146 for a review and summary). RCM and its des-glycinated metabolite are active in several different preclinical seizure tests.[147–150] They both inhibit sound-induced seizures in DBA/2 audiogenic mice. In addition, they are effective against tonic extension seizures induced by MES and 4-aminopyri-dine. In contrast, neither compound is active against clonic seizures induced by the chemoconvulsants PTZ, picrotoxin, bicuculline, or strychnine. Interestingly, both compounds are able to block seizures and death induced by the glutamate agonist NMDLA, whereas only RCM displayed activity against kainate-induced seizures and lethality. RCM is not active against fully kindled stage 5 seizures in corneal-kindled rats but does appear to suppress kindled seizures induced by rapid hippocampal stimulation.

The precise mechanism of action of RCM and its des-glycinated metabolite has yet to be clearly established; however, two putative mechanisms appear to contribute to their anticonvulsant and neuroprotectant properties (see Figure 1.1, Table 1.3). At relatively low concentrations, RCM (8 μmol/liter) and the des-glycinated metabolite (0.8 μmol/liter) inhibit sustained repetitive firing in cultured mouse spinal cord neurons, thereby suggesting an action at voltage-sensitive Na^+ channels.[151, 152] Consistent with this conclusion is the finding that both substances display a weak affinity for the batrachotoxin binding site on the Na^+ channel.[146]

In addition to inhibiting sustained repetitive firing, both substances appear to exert a unique ability to block excitatory neurotransmission mediated by the NMDA receptor. The observation that RCM and its metabolite blocks NMDA-evoked seizures and death provided the first evidence implicating the NMDA receptor.[150] In subsequent studies, both compounds were shown to inhibit [^{3}H] MK-801 binding and NMDA-evoked whole-cell currents.[153–155] In these studies, RCM displays a weak affinity for the NMDA channel compared with the des-glycinated metabolite. For example, the concentration at which it inhibits [^{3}H] MK-801 binding and NMDA-evoked currents is approximately eightfold higher than that which inhibits sustained repetitive firing. In contrast, the des-glycinated metabolite of RCM inhibits [3H] MK-801 binding in the same concentration range that it blocks sustained repetitive firing.

One limitation of drugs that act at the NMDA receptor is their potential to impair learning and memory and to produce phencyclidine (PCP)-like behavior. In a number of different acute and subacute studies, RCM appears to be relatively free of any deleterious effects on learning and memory.[156] Furthermore, in an open-field test, rodents treated with high doses of RCM (up to 30 times the oral MES ED50 dose) did not display PCP-like behavior.[153] Likewise, RCM did not substitute for PCP when it was administered to rats trained to discriminate for PCP. Furthermore, RCM, in contrast to PCP and MK-801, did not facilitate intracranial self-stimulation when administered to rats with chronic median forebrain bundle electrode implants.[157, 158]

In summary, RCM and its des-glycinated metabolite may represent a novel class of anticonvulsant drugs. It appears to exert its anticonvulsant effect through at least two mechanisms of action that may include an interaction with the voltage-sensitive Na^+ channel and the NMDA receptor. It is important to note that the results from behavioral studies conducted thus far tend to suggest that the nature of the interaction between RCM and the NMDA receptor is different from that observed with MK-801 and PCP. Whether RCM will ultimately benefit patients with epilepsy will have to await additional clinical investigation; however, the early clinical data have provided evidence of efficacy when RCM has been administered as adjunctive therapy to patients with refractory seizure disorders (see reference 146 for a discussion).

Zonisamide

ZNS (1,2-benzisoxazole-3-methanesulfonamide) was discovered as a result of routine biologic screening of 1,2-benzisoxazole derivatives. ZNS possesses a broad anticonvulsant profile in animal seizure models.[24, 159] It blocks MES-induced seizures in different species and restricts the spread of focal cortical seizures in cats. In addition, ZNS blocked tonic extension seizures in spontaneous epileptic rats and audiogenic seizures in DBA/2 mice.[104] It was as effective as, albeit less potent than, PHT and TPM. ZNS also has been found to suppress focal seizure activity in cats and rats induced by cortical freezing and tungstic acid gel, respectively. Moreover, ZNS suppresses subcortically evoked seizures in hippocampal-kindled rats, amygdala-kindled rats and cats, and photically induced myoclonus in geniculate-kindled cats. In spontaneous epileptic rats, ZNS did not affect spike-wave discharges.[104] Clinically, ZNS appears to possess efficacy against a number of seizure types, including partial and secondarily generalized seizures, generalized tonic-clonic, generalized tonic, atypical absence, atonic, and myoclonic seizures.[159]

The broad anticonvulsant profile of ZNS can likely be accounted for by a similarly broad mechanistic profile (Figure 1.1, Table 1.3). For example, it has been found to block sustained repetitive firing in cultured spinal cord neurons[160] through an effect on voltage-sensitive Na^+ channels.[161] In voltage-clamped *Myxicola* giant axons, ZNS retarded recovery from fast and slow Na^+ channel inactivation and produced a hyperpolarizing shift in the steady-state inactivation curve. ZNS has also been demonstrated to reduce voltage-dependent T-type calcium currents in cultured neurons.[162] ZNS has been reported to decrease [^{3}H]flunitrazepam and [^{3}H]muscimol binding to the BZD and $GABA_A$, respectively. Furthermore, [^{3}H]ZNS binding to rat whole-brain membranes was reduced by clonazepam and enhanced by GABA.[163] However, in electrophysiologic studies ZNS did not affect ion currents evoked by iontophoretically applied GABA.[160] Nonetheless, experimental and clinical studies demonstrating efficacy against myoclonic seizures support a GABAergic mechanism of action; however, additional experiments are required to resolve this apparent discrepancy.

It is apparent from the number of studies conducted thus far that ZNS possesses a broad anticonvulsant and mechanistic profile. Effects on voltage-sensitive Na^+ channels are likely to contribute to the ability of ZNS to block MES-induced tonic extension in animals and generalized tonic seizures in humans, whereas effects on low voltage-activated T currents and perhaps GABA receptors are more likely to correlate with its efficacy against generalized absence and myoclonic seizures, respectively.

SUMMARY AND CONCLUSIONS

In recent years many significant advances have contributed to a greater understanding of the intrinsic mechanisms underlying epileptiform events and seizure disorders. An increased appreciation of the underlying pathologic features has led to the rational design and development of several clinical candidates that were synthesized to enhance inhibition or diminish excitation. The GABA uptake inhibitor TGB and the GABA-T inhibitor VGB represent two examples wherein this approach has led to the successful development of clinically effective drugs. These two AEDs demonstrate that it is possible to enhance GABAergic neurotransmission by mechanisms other than direct allosteric modulation of the postsynaptic receptor and support the validity of the mechanistic approach. Despite an extensive understanding of the processes underlying excitatory neurotransmission, the drugs developed thus far to target specifically the NMDA-preferring glutamate receptor have not only lacked efficacy in the limited clinical trials conducted to date, but have also resulted in intolerable side effects. Increased understanding of the molecular biology of not only the NMDA receptor, but also the AMPA and kainate receptors may ultimately lead to the development of selective, less toxic, and clinically efficacious glutamate antagonists.

In contrast to the mechanistic approach, animal model–based screening programs have identified most of the new AEDs registered in the United States and abroad. Without any appreciation of their precise mechanism or mechanisms of action, these drugs have demonstrated considerable promise in clinical trials, and many are likely to be useful alternatives to the established AEDs in managing some refractory patients. For many of these new AEDs, results from subsequent preclinical investigations have led to a greater understanding of their molecular mechanisms. The newer AEDs appear to act through one or more of the three major mechanisms of action proposed for the established AEDs (see Table 1.3), and these effects appear to correlate with their preclinical and clinical anticonvulsant profiles. Thus, drugs effective against generalized tonic-clonic and partial seizures appear to reduce sustained repetitive firing by delaying the rate of recovery from channel inactivation. Drugs effective against generalized absence epilepsy exert an inhibitory effect on low-threshold T-type calcium currents, whereas drugs that are effective against myoclonic seizures appear to enhance $GABA_A$ receptor–mediated inhibition. However, these effects alone are probably not sufficient to account for the apparent efficacy of the newer AEDs in highly refractory seizure patients.

Many of the new AEDs appear to act through a combination of mechanisms that likely extend beyond effects on Na^+ and Ca^{2+} channels and GABA receptors. Indeed, three of the newer drugs (FBM, TPM, and RCM) appear to possess a unique ability to inhibit glutamate-mediated neurotransmission through an effect on NMDA (FBM and RCM) and AMPA/kainate (TPM) receptors. The finding that these drugs limit glutamatergic neurotransmission without producing the typical behavioral disturbances associated with selective glutamate antagonists may suggest that they target a different glutamate receptor subtype. It may be possible to address this issue in the near future with newly developed molecular biologic techniques.

Finally, mechanisms of action beyond the four discussed above are likely to contribute to the underlying efficacy of the new AEDs. A thorough understanding of the molecular mode of action of the currently available drugs and those AEDs still under development will indirectly provide important information concerning the underlying causes of seizure disorders. Ultimately, insights gained from these and other studies will undoubtedly assist in the rational design of newer, more effective, and less toxic drugs that not only inhibit acute seizures but also interfere with the pathologic processes that underlie the development of drug-resistant epilepsy. Only then will the search for the ideal AED come to an end.

REFERENCES

1. White HS, Woodhead JH, Franklin MR, et al. General Principles: Experimental Selection, Quantification, and Evaluation of Antiepileptic Drugs. In RH Levy, RH Mattson, BS Meldrum (eds), Antiepileptic Drugs (4th ed). New York: Raven, 1995;99.
2. White HS, Johnson M, Wolf HH, Kupferberg HJ. The early identification of anticonvulsant activity: role of the maximal electroshock and subcutaneous pentylenetetrazol seizure models. Ital J Neurol Sci 1995;16:73.
3. Goodman LS, Swinyard EA, Toman JEP. Laboratory technics for the identification and evaluation of potentially antiepileptic drugs. Proc Am Fed Clin Res 1945;2:100.
4. Everett GM, Richards RK. Comparative anticonvulsive action of 3,5,5-trimethyloxazolidine-2,4-dione (Tridione), Dilantin and phenobarbital. J Pharmacol Exp Ther 1944;81:402.
5. Lennox WG. The petit mal epilepsies. Their treatment with Tridione. JAMA 1945;129:1069.
6. McNamara JO. Development of new pharmacological agents for epilepsy: lessons from the kindling model. Epilepsia 1989;30:513.
7. McNamara JO, Byrne MC, Dasheiff RM, Fitz JG. The kindling model of epilepsy: a review. Prog Neurobiol 1980;15:139.
8. Mayer ML, Westbrook GL. The physiology of excitatory amino acids in the vertebrate central nervous system. Prog Neurobiol 1987;28:197.
9. Danysz W, Parsons CG, Bresink I, Quack G. Glutamate in CNS disorders. Drug News Perspect 1995;8:261.
10. Watkins JC, Evans RH. Excitatory amino acid transmitters. Annu Rev Pharmacol Toxicol 1981;21:165.
11. Pellegrini-Giampietro DE, Zukin RS, Bennett MVL, et al. Switch in glutamate receptor subunit gene expression in CA1 subfield of hippocampus following global ischemia in rats. Proc Natl Acad Sci U S A 1992;89:10499.
12. Brusa R, Zimmermann F, Koh D-S, et al. Early-onset epilepsy and postnatal lethality associated with an editing-deficient GluR-B allele in mice. Science 1995;270:1677.
13. Rogers SW, Twyman RE, Gahring LC. The role of autoimmunity to glutamate receptors in neurologic disease. Mol Med Today 1996;2:76.
14. Twyman RE, Gahring LC, Speiss J, Rogers SW. Glutamate receptor antibodies activate a subset of receptors and reveal an agonist binding site. Neuron 1995;17:755.
15. Heinemann U, Draguhn A, Ficker E, et al. Strategies for the development of drugs for pharmacoresistent epilepsies. Epilepsia 1994;35(Suppl 5):S10.
16. Hollmann M, Heinemann S. Cloned glutamate receptors. Annu Rev Neurosci 1994;17:31.
17. McBain CJ, Mayer ML. *N*-methyl-D-aspartic acid receptor structure and function. Physiol Rev 1994;74:723.
18. Wroblewski JT, Danysz W. Modulation of glutamate receptors: molecular mechanisms and functional implications. Annu Rev Pharmacol Toxicol 1989;29:441.
19. Löscher W. Basic aspects of epilepsy. Curr Opin Neurol Neurosurg 1993;6:223.
20. Meldrum BS. Neurotransmission in epilepsy. Epilepsia 1995;36(Suppl 1):S30.
21. Dichter MA. Emerging insights into mechanisms of epilepsy: implications for new antiepileptic drug development. Epilepsia 1994;35(Suppl 4):S51.
22. Macdonald RL, Meldrum BS. General Principles. Principles of Antiepileptic Drug Action. In RH Levy, RH Mattson, BS Meldrum (eds), Antiepileptic Drugs (4th ed). New York: Raven, 1995;61.
23. Macdonald RL, Kelly KM. Antiepileptic drug mechanisms of action. Epilepsia 1995;36(Suppl 2):S2.
24. Rogawski MA, Porter RJ. Antiepileptic drugs: pharmacological mechanisms and clinical efficacy with consideration of promising developmental stage compounds. Pharmacol Rev 1990;42:223.
25. Upton N. Mechanisms of action of new antiepileptic drugs: rational design and serendipitous findings. Trends Pharm Sci 1994;15:456.
26. Piredda SG, Woodhead JH, Swinyard EA. Effect of stimulus intensity on the profile of anticonvulsant activity of phenytoin, ethosuximide and valproate. J Pharmacol Exp Ther 1985;232:741.
27. Putnam TJ, Merritt HH. Experimental determination of the anticonvulsant properties of some phenyl derivatives. Science 1937;85:525.
28. Macdonald RL. Antiepileptic drug actions. Epilepsia 1989;30:S19.
29. McLean MJ, Macdonald RL. Carbamazepine and 10,11-epoxycarbamazepine produce use- and voltage-dependent limitation of rapidly firing action potentials of mouse central neurons in cell culture. J Pharmacol Exp Ther 1986;238:727.

30. Lang DG, Wang CM, Cooper BR. Lamotrigine, phenytoin and carbamazepine interactions on the sodium current present in N4TG1 mouse neuroblastoma cells. J Pharmacol Exp Ther 1993;266:829.
31. Willow M, Catterall WA. Inhibition of binding of [^{2}H]batrachotoxinin A20-a-benzoate to sodium channels by the anticonvulsant drugs diphenylhydantoin and carbamazepine. Mol Pharmacol 1982;22:627.
32. Willow M, Gonoi T, Catterall WA. Voltage clamp analysis of the inhibitory actions of diphenylhydantoin and carbamazepine on voltage-sensitive sodium channels in neuroblastoma cells. Mol Pharmacol 1985;27:549.
33. Willow M, Kuenzel EA, Catterall WA. Inhibition of voltage-sensitive sodium channels in neuroblastoma cells and synaptosomes by the anticonvulsant drugs diphenylhydantoin and carbamazepine. Mol Pharmacol 1984;25:228.
34. Schwarz JR, Grigat G. Phenytoin and carbamazepine: potential- and frequency-dependent block of Na currents in mammalian myelinated nerve fibers. Epilepsia 1989;30:286.
35. Tomaselli G, Marban E, Yellen G. Sodium channels from human brain RNA expressed in *Xenopus* oocytes basic electrophysiologic characteristics and their modifications by diphenylhydantoin. J Clin Invest 1989;83:1724.
36. Wakamori M, Kaneda M, Oyama Y, Akaike N. Effects of chlordiazepoxide, chlorpromazine, diazepam, diphenylhydantoin, flunitrazepam and haloperidol on the voltage-dependent sodium current of isolated mammalian brain neurons. Brain Res 1989;494:374.
37. Coulter DA, Huguenard JR, Prince DA. Calcium currents in rat thalamocortical relay neurones: kinetic properties of the transient low-threshold current. J Physiol 1989;44:587.
38. Coulter DA, Huguenard JR, Prince DA. Characterization of ethosuximide reduction of low threshold calcium current in thalamic neurons. Ann Neurol 1989;25:582.
39. Coulter DA, Huguenard JR, Prince DA. Differential effects of petit mal anticonvulsants and convulsants on thalamic neurones: calcium current reduction. Br J Pharmacol 1990;100:800.
40. McLean MJ, Macdonald RL. Sodium valproate but not ethosuximide, produces use- and voltage-dependent limitation of high frequency repetitive firing of action potentials of mouse central neurons in cell culture. J Pharmacol Exp Ther 1986;237:1001.
41. Capek R, Esplin B. Effects of valproate on action potentials and repetitive firing of CA1 pyramidal cells in the hippocampal slice. Soc Neurosci Abstr 1986;14:570.
42. Van Dongen AMJ, Van Erp MG, Voskuyl RA. Valproate reduces excitability by blockage of sodium and potassium conductance. Epilepsia 1986;27:177.
43. Zona C, Avoli M. Effects induced by the antiepileptic drug valproic acid upon the ionic currents recorded in rat neocortical neurons in cell culture. Exp Brain Res 1990;81:313.
44. Van den Berg RJ, Kok P, Voskuyl RA. Valproate and sodium currents in cultured hippocampal neurons. Exp Brain Res 1993;93:279.
45. Kelly KM, Gross RA, Macdonald RL. Valproic acid selectively reduces the low-threshold (T) calcium in rat nodose neurons. Neurosci Lett 1990;116:233.
46. Macdonald RL, Olsen RW. GABA$_A$ receptor channels. Annu Rev Neurosci 1994;17:569.
47. Olsen RW. The Gamma-aminobutyric Acid/Benzodiazepine/Barbiturate Receptor-Chloride Ion Channel Complex of Mammalian Brain. In GM Edelman, WE Gall, WM Cowan (eds), Synaptic Function. New York: Wiley, 1987;257.
48. Macdonald RL, Rogers CJ, Twyman RE. Barbiturate regulation of kinetic properties of the GABA$_A$ receptor channel of mouse spinal neurones in culture. J Physiology 1989;417:483.
49. Twyman RE, Rogers CJ, Macdonald RL. Differential regulation of gamma-aminobutyric acid receptor channels by diazepam and phenobarbital. Ann Neurol 1989;25:213.
50. Study RE, Barker JL. Diazepam and (-)-pentobarbital: fluctuation analysis reveals different mechanisms for potentiation of gamma-aminobutyric acid responses in cultured central neurons. Proc Natl Acad Sci U S A 1981;78:7180.
51. Vicini S, Mienville JM, Costa E. Actions of benzodiazepine and β-carboline derivatives on gamma-aminobutyric acid-activated Cl-channels recorded from membrane patches of neonatal rat cortical neurons in culture. J Pharmacol Exp Ther 1987;243:1195.
52. Rogers CJ, Twyman RE, Macdonald RL. Benzodiazepine and β-carboline regulation of single GABA$_A$ receptor channels of mouse spinal neurones in culture. J Physiol 1994;475:69.
53. Moss SJ, Smart TA, Porter NM, et al. Cloned GABA receptors are maintained in a stable cell line: allosteric and channel properties. Eur J Pharmacol 1990;189:177.
54. Verdoorn TA, Draguhn A, Ymer S, et al. Functional properties of recombinant rat GABA$_A$ receptors depend upon subunit composition. Neuron 1990;4:919.
55. Pritchett DB, Sontheimer H, Shivers BD, et al. Importance of a novel GABA$_A$ receptor subunit for benzodiazepine pharmacology. Nature 1989;338:582.

56. Doble A, Martin IL. Multiple benzodiazepine receptors—no reason for anxiety. Trends Pharmacol Sci 1992;13:76.
57. Macdonald RL. Benzodiazepines. Mechanisms of Action. In RH Levy, RH Mattson, BS Meldrum (eds), Antiepileptic Drugs (4th ed). New York: Raven, 1995;695.
58. Swinyard EA, Sofia RD, Kupferberg HJ. Comparative anticonvulsant activity and neurotoxicity of felbamate and four prototype antiepileptic drugs in mice and rats. Epilepsia 1986;27:27.
59. White HS, Wolf HH, Swinyard EA, et al. A neuropharmacological evaluation of felbamate as a novel anticonvulsant. Epilepsia 1992;33:564.
60. Sofia RD. Felbamate. Mechanisms of Action. In RH Levy, RH Mattson, BS Meldrum (eds), Antiepileptic Drugs (4th ed). New York: Raven, 1995;791.
61. Wallis RA, Panizzon KL, Fairchild MD, Wasterlain CG. Protective effects of felbamate against hypoxia in the rat hippocampal slice. Stroke 1992;23:547.
62. Wasterlain CG, Adams LM, Hattori H, Schwartz PH. Felbamate reduces hypoxic-ischemic brain damage in vivo. Eur J Pharmacol 1992;212:275.
63. Wasterlain CG, Adams LM, Schwartz PH, et al. Post-hypoxic treatment with felbamate is neuro-protective in a rat model of hypoxia-ischemia. Neurology 1994;43:2303.
64. Chronopoulos A, Stafstrom C, Thurber S, et al. Neuroprotective effect of felbamate after kainic acid–induced status epilepticus. Epilepsia 1993;34:359.
65. Theodore WH, Jensen PK, Kwan RMF. Felbamate. Clinical Use. In RH Levy, RH Mattson, BS Meldrum (eds), Antiepileptic Drugs (4th ed). New York: Raven, 1995;817.
66. Adusumalli VE, Wichmann JK, Kucharczyk N, Sofia RD. Distribution of the anticonvulsant felbamate to cerebrospinal fluid and brain tissue of adult and neonatal rats. Drug Metab Dispos 1993;21:1079.
67. McCabe RT, Wasterlain CG, Kucharczyk N, et al. Evidence for anticonvulsant and neuroprotectant action of felbamate mediated by strychnine-insensitive glycine receptors. J Pharmacol Exp Ther 1993;264:1248.
68. Adusumalli VE, Wichmann JK, Kucharczyk N, et al. Drug concentrations in human brain tissue samples from epileptic patients treated with felbamate. Drug Metab Dispos 1994;22:168.
69. Klein M, Musacchio JM. High affinity dextromethorphan binding sites in guinea pig brain. Effect of sigma ligands and other agents. J Pharmacol Exp Ther 1989;251:207.
70. Sofia RD, Gordon R, Gels M, Diamantis W. Comparative effects of felbamate and other compounds on N-methyl-D-aspartic acid-induced convulsions and lethality in mice. Pharmacol Res 1994;29:139.
71. Wamsley JK, Sofia RD, Faull RLM, et al. Interaction of felbamate with [^{3}H]DCKA-labeled strychnine-insensitive glycine receptors in human postmortem brain. Exp Neurol 1994;129:244.
72. White HS, Harmsworth WL, Sofia RD, Wolf HH. Felbamate modulates the strychnine-insensitive glycine receptor. Epilepsy Res 1995;20:41.
73. Wallis RA, Panizzon KL. Glycine reversal of felbamate hypoxic protection. Neuroreport 1993;4:951.
74. Panizzon KL, Wallis RA. Histidine, a glycine uptake inhibitor, blocks hypoxic protection with felbamate. Neurology 1993;43:A312.
75. Harmsworth WL, Wolf HH, Swinyard EA, White HS. Felbamate modulates glycine receptor function. Epilepsia 1993;34:92.
76. Coffin V, Cohen-Williams M, Barnett A. Selective antagonism of the anticonvulsant effects of felbamate by glycine. Eur J Pharmacol 1994;256:R9.
77. De Sarro G, Ongini E, Bertorelli R, et al. Excitatory amino acid neurotransmission through both NMDA and non-NMDA receptors is involved in the anticonvulsant activity of felbamate in DBA/2 mice. Eur J Pharmacol 1994;262:11.
78. Rho JM, Donevan DC, Rogawski MA. Mechanism of action of the anticonvulsant felbamate: opposing effects on NMDA and GABA$_A$ receptors. Ann Neurol 1994;35:229.
79. Ticku MK, Kamatchi GL, Sofia RD. Effect of anticonvulsant felbamate on GABA$_A$ receptor system. Epilepsia 1991;32:389.
80. Schmidt B. Potential Antiepileptic Drugs: Gabapentin. In RH Levy, FE Driefuss, RH Mattson, et al. (eds), Antiepileptic Drugs (3rd ed). New York: Raven, 1989;925.
81. Bartoszyk GD, Meyerson N, Reimann W, et al. Gabapentin. In BS Meldrum, RJ Porter (eds), Current Problems in Epilepsy: New Anticonvulsant Drugs. London: John Libbey, 1986;147.
82. Taylor CP. Gabapentin. Mechanisms of Action. In RH Levy, RH Mattson, BS Meldrum (eds), Antiepileptic Drugs (4th ed). New York: Raven, 1995;829.
83. Welty DF, Schielke GP, Vartanian MG, Taylor CP. Gabapentin anticonvulsant action in rats: disequilibrium with peak drug concentrations in plasma and brain microdialysate. Epilepsy Res 1993;16:175.
84. Wamil AW, McLean MJ. Limitation by gabapentin of high frequency action potential firing by mouse central neurons in cell culture. Epilepsy Res 1994;7:1.

85. Löscher W, Honack D, Taylor CP. Gabapentin increases aminooxyacetic acid-induced GABA accumulation in several regions of rat brain. Neurosci Lett 1991;128:150.
86. Kocsis JD, Honmou O. Gabapentin increases GABA-induced depolarization in rat neonatal optic nerve. Neurosci Lett 1994;169:181.
87. Ochi S, Lim JY, Rand MN, et al. Transient presence of GABA in astrocytes of the developing optic nerve. Glia 1993;9:188.
88. Honmou O, Kocsis JD, Richerson GB. Gabapentin potentiates the conductance increase induced by nipecotic acid in CA1 pyramidal neurons in vitro. Epilepsy Res 1995;20:193.
89. Petroff OAC, Rothman DL, Behar KL, et al. Gabapentin increases brain gamma-aminobutyric acid levels in patients with epilepsy. Ann Neurol 1995;38:295.
90. Suman-Chauhan N, Webdale L, Hill DR, Woodruff GN. Characterization of [^{3}H]-gabapentin binding to a novel site in rat brain: homogenate binding studies. Eur J Pharmacol 1993;244:293.
91. Thurlow RJ, Brown JP, Gee NS, et al. [^{3}H]-gabapentin binding may label a system-L like neutral amino acid carrier in brain. Eur J Pharmacol 1993;247:341.
92. Reynolds EH, Milner G, Matthews DM, Chanarin I. Anticonvulsant therapy, megaloblastic haemopoiesis and folic acid metabolism. QJM 1966;35:521.
93. Hommes OR, Obbens EAMT. The epileptogenic action of sodium folate in the rat. J Neurol Sci 1972;20:269.
94. Miller AA, Wheatley P, Sawyer DA, et al. Pharmacological studies on lamotrigine, a novel potential antiepileptic drug. I: Anticonvulsant profile in mice and rats. Epilepsia 1986;27:483.
95. Wheatley P, Miller AA. Effects of lamotrigine on electrically induced after discharge duration in anaesthetized rat, dog and marmoset. Epilepsia 1989;30:34.
96. Leach JP, Brodie MJ. Lamotrigine. Clinical Use. In RH Levy, RH Mattson, BS Meldrum (eds), Antiepileptic Drugs (4th ed). New York: Raven, 1995;889.
97. Leach MJ, Marden CM, Miller AA. Pharmacological studies on lamotrigine, a novel potential antiepileptic drug. II: Neurochemical studies on the mechanism of action. Epilepsia 1986;27:490.
98. Cheung H, Kamp D, Harris E. An in vitro investigation of the action of lamotrigine on neuronal voltage-activated sodium channels. Epilepsy Res 1992;13:107.
99. Lees G, Leach MJ. Studies on the mechanism of action of the novel anticonvulsant lamotrigine (Lamictal) using primary neuroglial cultures from rat cortex. Brain Res 1993;612:190.
100. Riddall DR, Clackers M, Leach MJ. Correlation of inhibition of veratrine evoked [^{14}C] guanidine uptake with inhibition of veratrine evoked release of glutamate by lamotrigine and its analogues. Can J Neurol Sci 1993;20(Suppl 4):S181.
101. Shank RP, Gardocki JF, Vaught JL, et al. Topiramate: preclinical evaluation of a structurally novel anticonvulsant. Epilepsia 1994;35(Suppl 2):450.
102. Wauquier A, Zhou S. Topiramate: a potent anticonvulsant in the amygdala-kindled rat. Epilepsy Res 1996;24:73.
103. Nakamura J, Tamura S, Kanda T, et al. Inhibition by topiramate of seizures in spontaneously epileptic rats and DBA/2 mice. Eur J Pharmacol 1994;254:83.
104. Espe-Lillo J, Ritter FJ, Frost MD, et al. Topiramate in childhood epilepsy: titration, adverse events, and efficacy in multiple seizure types. Epilepsia 1995;36(Suppl 4):56.
105. Coulter DA, Sombati S, DeLorenzo RJ. Selective effects of topiramate on sustained repetitive firing and spontaneous bursting in cultured hippocampal neurons. Epilepsia 1993;34(Suppl 2):123.
106. Zona C, Barbarosie M, Kawasaki H, Avoli M. Effects induced by the anticonvulsant drug topiramate on voltage-gated sodium currents generated by cerebellar granule cells in tissue culture. Epilepsia 1996;37(Suppl 5):24.
107. Severt L, Coulter DA, Sombati S, DeLorenzo RJ. Topiramate selectively blocks kainate currents in cultured hippocampal neurons. Epilepsia 1995;36(Suppl 4):S38
108. Brown SD, Wolf HH, Swinyard EA, et al. The novel anticonvulsant topiramate enhances GABA-mediated chloride flux. Epilepsia 1993;34(Suppl 2):122.
109. White HS, Brown D, Skeen GA, et al. The anticonvulsant topiramate displays a unique ability to potentiate GABA-evoked chloride currents. Epilepsia 1995;36(Suppl 3):S39.
110. Jung MJ, Palfreyman MG. Vigabatrin. Mechanisms of Action. In RH Levy, RH Mattson, BS Meldrum (eds), Antiepileptic Drugs (4th ed). New York: Raven, 1995;903.
111. Meldrum BS, Murugaiah K. Anticonvulsant action in mice with sound-induced seizures of the optical isomers of gamma vinyl GABA. Eur J Pharmacol 1983;89:149.
112. Schechter PJ, Tranier Y, Jung MJ, Bohlen P. Audiogenic seizure protection by elevated brain GABA concentration in mice: effects of gamma-acetylenic GABA and gamma-vinyl GABA, two irreversible GABA-T inhibitors. Eur J Pharmacol 1977;45:319.

113. Meldrum BS, Horton R. Blockade of epileptic responses in photosensitive baboon *Papio papio* by two irreversible inhibitors of GABA-transaminase, gamma-acetylenic GABA (4-amino-hex-5-ynoic acid) and gamma-vinyl GABA (4-amino-hex-5-enoic acid). Psychopharmacologia 1978;59:47.

114. Löscher W, Czuczwar SJ, Jackel R, Schwarz M. Effect of microinjections of gamma-vinyl GABA or isoniazid into substantia nigra on the development of amygdala kindling in rats. Exp Neurol 1987;95:622.

115. Shin C, Rigsbee LC, McNamara JO. Anti-seizure and anti-epileptogenic effect of gamma-vinyl gamma-aminobutyric acid in amygdaloid kindling. Brain Res 1986;398:370.

116. Kalichman MW, Burnham WM, Livingstone KE. Pharmacological investigation of gamma-aminobutyric acid (GABA) and fully developed generalized seizures in the amygdala-kindled rat. Neuropharmacology 1982;21:127.

117. Liu Z, Vergnes M, Depaulis A, Marescaux C. Evidence for a critical role of GABAergic transmission within the thalamus in the genesis and control of absence seizures. Brain Res 1991;545:1.

118. Marescaux C, Micheletti G, Vergnes M, et al. Diazepam antagonizes GABAmimetics in rats with spontaneous petit mal-like epilepsy. Eur J Pharmacol 1985;113:19.

119. Jung MJ, Lippert B, Metcalf B, et al. Gamma-vinyl GABA (4-amino-hex-5-enoic acid), a new irreversible inhibitor of GABA-T: effects on brain GABA metabolism in mice. J Neurochem 1977;29:797.

120. Chapman AG, Riley K, Evans MC, Meldrum BS. Acute effects of sodium valproate and gamma-vinyl GABA on regional amino acid metabolism in the rat brain: incorporation of 2-[^{14}C]glucose into amino acids. Neurochem Res 1982;7:1089.

121. Ben-Menachem E. Pharmacokinetic effects of vigabatrin on cerebrospinal fluid amino acids in humans. Epilepsia 1989;30(Suppl 3):S12.

122. Grove J, Schechter PJ, Tell G, et al. Increased gamma-aminobutyric acid (GABA), homocarnosine and β-alanine in cerebrospinal fluid of patients treated with gamma-vinyl GABA (4-amino-hex-5-enoic acid). Life Sci 1981;28:2431.

123. Schechter PJ, Hanke NFJ, Grove J, et al. Biochemical and clinical effects of gamma-vinyl GABA in patients with epilepsy. Neurology 1984;34:182.

124. Sarhan S, Seiler N. Metabolic inhibitors and subcellular distribution of GABA. J Neurosci Res 1979;4:399.

125. Suzdak PD, Jansen JA. A review of the preclinical pharmacology of tiagabine: a potent and selective anticonvulsant GABA uptake inhibitor. Epilepsia 1995;36:612.

126. Crawford PM, Engelsman M, Brown SW, et al. Tiagabine: phase II study of efficacy and safety in adjunctive treatment of partial seizures. Epilepsia 1993;34(Suppl 2):182.

127. Richens A, Chadwick D, Duncan J. Safety and efficacy of tiagabine as adjunctive treatment for complex partial seizures. Epilepsia 1992;33(Suppl 3):119.

128. Rowan AJ, Ahmann P, Wannamaker B, et al. Safety and efficacy of three dose levels of tiagabine HCl versus placebo as adjunctive treatment for complex partial seizures. Epilepsia 1993;34(Suppl 2):157.

129. Braestrup C, Nielsen EB, Sonnewald U, et al. NO-328 binds with high affinity to the brain GABA uptake carrier. J Neurochem 1990;54:639.

130. Fink-Jensen A, Suzdak PD, Swedberg MBD, et al. The GABA uptake inhibitor tiagabine increases extracellular brain levels of GABA in awake rats. Eur J Pharmacol 1992;220:197.

131. During M, Mattson R, Scheyer R, et al. The effect of tiagabine HCl on extracellular GABA levels in the human hippocampus. Epilepsia 1992;33(Suppl 3):83.

132. Rekling JC, Jahnsen H, Laursen AM. The effect of two lipophilic GABA uptake blockers in CA1 of the rat hippocampal slice. Br J Pharmacol 1990;99:103.

133. Roepstorff A, Lambert JDC. Comparison of the effect of the GABA uptake blockers tiagabine and nipecotic acid on inhibitory synaptic efficacy in hippocampal CA1 neurons. Neurosci Lett 1992;146:131.

134. Thompson SM, Gahwiler BH. Effects of the GABA uptake blocker tiagabine on inhibitory synaptic potentials in rat hippocampal slice cultures. J Neurophysiol 1992;67:1698.

135. Dam M, Østergaard LH. Other Antiepileptic Drugs. Oxcarbazepine. In RH Levy, RH Mattson, BS Meldrum (eds), Antiepileptic Drugs (4th ed). New York: Raven, 1995;987.

136. Dam M, Ekberg R, Loyning Y, et al. A double-blind study comparing oxcarbazepine and carbamazepine in patients with newly diagnosed, previously untreated epilepsy. Epilepsy Res 1989;3:70.

137. Gram L, Philbert A. Oxcarbazepine. In BS Meldrum, RJ Porter (eds), New Anticonvulsant Drugs. London: John Libbey, 1986;229.

138. Houtkooper MA, Lammertsma A, Meyer JMA, et al. Oxcarbazepine (GP 47.680): a possible alternative to carbamazepine? Epilepsia 1987;28:693.

139. Reinikainen KJ, Keranen T, Halonen T, et al. Comparison of oxcarbazepine and carbamazepine: a double-blind study. Epilepsy Res 1987;1:284.

140. Jensen PK, Gram L, Schmutz M. Oxcarbazepine. Epilepsy Res 1991;3:135.
141. Schmutz M, Ferret T, Heckendorn R, et al. GP 47779, the main human metabolite of oxcarbazepine (Trileptal), and both enantiomers have equal anticonvulsant activity. Epilepsia 1993;34(Suppl 2):122.
142. Baltzer V, Schmutz M. Experimental Anticonvulsant Properties of GP 47680 and of MHD, Its Main Human Metabolite: Compounds Related to Carbamazepine. In H Meinardi, AJ Rowan (eds), Advances in Epileptology. Amsterdam: Swets & Zeitlinger, 1978;295.
143. Kubova H, Mares P. Anticonvulsant action of oxycarbazepine, hydroxycarbamazepine, and carbamazepine against Metrazol-induced motor seizures in developing rats. Epilepsia 1993;34:188.
144. McLean MJ, Schmutz M, Wamil AW, et al. Oxcarbazepine: mechanisms of action. Epilepsia 1994;35(Suppl 3):S5.
145. Wamil AW, Porter C, Jensen PK, et al. Oxcarbazepine and its monohydroxy metabolite limit action potential firing by mouse central neurons in cell culture. Epilepsia 1991;32(Suppl 3):65.
146. Clark B, Hutchison JB, Jamieson V, et al. Potential Antiepileptic Drugs. Remacemide Hydrochloride. In RH Levy, RH Mattson, BS Meldrum (eds), Antiepileptic Drugs (4th ed). New York: Raven, 1995;1035.
147. Cramer CL, Stagnitto ML, Knowles MA, Palmer GC. Kainic acid and 4-aminopyridine seizure models in mice: evaluation of efficacy of antiepileptic agents and calcium antagonists. Life Sci 1994;54:P1271.
148. Garske JE, Palmer GC, Napier JJ, et al. Preclinical profile of the anticonvulsant remacemide and its enantiomers in the rat. Epilepsy Res 1991;9:161.
149. Palmer GC, Murray RJ, Wilson JCM, et al. Biological profile of the metabolites and potential metabolites of the anticonvulsant remacemide. Epilepsy Res 1992;12:9.
150. Stagnitto ML, Palmer GC, Ordy MJ, et al. Preclinical profile of remacemide: a novel anticonvulsant effective against maximal seizures in mice. Epilepsy Res 1990;7:11.
151. Cheung H, Wamil AW, Harris EW, et al. Effects of remacemide hydrochloride, its desglycinated metabolite and isomers on sustained repetitive firing in mouse spinal cord cultured neurones. FASEB J 1992;6:A1879.
152. Wamil AW, McLean MJ, Cheung H, Harris E. Remacemide and its desglycinated metabolite limit sustained high-frequency repetitive firing of action potentials of mouse central neurons in-vitro. Epilepsia 1992;33(Suppl 3):84.
153. Palmer GC, Clark B, Hutchison JB. Antiepileptic and neuroprotective potential of remacemide hydrochloride. Drugs Future 1993;18:1021.
154. Subramaniam S, Donevan SD, Rogawski MA. 1,2-Di-phenyl-2-propylamine, a major metabolite of the anticonvulsant remacemide hydrochloride, produces a stereoselective block of NMDA receptor currents. Soc Neurosci 1993;19:717.
155. Subramaniam S, Donevan SD, Rogawski MA. Block of the *N*-methyl-D-aspartate receptor by remacemide and its des-glycine metabolite. J Pharmacol Exp Ther 1996;276:161.
156. Ordy JM, Volpe B, Murray R, et al. Pharmacological Effects of Remacemide and MK-801 on Memory and Hippocampal CA1 Damage in the Rat Four-Vessel Occlusion (4-VO) Model of Global Ischemia. In MY-T Globus, WD Dietrich (eds), The Role of Neurotransmitters in Brain Injury. New York: Plenum, 1992;89.
157. Corbett D. Possible abuse potential of the NMDA antagonist MK801. Behav Brain Res 1989;34:239.
158. Corbett D, McKay K, Evans SJ. Lack of abuse potential of the novel NMDA antagonist, remacemide hydrochloride. Soc Neurosci 1993;19:830.
159. Seino M, Naruto S, Ito T, Miyazaki H. Other Antiepileptic Drugs. Zonisamide. In RH Levy, RH Mattson, BS Meldrum (eds), Antiepileptic Drugs (4th ed). New York: Raven, 1995;1011.
160. Rock DM, Macdonald RL, Taylor CP. Blockade of sustained repetitive action potentials in cultured spinal cord neurons by zonisamide (AD 810, CI 912), a novel anticonvulsant. Epilepsy Res 1989;3:138.
161. Schauf CL. Zonisamide enhances slow sodium inactivation in Myxicola. Brain Res 1987;413:185.
162. Suzuki S, Kawakami K, Nishimura S, et al. Zonisamide blocks T-type calcium channel in cultured neurons of rat cerebral cortex. Epilepsy Res 1992;12:21.
163. Mimaki T, Suzuki Y, Tagawa T, et al. [^{3}H]Zonisamide binding in rat brain. Jpn J Psychiatry Neurol 1988;42:640.

2
Mechanisms of Generalized Spike-Wave Epilepsy*

Massimo Avoli

HISTORICAL BACKGROUND

The generalized 3-hertz (Hz) spike and wave (SW) discharge that occurs during a clinical absence attack is one of the most dramatic patterns seen in clinical electroencephalography and represents the prototype of nonconvulsive generalized seizures. First described in epileptic patients by Gibbs et al.,[1] the generalized SW discharge was produced experimentally for the first time in 1946 by Jasper and Droogleever-Fortuyn using low-frequency stimulation of the midline and intralaminar nuclei of the thalamus in cats.[2] This finding strongly supported a subcortical (then termed *centrencephalic*) origin of the generalized 3-Hz SW seizure discharge. This mechanism, however, was not universally accepted because it could not be consistently reproduced (see review in reference 3). Thus, some years later, Marcus and Watson[4, 5] provided experimental evidence for a cortical origin of bilaterally synchronous SW discharges by demonstrating that bilateral application of convulsant drugs to the frontal cortex of cats and monkeys could suffice for the appearance of such an epileptiform pattern. Arguments in favor of a cortical origin of primary generalized epilepsy could also be obtained from observations in the Senegalese baboon *Papio papio*, a primate that presents a genetically transmitted photosensitive generalized epilepsy (see for a review references 6 and 7). In the late 1960s, Gloor[8-10] proposed the term *generalized corticoreticular epilepsy* to group under one heading all generalized seizures exhibiting SW discharges in the electroencephalographic (EEG) tracing. By using this new term, an attempt was made to reconcile the *centrencephalic* and the *diffuse cortical* mechanisms of 3-Hz generalized SW discharges.

This new concept, which assigned essential roles to the cortex and the *reticular system* of the thalamus and brain stem, has been widely tested during the last

*This chapter is dedicated to Dr. Pierre Gloor, my long-time teacher and friend.

2 decades in the feline generalized penicillin epilepsy (FGPE) model. This model, discovered by Prince and Farrell,[11] is produced by giving large intramuscular doses of penicillin to cats. FGPE is a valid model for human primary generalized epilepsy characterized clinically by absence attacks and electroencephalographically by bilaterally synchronous 3-Hz SW discharges. In addition to an EEG pattern that is similar to that seen in absence attacks (Figure 2.1), cats exhibit behavioral manifestations consisting of rhythmic blinking and facial twitching. As in humans, a generalized SW discharge induced by parenteral penicillin is also associated with an abrupt and pronounced drop in responsiveness to stimuli presented during SW discharge in an operant conditioning procedure and arrest of self-paced motor behavior.[12] The responsiveness profile of the penicillin-induced generalized SW discharges to anticonvulsant drugs is similar to that found in human absence epilepsy: ethosuximide and valproate are effective in reducing generalized SW activity, whereas phenytoin is not.[13, 14]

This chapter describes the thalamocortical mechanisms that are involved in the 3-Hz SW discharge and considers the neocortical cellular events that underlie such activity. Moreover, the mechanisms of action of antiabsence drugs are discussed in the context of the mechanisms that appear to be responsible for the rhythmic behavior of thalamic and cortical neurons during a 3-Hz SW discharge. Much of this review is devoted to experimental findings obtained in the model of FGPE; however, results originating from other experimental studies are also considered whenever appropriate.

THALAMOCORTICAL MECHANISM AND SPIKE-WAVE EPILEPSY

Our studies have demonstrated that SW discharges of FGPE evolve from spindles and therefore are presumably mediated by a common thalamocortical mechanism. The transformation of spindles into SW discharges of FGPE results from an increased excitability of cortical neurons that follows the intramuscular injection of penicillin and is responsible for the secondary recruitment of a powerful, and at least in part recurrent, intracortical inhibitory mechanism.[15–17] Therefore, the *spike* of the SW complex represents an exaggerated spindle-wave that results from summed cortical excitatory postsynaptic potentials (EPSPs) induced by thalamocortical volleys. By contrast, the *slow-wave* component is associated with a 200–300 ms hyperpolarization (Figure 2.2)[18] and thus reflects the summation of intracortical inhibitory postsynaptic potentials (IPSPs) of gamma-aminobutyric acid $(GABA)_A$ and $GABA_B$ types. In keeping with such a sequence of neuronal potentials, the pattern of a SW discharge correlates at the cellular level with a striking oscillation between marked increases in firing probability of cortical neurons during the *spike* and a reduction of this probability of firing to virtually zero during the *slow-wave* component of the SW complex (see Figures 2.5 and 2.6).

The cortex and the thalamus are both required for the occurrence of generalized SW discharges that are recorded in cats injected with intramuscular penicillin. If the thalamic activity is transiently depressed by a local microinjection of KCl, SW discharges in thalamus and cortex are abolished (Figure 2.3).[19] On

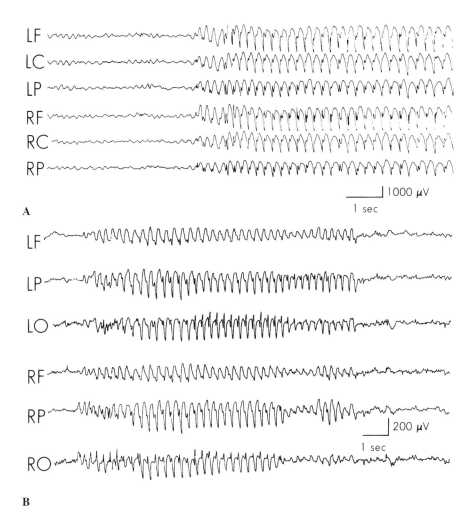

Figure 2.1 Electroencephalographic (EEG) patterns of a generalized spike and wave (SW) discharge recorded (A) in a 9-year-old boy during an absence attack and (B) in a cat after a large dose of intramuscular penicillin. Note the similarity of the EEG patterns observed in human and cat generalized SW discharges. (L = left; R = right; F = frontal; P = parietal; O = occipital; C = central.) (A is reprinted with permission from P Gloor, R Fariello. Generalized epilepsy: some of its cellular mechanisms differ from those of focal epilepsy. Trends Neurosci 1988;11:63. B is reprinted with permission from A Guberman, P Gloor, AL Sherwin. Response of generalized penicillin epilepsy in the cat to ethosuximide and diphenylhydantoin. Neurology 1975;25:758.)

the other hand, when the thalamus is deprived of inputs from and outputs toward the cortex, a SW discharge is not seen. As illustrated in Figure 2.4, the thalamus of a decorticated cat does not generate SW discharges after large doses of intramuscular penicillin.[20] Under these conditions, spindles are recorded from different thalamic nuclei before and after penicillin. Moreover, thalamic SWs in the

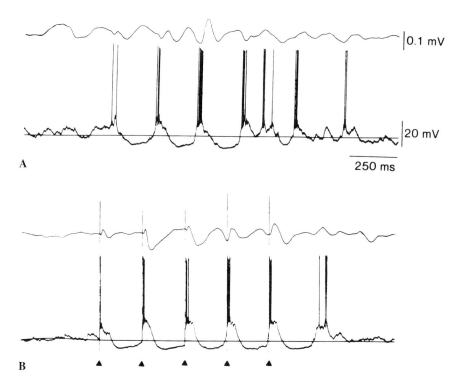

Figure 2.2   Similarities in the electroencephalographic (upper trace) and intracellular (lower trace) recordings between (A) penicillin-induced spike and wave discharges and (B) thalamocortical responses induced by repetitive stimuli (triangles) delivered to the nucleus ventralis lateralis of the thalamus. (Reprinted with permission from D Giaretta, M Avoli, P Gloor. Intracellular recordings in pericruciate neurons during spike and wave discharges of feline generalized penicillin epilepsy. Brain Res 1987;405:68.)

intact brain are replaced by spindles when the cortex is inactivated bilaterally by spreading depression.[20] The involvement in FGPE of a thalamocortical mechanism that is operant under normal physiologic conditions is supported by the similarities shared by incrementing cortical responses induced by low-frequency repetitive stimuli delivered in the thalamus and spontaneous SW discharges occurring after an intramuscular injection of penicillin (see Figure 2.2).

In the model of FGPE, the thalamus is secondarily but very quickly recruited into this oscillatory pattern via corticothalamic pathways. Accordingly, electrophysiologically identified corticothalamic neurons fire bursts of action potentials during the *spike* of the SW discharge[21] and thus provide the excitatory inputs that impose on thalamic neurons the oscillatory modality of firing that is characteristic of SW discharge; in turn, many of these cells are thalamocortical neurons that project back to the neocortex.

Interhemispheric synchronization of 3-Hz SW discharges is mainly caused by the corpus callosum. Accordingly, surgical sectioning of the corpus callosum and

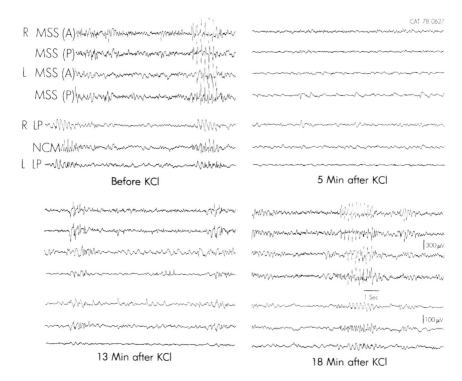

R MSS (A)
   MSS (P)
L MSS (A)
   MSS (P)

R LP
   NCM
L LP

Before KCl

CAT 78 0627

5 Min after KCl

13 Min after KCl

18 Min after KCl

300 μV

1 Sec

100 μV

Figure 2.3   Effects exerted on the spontaneous thalamic and cortical electroencephalographic activity by a thalamic microinjection of 10 ml 25% KCl into the left thalamic nucleus lateralis posterior (L LP). Note that cortical and thalamic spike and wave discharges of feline generalized penicillin epilepsy disappear and recover together with the return of normal thalamic activity, which is depressed most markedly at the site of the microinjection. (MSS = middle suprasylvian gyrus; NCM = nucleus centralis medialis; R = right; L = left; (A) = anterior; (P) = posterior.) (Reprinted with permission from M Avoli, P Gloor. The effects of transient functional depression of the thalamus on spindles and on bilateral synchronous discharges of feline generalized penicillin epilepsy. Epilepsia 1981;22:443.)

of the anterior commissure disrupts the bilateral synchrony of SW discharges, whereas sectioning of the massa intermedia does not.[22] Similar findings have been obtained in the Strasbourg Wistar model[23] as well as in the *Papio papio* photosensitive epilepsy.[7]

The mechanism of interaction between the thalamus and cortex in SW discharges has also been studied by recording cortical and thalamic EEG findings as well as the firing of a pair of neurons (one in the cortex, the other in the thalamus). In these experiments, we used EEG averaging and time histogram computation techniques (Figures 2.5 and 2.6). The essential features that were revealed by these studies can be summarized as follows.[24] First, the cortical and thalamic neurons within a thalamocortical sector (most often in the middle suprasylvian gyrus and the nucleus lateralis posterior) fire in an oscillatory fashion in a tightly phase-locked manner. Second, the oscillatory pattern in each burst of SW

Bilateral Decortication

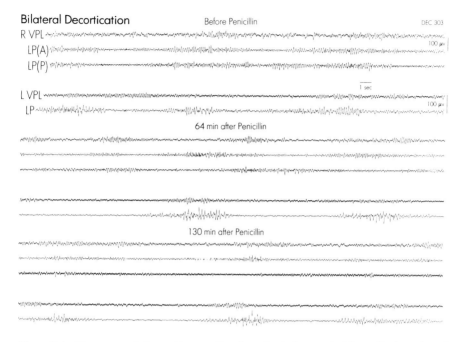

Figure 2.4   Electroencephalographic recording from the thalamus of a bilaterally decorticated cat before and after intramuscular injection of 350,000 IU/kg penicillin. (LP = nucleus lateralis posterior; VPL = nucleus ventroposterolateralis; R = right; L = left; (A) = anterior; (P) = posterior.) (Reprinted with permission from M Avoli, P Gloor. Role of the thalamus in generalized penicillin epilepsy: observations on decorticated cats. Exp Neurol 1982;77:386.)

discharge appears to be initiated by the cortex and entrains the thalamus secondarily. Third, most thalamic neurons reach the peak of their firing probability at the time of the cortical and thalamic *spike* component of the SW complex (see Figures 2.5 and 2.6), while a small number of thalamic cells, which were not identified electrophysiologically, fire 180 degrees out of phase with the others, i.e., in coincidence with the *slow-wave* component of the SW complex. Further experiments have demonstrated that the oscillatory pattern in the thalamus is seen more clearly in neurons of the *specific* nuclei than in those of *nonspecific* nuclei.[25] Furthermore, following intramuscular injection of penicillin, the oscillatory pattern of thalamic neurons appears earlier in *specific* than in *nonspecific* thalamic nuclei.

Our data therefore indicated that although a SW discharge is initiated in the cortex, the thalamus plays an active role in FGPE. Hence, it becomes meaningless once the thalamocortical oscillation is established to ask whether the cortex or the thalamus paces the SW rhythm. Both structures are essential, and the functional and anatomic integrity of each of them is required to maintain the SW discharge. SW discharges in other experimental models of generalized epilepsy (e.g., some rodent models) appear to be initiated from thalamic structures rather than the cortex. For instance, SW discharges in the Strasbourg Wistar model often

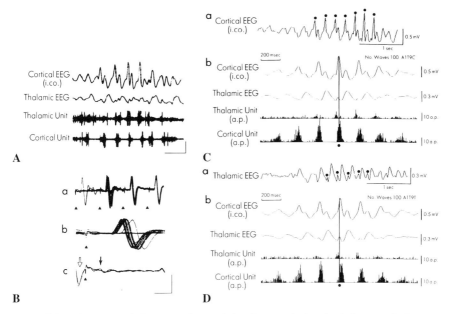

Figure 2.5 Electroencephalogram-unit correlation for a cortical and a thalamocortical neuron that projects to the cortical area containing the recorded cortical neuron during a generalized spike and wave (SW) discharge in feline generalized penicillin epilepsy. A. Raw data: cortical and thalamic electroencephalographic (EEG) (upper traces) recordings and respective single unit activity (lower traces). B. Identification of the thalamic neuron analyzed in C and D as a thalamocortical cell by virtue of its antidromic activation from the cortex (a and b) and collision test (c); triangles indicate cortical stimuli. C, D. EEG averages and histograms of single unit activity of a cortical neuron in the middle suprasylvian gyrus and of the antidromically activated thalamic neuron shown in B. In C, EEG averages and histograms of single unit activity were triggered by the negative peaks of *spikes* of intracortically recorded SW discharges (as shown in sample a). In D, EEG averages and histograms of single unit activity were triggered by the negative peaks of *spikes* of SW discharges recorded in the thalamus (as shown in sample a). Spikes of SW complexes are associated with increased slow waves with a decreased firing probability of cortical and thalamic neurons. Note that during the SW sequences, the alternating firing pattern characteristic of SW discharges develops earlier in the cortex than in the thalamus, but once it is fully developed, the thalamic unit tends to fire before the cortical unit. These features emerge regardless of whether the cortical or the thalamic spikes of SWs are used as triggers. Calibrations in Figure 2.5A are 0.5 mV and 500 ms; in Figure 2.5B: a, 4 ms; b, 1 ms; c, 2 mV. (i. co. = intracortical; a.p. = action potentials.)

start in the thalamus and then seem to entrain the cortex.[26] However, this evidence is based solely on EEG recordings. Moreover, in this genetic model of generalized SW seizures a tightly interlocked thalamocortical mechanism is present. In the Strasbourg Wistar model, as well as in two other pharmacologic rodent models, the thalamus and cortex are required for generalized SW seizures to occur. Neither structure alone can sustain bilateral SW discharges.[27] Hence, in different models the SW rhythm may be initiated from the cortex or the thalamus, but this point is relatively trivial compared with the importance of the role of the oscil-

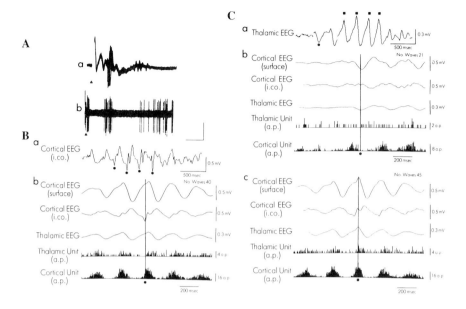

Figure 2.6   Relationship between the firing of a cortical neuron and a thalamic neuron receiving corticothalamic inputs from the area containing the recorded cortical neuron. A. Evidence for orthodromic activation by cortical stimulation of the thalamic neuron (analyzed in B and C) in which the latency of the response to cortical stimulation is variable. Triangles indicate cortical stimuli (0.08 ms, 0.4 mA). Calibrations: a, 4 ms; b, 20 ms, 2 mV. B and C. Electroencephalographic (EEG) averages and histograms of single unit activity are triggered by positive peaks of spikes of intracortically recorded spike and wave discharges (as shown in sample a of B). C. Negative peaks of sharp waves recorded in the thalamus (as shown in sample a of C). The thalamic neuron tends to fire after the cortical neurons. (i. co. = intracortical; a.p. = action potentials.) (Reprinted with permission from M Avoli, P Gloor, G Kostopoulos, J Gotman. An analysis of penicillin-induced generalized spike and wave discharges using simultaneous recording of cortical and thalamic single units. J Neurophysiol 1983;50:819.)

lation of the thalamocorticothalamic loop in the elaboration and maintenance of generalized SW discharges.

How is the frequency of oscillation in this thalamocortical network reduced to about one-half as spindles evolve into SWs?[16] Our own studies have not addressed this problem, but it is likely that the mechanisms responsible for intrathalamic oscillations that have recently been described by several authors[28–31] are also involved in the linkage between corticothalamic and thalamocortical mechanisms operant in SW seizures. In the spindle stage the frequency of oscillation in thalamocortical networks depends on the deinactivation of a Ca^{2+} conductance (termed *low-threshold*) of thalamocortical neurons paced by rhythmic GABAergic inputs from neurons that are located in the thalamic reticular nucleus; these cells cause pronounced hyperpolarizations in thalamocortical neurons and these IPSPs are required to deinactivate the Ca^{2+} conductance.

Two possible explanations can be envisaged as to how the thalamocortical neurons, which sustain spindles, and the SW discharge respond to cortical inputs by an oscillation that after penicillin injection has a frequency that is only one-half that of the spindle rhythm. The first explanation relates solely to an intrathalamic change and is based on the fact that penicillin is a weak $GABA_A$ antagonist. Penicillin may therefore weaken $GABA_A$-mediated inhibition and thus increase the excitability of the reticular nucleus, while leaving the $GABA_B$-mediated mechanism intact and augmented. According to von Krosigk et al.,[31] in an in vitro slice preparation, blockage of $GABA_A$ action shifts the oscillation in the network connecting the reticular nucleus to thalamic relay cells to a slower frequency that is within the range of the SW rhythm. This explanation, however, might not be fully satisfactory, as one would expect the thalamus of a decorticated cat to produce a SW rhythm instead of spindles when doses sufficient or exceeding those required to produce SW discharge are injected in an intact cat. However, this is not the case. The thalamus continues to produce spindles under these conditions (see Figure 2.4).[20] The second explanation is based on the fact that the cortical output through corticothalamic volleys becomes more powerful as spindles evolve into SWs.[15] Thus, the reticular nucleus is more powerfully stimulated through corticothalamic volleys and hence produces a more powerful inhibitory output to thalamocortical neurons, which therefore will generate hyperpolarizations that are of larger amplitude and longer duration. This process may shift the membrane potential of thalamocortical neurons into the region where the slow delta oscillator described by Steriade et al.[30] becomes activated and supersedes the spindle oscillation. The frequency of this slower oscillation is within the range of the SW rhythm. This hypothesis, which required a change in cortical excitability, is more attractive in the light of the experiments on decorticate cats mentioned above. However, a coexistence of the two mechanisms should not be excluded, as they would both explain the switch from the spindle to the SW rhythm.

Thalamocortical projections represent an important link in the final processing of sensory information coming from the periphery. The tight synchronization between thalamus and cortex that occurs during SW discharges might interfere with this information processing and thus account for the marked impairment of such processing during an absence attack. To test this hypothesis, somatosensory responses were recorded with an extracellular recording microelectrode positioned in the somatosensory area of the neocortex while the contralateral radial nerve was stimulated with electrical shocks (2 Hz) during SW discharges induced by penicillin. As illustrated in Figure 2.7, when stimuli occurred between one SW burst and the next, the somatosensory neocortical cell discharge showed a prominent response to electrical radial nerve stimulation. By contrast, this response was greatly reduced when the stimuli occurred during the SW discharge. This markedly reduced response to a sensory stimulus during SW discharges coupled with its preservation in the inter–SW-burst interval dovetails with the marked reduction of behavioral responsiveness during SW discharges in cats subject to FGPE and contrasts with its full preservation between SW bursts.[12] This condition mimics quite closely the situation that is seen in human absence attacks. These findings therefore indicate that during SW activity, the pattern of cortical neuronal discharge is highly disruptive of integrated cortical function. They thus explain the deficit in cognitive functions that characterizes absence attacks.[32]

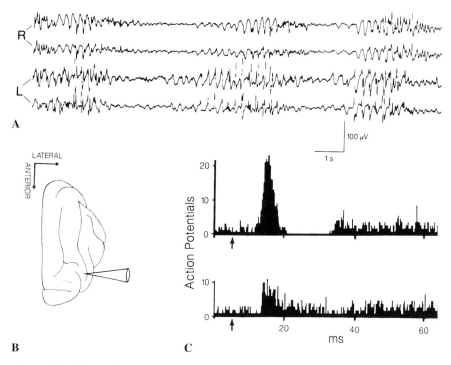

Figure 2.7   Spike and wave (SW) discharges depress the response of a neocortical cell in the contralateral somatosensory area to electrical stimuli delivered at 2 hertz to the radial nerves. A. SW discharges recorded from the anterior and posterior suprasylvian gyrus of both hemispheres. B. Schematic drawing of a cat brain seen from above shows position of the recording microelectrode. C. Upper panel shows peristimulation histogram that was constructed by selecting stimuli occurring between SW discharges; the lower histogram was made from stimuli delivered during SW discharge. (R = right; L = left.) (Based on unpublished data from P White, R Dykes, M Avoli, and P Gloor.)

INTRACORTICAL INHIBITION AND GENERALIZED SEIZURE ACTIVITY

A hallmark of generalized SW discharges in FGPE is the "preservation" of $GABA_A$- and $GABA_B$-mediated intracortical inhibitory mechanisms that underlie the slow-wave component of the SW complex.[18] This conclusion is further supported by experiments in which two well-known GABA-mediated inhibitory mechanisms (i.e., cerebral peduncle and cortical shock-induced IPSPs) were shown to be unchanged after intramuscular penicillin up to and beyond the appearance of fully developed SW activity (Figure 2.8A and B).[17, 33] Doses of penicillin similar to those present in the brains of cats after injection of penicillin, when applied to rat hippocampal slices, induce an increase of EPSP without any measurable decrease of the amplitude of the recurrent IPSP induced by alvear stimuli (Figure 2.8C).[34]

However, as illustrated in Figure 2.9, cortical IPSPs disappear shortly before the onset of as well as during the EEG pattern that is commonly associated with

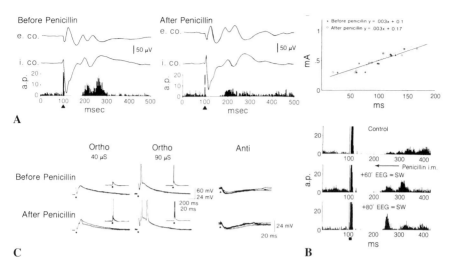

Figure 2.8   A. Lack of changes in recurrent inhibition induced by electrical stimulation of the cerebral peduncle (triangle) before and after an intramuscular injection of penicillin sufficient to induce a generalized spike and wave discharge. In each panel, upper traces are averages of the field potentials recorded from the cortical surface (e. co.) and the intracortical (i. co.) layers of the pericruciate gyrus; lower traces are single unit peristimulus time histograms of the activity of a cortical cell antidromically activated from the cerebral peduncle. The duration of the inhibitory pause is unchanged after intramuscular penicillin. B. Upper part: relationship between the intensity of the direct cortical shock (mA) and the duration of the inhibitory period (ms) before (solid line) and after intramuscular penicillin. Lower part: peristimulus time histograms of a neuron of the middle suprasylvian gyrus in response to direct cortical shock at the indicated time after intramuscular penicillin. The length of the inhibitory pause was unchanged. C. In a CA1 pyramidal cell of a rat hippocampal slice, low concentrations of penicillin (0.34 mmol/liter) induce an increase in the amplitude and half-width of the excitatory postsynaptic potential as well as the discharge of two action potentials (a.p.) after orthodromic stimuli without changing the amplitude or the duration of the recurrent inhibitory postsynaptic potential. (A is reprinted with permission from G Kostopoulos, M Avoli, P Gloor. Participation of cortical recurrent inhibition in the genesis of the spike and wave discharges in feline generalized penicillin epilepsy. Brain Res 1983;267:101. B is reprinted with permission from D Giaretta, G Kostopoulos, P Gloor, M Avoli. Intracortical inhibitory mechanisms are preserved in feline generalized penicillin epilepsy. Neurosci Lett 1984;59:203. C is reprinted with permission from M Avoli. Penicillin-induced hyperexcitability in the "in vitro" hippocampal slice can be unrelated to impairment of somatic inhibition. Brain Res 1984;323:154.)

generalized tonic-clonic convulsions.[17] EEG tonic-clonic convulsions are commonly seen in cats with reticular-formation lesions or after several hours of SW discharge. Therefore, the transition from generalized 3-Hz SW discharges of an absence attack to generalized convulsive seizures is accompanied and possibly caused by the breakdown of one or more hyperpolarizing inhibitory potentials in the cortex. This view is in keeping with the observation that in the neocortex of a cat that had received a topical application of penicillin, post-paroxysmal depolarizing shift hyperpolarizations disappear before the onset of focal ictal

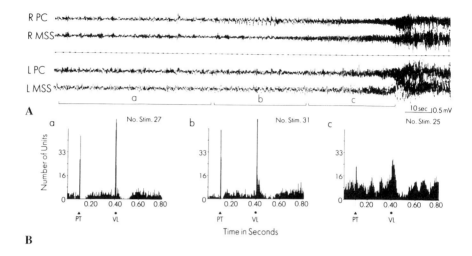

Figure 2.9   Peristimulus time histograms (panel B) of an identified pyramidal tract cell recorded at a stage when spike and wave discharges were cyclically turning into convulsive seizure activity (panel A). Computation of each histogram was limited to the period associated with one of the three different patterns of electroencephalographic activity shown in panel A. Note the gradual disappearance of the inhibitory pause after antidromic pyramidal tract (PT) or orthodromic thalamic (VL) stimulation as the convulsive seizure activity approaches. (R = right; L = left; PC = pericruciate; MSS = middle suprasylvian gyrus.) (Reprinted with permission from M Avoli. GABAergic Mechanisms and Epileptic Discharges. In M Avoli, TA Reeder, RW Dykes, P Gloor [eds] Neurotransmitters and Cortical Function: From Molecules to Mind. New York: Plenum, 1988;187.)

discharge and are barely observed during such discharge.[35] A breakdown of GABAergic potentials has also been reported for epileptiform responses evoked in the hippocampus of rats,[36] in the human neocortex maintained in vitro[37] by repetitive electrical stimulation, and in the slices of the in vitro olfactory cortex during seizure-like activity induced by application of 4-aminopyridine.[38]

Several cellular phenomena might cause the decreased efficacy and eventual disappearance of GABA-mediated potentials observed immediately before the onset and during the tonic-clonic ictal discharge. These include a use-dependent depression of inhibitory potentials, which can occur pre- and post-synaptically,[39] and a decreased efficacy of GABAergic potentials resulting from the changes in the ionic composition of the extracellular environment that accompany epileptiform discharges. For instance, as has been documented in several models of epilepsy, $[K^+]_o$ increases from a baseline of 3 mmol/liter up to 15–20 mmol/liter during seizure activity.[37, 40, 41] This change in $[K^+]_o$ can influence the efficacy of GABAergic conductances by causing a shift of the Cl⁻ equilibrium potential in the positive direction and thus a decrease in the drive of the hyperpolarizing IPSPs mediated through $GABA_A$ receptors. Furthermore, an increase in $[K^+]_o$ will diminish the chemical gradient for this cation and thus it will influence the K⁺ outward current caused by the activation of the $GABA_B$ receptor.

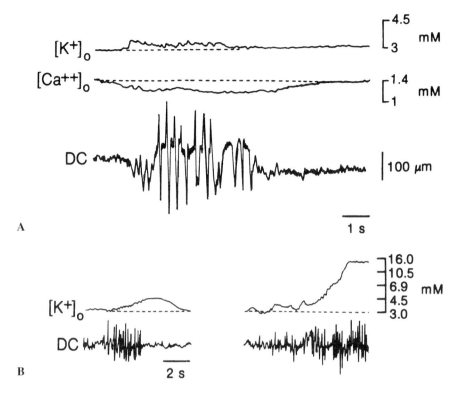

Figure 2.10   A. Measurement of $[K^+]_o$ and $[Ca^{2+}]_o$ during a spike and wave (SW) discharge (DC) recorded in the middle suprasylvian gyrus of a cat given an intramuscular injection of penicillin. B. Changes in $[K^+]_o$ during a SW discharge (left panel) and "tonic-clonic" activity (right panel). (Based on unpublished data from G Kostopoulos, C Drapeau, and M Avoli.)

$[K^+]_o$ increases only by 1.2–1.8 mmol/liter during the SW discharges of FGPE (Figure 2.10A and 2.10B, left sample), while it can reach values as high as 16 mmol/liter during the tonic-clonic activity recorded in this model (Figure 2.10, right sample). Concomitant analysis of $[Ca^{2+}]_o$ during the two types of discharges in cats injected with penicillin has also shown that Ca^{2+} only decreases by 0.2–0.4 mmol/liter during SW discharges but can drop by 1 mmol/liter during the tonic-clonic activity (G. Kostopoulos, C. Drapeau, and M. Avoli, unpublished observations). This is in agreement with the observation made by Pumain et al.[42] in photosensitive baboons, where the drop in $[Ca^{2+}]_o$ was minimal during photically evoked SW discharges but became large when the convulsive seizure appeared. Such a decrease in $[Ca^{2+}]_o$ can exert a depressant effect on the IPSP[42, 43] by diminishing the release of GABA and thus the efficacy of the IPSP. Connor et al.[44] have shown that in response to glutamate-induced depolarization, Ca^{2+} enters the cell, and, after repeated glutamate pulses, its intracellular concentration may continue to rise. This may be an additional factor in decreasing the response to GABA.[45]

The differences in the cellular mechanisms underlying generalized SW discharges and tonic-clonic discharges might explain some differences in the clinical consequences of pure absence epilepsy with generalized SW discharge compared with seizure disorders associated with generalized convulsive or partial seizures.[46] Absence epilepsy uncomplicated by generalized convulsions is one of the most benign forms of epilepsy.[47–49] Its EEG manifestation (i.e., the generalized SW discharge), is a nonevolving seizure pattern that is not followed by any postictal depression electrographically or clinically, indicating the likely lack of any deleterious after effects of the discharge. Pure absence epilepsy uncomplicated by convulsive seizures tends to have a benign course, since it often remits spontaneously or under treatment.[46] By contrast, the EEG pattern of tonic-clonic seizures is followed by EEG and clinical signs of postictal depression. These seizures are more resistant to therapy and may have short or more enduring deleterious consequences.

The experiments reviewed here indicate that during generalized SW discharges induced in cats by the intramuscular injection of penicillin, hyperpolarizing mechanisms mediated through GABA receptors are preserved. One important implication that derives from the preservation of hyperpolarizing GABAergic mechanisms is that in the experimental model of a generalized SW discharge the ionic conductance changes caused by activation of the N-methyl-D-aspartate (NMDA) receptor through the action of the excitatory amino acids glutamate and aspartate are relatively limited. The NMDA receptor is coupled with an ionophore that displays a voltage-dependent block exerted by extracellular Mg^{2+} and is permeable to Ca^{2+}.[50] Such a condition changes when inhibition breaks down, as in the case of the transition from interictal to ictal epileptiform activity in partial (focal) epilepsy or from a generalized SW discharge to generalized convulsive seizure activity. The breakdown of inhibitory hyperpolarizing mechanisms as it occurs during the transition from one state to the other in these two types of seizures might lead to membrane depolarization and thus may relieve the blockade of the NMDA channel exerted by Mg^{2+}. Hence, the NMDA-ionophore will become fully permeant to cations and in particular to Ca^{2+}. Consequently, during seizures in which a breakdown of GABA-mediated inhibitory mechanisms occurs, a large amount of Ca^{2+} will enter the intracellular compartment as shown by extracellular measurements of the Ca^{2+} activity.

The Ca^{2+} influx into neurons that occurs during the ictal stage of seizures, with the exception of absence attacks, will undoubtedly cause a number of intracellular responses, some of which are mediated directly by Ca^{2+}, others indirectly through the activation of one or several second messenger systems. In most instances these effects are probably only temporary and relatively benign, expressing themselves by the well-known postictal depression evident in the EEG recording in the form of slow waves or clinically in the form of Todd's paralysis, mental confusion, or postictal amnesia. Plastic neuronal changes analogous to those underlying kindling may also occur and could cause the seizure tendency to become more firmly entrenched in the brain. This may explain the relative therapy resistance of long-standing seizure disorders.[51] Prolonged and massive entry of Ca^{2+} as it occurs during major seizures may exert deleterious consequences that may include reversible or irreversible cell damage and even cell death. None of these deleterious consequences is known to occur in pure absence epilepsy characterized by generalized SW discharges.[46]

MECHANISMS OF ACTION OF ANTIABSENCE DRUGS

An important role in the oscillatory behavior seen during SW discharges is played by ionic mechanisms that are intrinsic to neurons in the thalamus and probably in the neocortex. One of these, the so-called low-threshold Ca^{2+} conductance, is deinactivated by membrane hyperpolarization and is particularly prominent in the thalamic structures. It might therefore play a role in the rhythmic behavior of neurons located in the thalamus that participate in SW discharges.[28, 30, 31, 52–54] This type of ionic conductance is diminished and eventually blocked by the antiabsence drug ethosuximide.[28, 55, 56] On the other hand, as the membrane hyperpolarization seen during the slow wave of SW discharge is necessary for deinactivating the Ca^{2+} current, drugs that antagonize the synaptic mechanism responsible for this hyperpolarization might be effective as antiabsence agents. This is the case for the $GABA_B$ antagonist CGP35348, which is capable of decreasing SW discharges in the Strasbourg Wistar rat model.[57] Similar findings have been obtained in the lethargic mouse, which represents a model of primary generalized absence seizures.[58]

An in vitro study has also shed light on the beneficial actions of the benzodiazepine clonazepam on the generalized SW discharges of absence attacks.[59] According to this study, clonazepam appears to reduce the $GABA_B$ component of the hyperpolarization generated by thalamocortical cells, an effect that is presumably secondary to an action of this benzodiazepine on inhibitory circuits of the reticular nucleus. Thus, the final effect of clonazepam is to decrease the late hyperpolarization necessary for deinactivating the low-threshold Ca^{2+} current.

A different mechanism of action should be considered for valproate, which is effective in controlling absence attacks as well as generalized tonic-clonic seizures. Valproate is able to reduce voltage-gated Na^+ currents in cortical cells,[60] which is a mechanism that is of obvious relevance for reducing the sustained depolarizations and action-potential discharges that are seen in generalized tonic-clonic activity. However, the site of action of valproate for controlling absence attacks remains unknown. A clue for this latter mechanism might come from recent data obtained in subicular neurons, which have indicated that a Na^+ current might be responsible for the brief bursts generated by these cells.[61] This burst shares some similarities with the bursts generated by thalamic neurons, including the occurrence at the end of a hyperpolarizing pulse (the so-called postanodal exaltation). However, whether this Na^+ mechanism is present in neocortical cells still remains to be elucidated.

Acknowledgments

This work was supported by MRC of Canada Grant MT-8109. I thank Mr V. Epp for secretarial assistance.

REFERENCES

1. Gibbs FA, Davis H, Lennox WG. The electroencephalogram in epilepsy and in conditions of impaired consciousness. Arch Neurol Psychiatry 1935;34:1133.

2. Jasper HH, Droogleever-Fortuyn J. Experimental studies on the functional anatomy of petit mal epilepsy. Res Publ Assoc Nerv Ment Dis 1946;26:272.
3. Gloor P. Evolution of the Concept of the Mechanism of Generalized Epilepsy with Bilateral Spike and Wave Discharge. In JA Wada (ed), Modern Perspectives in Epilepsy. Montreal: Eden Press, 1978:99.
4. Marcus EM, Watson CW. Bilateral synchronous spike wave electrographic patterns in the cat. Arch Neurol 1966;14:601.
5. Marcus EM, Watson CW. Symmetrical epileptogenic foci in monkey cerebral cortex: mechanisms of interaction and regional variations in capacity for synchronous discharges. Arch Neurol 1968;18:99.
6. Ménini C, Naquet R. Generalized Photosensitive Epilepsy in the Senegalese Baboon "*Papio papio.*" In R Canger, F Angeleri, JK Penry (eds), XIth Epilepsy International Symposium. New York: Raven, 1980:265.
7. Naquet R, Ménini C, Catier J. Photically-Induced Epilepsy in *Papio papio*: The Initiation of Discharges and the Role of the Frontal Cortex and the Corpus Callosum. In MAB Brazier, H Petsche (eds), Synchronization of the EEG in the Epilepsies. Vienna: Springer-Verlag, 1972;347.
8. Gloor P. Generalized cortico-reticular epilepsies. Some considerations on the pathophysiology of generalized bilaterally synchronous spike and wave discharge. Epilepsia 1968;9:249.
9. Gloor P. Neurophysiological Bases of Generalized Seizures Termed Centrencephalic. In H Gastaut, H Jasper, J Bancaud (eds), The Physiopathogenesis of the Epilepsies. Springfield, IL: Thomas, 1969;209.
10. Gloor P. Generalized Spike and Wave Discharges: A Consideration of Cortical and Subcortical Mechanisms of Their Genesis and Synchronization. In H Petsche, MAB Brazier (eds), Synchronization of EEG Activity in Epilepsies. New York: Springer-Verlag, 1972;382.
11. Prince DA, Farrell D. "Centrencephalic" spike-wave discharges following parenteral penicillin injection in the cat. Neurology 1969;19:309.
12. Taylor-Courval D, Gloor P. Behavioral alterations associated with generalized spike and wave discharges in the EEG of the cat. Exp Neurol 1984;83:167.
13. Guberman A, Gloor P, Sherwin AL. Response of generalized penicillin epilepsy in the cat to ethosuximide and diphenylhydantoin. Neurology 1975;25:758.
14. Pellegrini A, Gloor P, Sherwin AL. Effect of valproate sodium on generalized penicillin epilepsy in the cat. Epilepsia 1978;19:351.
15. Kostopoulos G, Gloor P, Pellegrini A, Gotman J. A study of the transition from spindles to spike and wave discharge in feline generalized penicillin epilepsy: microphysiological features. Exp Neurol 1981;73:55.
16. Kostopoulos G, Gloor P, Pellegrini A, Siatitsas I. A study of the transition from spindles to spike and wave discharge in feline generalized penicillin epilepsy: EEG features. Exp Neurol 1981;73:43.
17. Kostopoulos G, Avoli M, Gloor P. Participation of cortical recurrent inhibition in the genesis of the spike and wave discharges in feline generalized penicillin epilepsy. Brain Res 1983;267:101.
18. Giaretta D, Avoli M, Gloor P. Intracellular recordings in pericruciate neurons during spike and wave discharges of feline generalized penicillin epilepsy. Brain Res 1987;405:68.
19. Avoli M, Gloor P. The effects of transient functional depression of the thalamus on spindles and on bilateral synchronous discharges of feline generalized penicillin epilepsy. Epilepsia 1981;22:443.
20. Avoli M, Gloor P. Interaction of cortex and thalamus in spike and wave discharges of feline generalized penicillin epilepsy. Exp Neurol 1982;76:196.
21. Avoli M, Kostopoulos G. Participation of corticothalamic cells in penicillin induced spike and wave discharges. Brain Res 1982;247:159.
22. Musgrave J, Gloor P. The role of the corpus callosum in bilateral interhemispheric synchrony of spike and wave discharge in feline generalized penicillin epilepsy. Epilepsia 1980;21:369.
23. Vergnes M, Marescaux C, Depaulis A, et al. Spontaneous Spike-and-Wave Discharges in Wistar Rats: A Model of Genetic Generalized Convulsive Epilepsy. In M Avoli, P Gloor, G Kostopoulos, R Naquet (eds), Generalized Epilepsy: Neurobiological Approaches. Boston: Birkhäuser, 1990;238.
24. Avoli M, Gloor P, Kostopoulos G, Gotman J. An analysis of penicillin-induced generalized spike and wave discharges using simultaneous recording of cortical and thalamic single units. J Neurophysiol 1983;50:819.
25. McLachlan RS, Gloor P, Avoli M. Differential participation of some "specific" and "non-specific" thalamic nuclei in generalized spike and wave discharges of feline generalized penicillin epilepsy. Brain Res 1984;307:277.
26. Vergnes M, Marescaux C, Depaulis A, et al. Spontaneous spike and wave discharges in thalamus and cortex in a rat model of genetic petit mal–like seizures. Exp Neurol 1987;96:127.

27. Snead OC. γ-Hydroxybutyrate model of generalized absence seizures: further characterization and comparison with other absence models. Epilepsia 1988;29:361.
28. Huguenard MR, Prince DA. Intrathalamic rhythmicity studied in vitro: nominal T-current modulation causes robust antioscillatory effects. J Neurosci 1994;14:5485.
29. Llinás R, Jansen H. Electrophysiology of mammalian thalamic neurons "in vitro." Nature 1982;297:406.
30. Steriade M, McCormick DA, Sejnowski TJ. Thalamocortical oscillations in the sleeping and aroused brain. Science 1993;262:679.
31. von Krosigk M, Bal T, McCormick DA. Cellular mechanisms of a synchronized oscillation in the thalamus. Science 1993;261:361.
32. Gloor P. Generalized epilepsy with spike and wave discharge: a reinterpretation of its electrographic and clinical manifestations. Epilepsia 1979;20:571.
33. Giaretta D, Kostopoulos G, Gloor P, Avoli M. Intracortical inhibitory mechanisms are preserved in feline generalized penicillin epilepsy. Neurosci Lett 1985;59:203.
34. Avoli M. Penicillin-induced hyperexcitability in the "in vitro" hippocampal slice can be unrelated to impairment of somatic inhibition. Brain Res 1984;323:154.
35. Matsumoto H, Ajmone-Marsan C. Cortical cellular phenomena in experimental epilepsy: ictal manifestations. Exp Neurol 1964;9:305.
36. Ben Ari Y, Krnjevic K, Reiffenstein RJ, Rehinhardt W. Inhibitory conductance changes and action of GABA in rat hippocampus. Neuroscience 1981;6:2445.
37. Avoli M, Louvel J, Drapeau C, et al. $GABA_A$-mediated inhibition and in vitro epileptogenesis in the human neocortex. J Neurophysiol 1995;73:468.
38. Galvan M, Grafe P, ten Bruggencate G. Convulsant actions of 4-aminopyridine on the guinea pig olfactory cortex slice. Brain Res 1982;241:75.
39. McCarren M, Alger BE. Use-dependent depression of IPSPs in rat hippocampal pyramidal cells in vitro. J Neurophysiol 1985;53:557.
40. Lücke A, Nagao T, Köhling R, Avoli M. Synchronous potentials and elevations in $[K^+]_o$ in the adult rat entorhinal cortex maintained in vitro. Neurosci Lett 1995;185:155.
41. Lux HD, Heinemann U, Dietzel I. Ionic Changes and Alterations in the Size of the Extracellular Space During Epileptic Activity. In AV Delgado-Escueta, AAJ Ward, DM Woodbury, RJ Porter (eds), Advances in Neurology. New York: Raven, 1986;619.
42. Pumain R, Menini C, Heinemann U, et al. Chemical synaptic transmission is not necessary for epileptic seizures to persist in the baboon *Papio papio*. Exp Neurol 1985;89:250.
43. Heinemann U, Lux HD, Gutnick MJ. Extracellular free calcium and potassium during paroxysmal activity in the cerebral cortex of the cat. Exp Brain Res 1977;27:237.
44. Connor JA, Wadman WJ, Hodeberger PE, Wong RKS. Sustained dendritic gradients of Ca^{2+} induced by excitatory amino acids in CA1 hippocampal neurons. Science 1988;240:649.
45. Stelzer A, Kay AR, Wong RKS. $GABA_A$-receptor function in hippocampal cell is maintained by phosphorylation factors. Science 1988;241:339.
46. Gloor P. Epilepsy: relationships between electrophysiology and intracellular mechanisms involving second messengers and gene expression. Can J Neurol Sci 1989;16:8.
47. Berkovic SF, Andermann F, Andermann E, Gloor P. Concepts of absence epilepsies: discrete syndromes or biological continuum. Neurology 1987;37:993.
48. Dalby MA. Epilepsy and 3 per second spike and wave rhythms. A clinical, electroencephalographic and prognostic analysis of 346 patients. Acta Neurol Scand 1969;45(Suppl 40):183.
49. Lennox WG, Lennox MA. Epilepsy and Related Disorders. Boston: Little, Brown, 1960.
50. Nowak L, Bregestovski P, Ascher P, et al. Magnesium gates glutamate-activated channels in mouse central neurons. Nature 1984;307:462.
51. Reynolds EH, Elwes RDC, Shorvon SD. Why does epilepsy become intractable? Lancet 1983;2:952.
52. Deschênes M, Roy JP, Steriade M. Thalamic bursting mechanism: an inward slow current revealed by membrane hyperpolarization. Brain Res 1982;239:289.
53. Jahnsen H, Llinás R. Electrophysiological properties of guinea-pig thalamic neurones: an in vitro study. J Physiol (Lond) 1984;349:205.
54. Steriade M. Spindling, Incremental Thalamocortical Responses, and Spike-Wave Epilepsy. In M Avoli, P Gloor, G Kostopoulos, R Naquet (eds), Generalized Epilepsy: Neurobiological Approaches. Boston: Birkhäuser, 1990;161.
55. Coulter DA, Huguenard JR, Prince DA. Specific petit mal anticonvulsants reduce calcium currents in thalamic neurons. Neurosci Lett 1989;98:74.
56. Coulter DA, Huguenard JR, Prince DA. Cellular Actions of Petit Mal Anticonvulsants: Implication of Thalamic Low-Threshold Calcium Current in Generation of Spike-Wave Discharge. In M Avoli,

P Gloor, G Kostopoulos, R Naquet (eds), Generalized Epilepsy: Neurobiological Approaches. Boston: Birkhäuser, 1990;425.

57. Marescaux C, Vergnes M, Bernasconi R. Generalized nonconvulsive epilepsy: focus on $GABA_B$ receptors. J Neural Transm 1992;(Suppl 35).

58. Hosford DA, Clark S, Cao F, et al. The role of $GABA_B$ receptor activation in absence seizures of lethargic (lh/lh) mice. Science 1992;257:398.

59. Huguenard JR, Prince DA. Clonazepam suppresses $GABA_B$-mediated inhibition in thalamic relay neurons through effects in nucleus reticularis. J Neurophysiol 1994;71:2576.

60. Zona C, Avoli M. Effects induced by the antiepileptic drug valproic acid upon the ionic currents recorded in rat neocortical neurons in cell culture. Exp Brain Res 1990;81:313.

61. Mattia D, Hwa GGC, Avoli M. Membrane properties of rat subicular neurons in vitro. J Neurophysiol 1993;70:1244.

3
Epilepsy and the New Genetics

Frances Elmslie and R. M. Gardiner

A genetic contribution to etiology has been estimated to be present in about 20% of patients with epilepsy. The genetic control of neuronal synchrony may be direct or indirect, and the various approaches to the classification of genetic epilepsies reflect this.

It is useful in the first instance to categorize genetic epilepsies according to the mechanisms of inheritance involved. This method identifies three major groups: (1) mendelian disorders in which a single major locus can account for segregation of the disease trait; (2) nonmendelian or "complex" diseases in which the pattern of familial clustering can be accounted for by the interaction of several loci together with environmental factors or by the maternal inheritance pattern of mitochondrial deoxyribonucleic acid (mtDNA); and (3) chromosomal disorders in which a gross cytogenetic abnormality is present. A second useful distinction is between those epilepsies in which recurrent seizures are merely one component of a multifaceted neurologic phenotype, and those in which recurrent seizures occur in individuals who are otherwise neurologically and cognitively intact and who have no detectable anatomic or metabolic abnormality.

There are more than 100 mendelian diseases that include epilepsy as part of the phenotype. Most are associated with obvious structural lesions—tuberous sclerosis, for example—or generalized metabolic changes that can be assumed to generate neuronal hyperexcitability. A small number are "pure" epilepsy syndromes, and these may be generalized epilepsies (e.g., benign familial neonatal convulsions [BFNC]) or partial epilepsies (e.g., autosomal dominant nocturnal frontal lobe epilepsy). Although numerous, the mendelian epilepsies are individually rare and probably account for no more than 1% of patients.

The common familial epilepsies tend to display "complex" inheritance. They include fairly well characterized entities, such as juvenile myoclonic epilepsy, childhood absence epilepsy, and benign childhood epilepsy with centrotemporal spikes. Several gross chromosomal aberrations are associated with epilepsy, including Down syndrome and trisomy 12p.

The molecular basis of the genetic epilepsies has until recently been entirely obscure. It is likely, of course, that this is heterogenous, as seizures may be the endpoint of myriad molecular aberrations that ultimately disturb neuronal synchrony. The methods now exist for elucidating the molecular genetics of the epilepsies, and the recent demonstration of a mutation in the gene encoding the α4 subunit of the neuronal nicotinic acetylcholine receptor in a family segregating autosomal dominant nocturnal frontal lobe epilepsy is an encouraging step in that direction.

MENDELIAN EPILEPSIES

Epilepsy forms part of the phenotype of a number of mendelian diseases, including tuberous sclerosis, fragile X syndrome, neurofibromatosis, and an array of metabolic disorders, all of which are individually rare. In these diseases, seizures are symptomatic of underlying neurologic involvement and may be accompanied by other neurologic signs, such as mental retardation or developmental regression. However, there are a few primary epilepsies that are inherited in a mendelian fashion. They are rare and together account for only a small fraction of all epilepsy, but they form an important group because recognition of the characteristic features and presence of a family history will enable the correct diagnosis to be made.

"Primary" Mendelian Epilepsies

Benign Familial Neonatal Convulsions

BFNC is a rare form of idiopathic primary epilepsy that is inherited in an autosomal dominant fashion. It is characterized by the onset of seizures in the first few days of life, with remission occurring commonly by 6 weeks. The seizures are usually brief and generalized with tonic and clonic phases. However, they may be accompanied by motor automatisms, ocular manifestations, and apnea. Subsequent neurodevelopment is normal, although about 10% of individuals will continue to have epilepsy in adult life.

A gene for BFNC was localized by linkage analysis to the long arm of chromosome 20 in a single three-generation family in 1989,[1] and the locus was designated EBN1. A maximum two-point logarithm of odds (lod) score of 3.12 at θ = 0.003 was obtained at the telomeric marker D20S20 (RNR6). In this family, no recombination was detected between either of the markers D20S19 (CMM6) or D20S20 and the trait. The results were subsequently confirmed in six French pedigrees.[2] However, an additional study of two North American families suggested the presence of clinical and genetic heterogeneity.[3] In a family of northern European origin, 4 of 15 individuals experienced seizures persisting beyond 12 months and one continued to have epilepsy into adolescence. The results of linkage analysis were suggestive of linkage between the BFNC trait and chromosome 20 markers. In the other family of Mexican-American extraction (family 1) seizures had ceased in all family members by the age of 2 months and none went on to develop epilepsy later. Linkage to D20S20 and D20S19 was excluded in this family. Subsequently, a lod score of 4.43 was obtained in family 1 between the disease trait and the markers D8S284 and D8S256, suggesting that a second locus (EBN2) exists on chromosome 8q.[4] Further evidence for a locus on chromosome 8q has been obtained in a German family.[5]

The region to which EBN1 maps contains the gene encoding the α4 subunit of the nicotinic acetylcholine receptor CHRNA4. A mutation has been found in CHRNA4 in a family with autosomal dominant frontal lobe epilepsy.[6] It therefore represents a likely candidate gene for BFNC, although to date no mutations have been found in CHRNA4 in families with BFNC.

Benign Familial Infantile Convulsions

The syndrome of benign familial infantile convulsions (BFIC) was described as a distinct clinical condition by Vigevano and colleagues in 1992.[7] The onset of seizures occurs usually at age 4–7 months in infants who are otherwise neurologically and developmentally normal. Some individuals have generalized tonic-clonic seizures, but in the majority complex partial seizures occur. Typically, seizures occur in clusters over a few days and may be followed by a seizure-free period of several days or weeks. Seizures remit before the age of 18 months, and follow-up has revealed normal neurologic and developmental outcome. Investigations including cranial imaging produce normal findings, although the interictal electroencephalographic (EEG) recording may reveal focal slow waves and spikes.

The inheritance pattern is autosomal dominant. The mode of inheritance, benign outcome, and early age of onset are similar to those of BFNC. These similarities led to the suggestion that BFIC may represent an allelic variant of BFNC. However, linkage studies performed in eight families using the markers D20S19 and D20S20 gave total pairwise lod scores of -18.4 and -4.02 at $\theta = 0$, respectively, therefore excluding chromosome 20q as the site of a locus predisposing to BFIC.[8]

Autosomal Dominant Nocturnal Frontal Lobe Epilepsy

Very recently, six families from Australia, the United Kingdom, and Canada with an autosomal dominantly inherited form of partial epilepsy were described.[9, 10] Seizures occurred during sleep and had frequently been misdiagnosed as nightmares, night terrors, hysteria, sleep paralysis, and paroxysmal nocturnal dystonia. The familial nature of the condition had therefore gone unrecognized. Seizures begin predominantly in childhood and persist into adulthood. They occur in clusters of four to 11 episodes a night, usually soon after the patient falls asleep or before awakening. Several individuals report an aura that may be sensory, somatosensory, or psychic. Episodes are brief, usually lasting about 60 seconds, beginning with vocalization and followed by motor activity, either thrashing movements or tonic stiffening with or without a clonic phase. The majority of subjects are aware throughout the seizure, although many develop secondarily generalized seizures at some time. Affected individuals are neurologically and intellectually normal. The interictal EEG recording usually appears normal, although the ictal EEG recording may show sharp and slow wave activity in the anterior quadrants bilaterally. The results of neuroimaging are also normal. The treatment of choice is carbamazepine.

Segregation analysis performed in the five families described supported autosomal dominant inheritance with 69% penetrance and variable expression. Linkage studies performed in a single large Australian pedigree assigned the gene to chromosome 20q13.2, the same region to which EBN1 maps.[11] However, the remaining families do not appear to be linked to chromosome 20q, indicating the presence of genetic heterogeneity. This region of chromosome 20q contains a candidate gene, CHRNA4, which encodes the α4 subunit of the nicotinic acetylcholine receptor. A missense mutation that replaces a serine with phenylalanine at codon 248 has recently been demonstrated in CHRNA4 in the chromosome 20-linked family.[6] This highly conserved amino acid lies in the second transmembrane domain, and it is likely that mutation at this site would cause disease. Moreover, the mutation has been demonstrated in 21 affected family members and four obligate carriers but not in 333 healthy controls. It therefore appears that mutation in CHRNA4 is the first genetic defect known to result in an idiopathic epilepsy.

Partial Epilepsy with Auditory Symptoms

In a large study of the genetic contribution to epilepsy, a family in which 11 individuals over three generations had idiopathic partial epilepsy was identified.[12] Ten of the affected family members had simple partial or complex partial seizures with secondarily generalized tonic-clonic seizures. Six individuals also reported auditory disturbance, such as a hum or a ringing that grew gradually louder as part of the seizure. The age of onset was 8–19 years. The interictal EEG recording appeared normal in all cases and neurologic examination findings were also normal in those who were examined. Three members of the family had symptomatic epilepsy and three more had acute symptomatic seizures. In two members, epilepsy was suspected, but insufficient information was available for a definitive diagnosis to be made. All these individuals were classified as unknown for the purposes of linkage analysis. Linkage analysis was performed assuming autosomal dominant inheritance with a penetrance of 71% in those older than 20. A maximum two-point lod score of 3.99 was obtained at $\theta = 0$ with the marker D10S192. All living affected individuals shared a haplotype for seven markers spanning 10 cM of chromosome 10q, placing the gene somewhere between the markers D10S185 and D10S566. Further refinement of the localization of the gene will be difficult in the absence of more chromosome 10q–linked families. This locus could represent a susceptibility gene for a very specific type of epilepsy in which auditory features form part of the phenotype, as in this family. Alternatively, allelic heterogeneity at the same locus may predispose individuals to other forms of epilepsy. Certainly, this locus will be a candidate for involvement in the predisposition to seizures in other large epilepsy families under investigation.

Mendelian Disorders in Which Epilepsy Forms Part of the Phenotype

Tuberous Sclerosis Complex

The classical triad of epilepsy, mental retardation, and facial angiofibromas was first described in 1880 by Bournville.[13] However, individuals with tuberous sclerosis complex (TSC) show extreme variability of expression, and none of these features is universally present. Diagnostic criteria have emerged and certain features, including facial angiofibromas, ungual fibromas, retinal phakomas, multiple cortical tubers, subependymal glial nodules, and bilateral renal angiomyolipomas, are considered to be pathognomonic. Numerous other features in the presence of an affected first-degree relative will also suggest the diagnosis. The prevalence of TSC is unknown but may be as high as 1 in 6,000. It is inherited in an autosomal dominant manner; two-thirds of cases are fresh mutations.

Estimates of the incidence of seizures and intellectual impairment in individuals with TSC have been confounded by ascertainment bias. The largest unbiased study of 138 individuals with TSC found that about 62% had seizures and 38% had learning difficulties of various degrees. All those with learning difficulties had seizures, and the seizures occurred at an earlier age than in individuals with normal intellect.[14] A study of individuals with TSC in the western part of Scotland found that infantile spasms and partial seizures occurred with equal frequency as the initial seizure type. Those with infantile spasms frequently developed other seizure types, including complex partial seizures, tonic, myoclonic, and generalized tonic-clonic seizures, and were more likely to be intellectually impaired.[15] Between 10% and 25% of children presenting with infantile spasms will have TSC.[16, 17] One study suggested that the outcome for children diagnosed as having TSC was worse than that for those who had idiopathic or another neurologic cause of infantile spasms.[17]

The relationship between seizures, intellectual disability, and the position and number of cortical tubers is unclear. In a study of cerebral magnetic resonance imaging (MRI) findings in 75 patients with TSC, those who presented with infantile spasms had more tubers than subjects presenting with other types of generalized seizure or partial seizures. Similarly, those with onset of seizures before the age of 1 year and more pronounced intellectual disability had more tubers.[18] Large tubers may correlate with the number of EEG foci. In addition, lesions in the occipital lobe seem to correlate best with interictal EEG abnormalities.[19] Surgery has been performed on individuals with TSC to remove cortical tubers or hamartomas thought to be acting as epileptic foci, and even in the presence of multifocal abnormalities a significant reduction in seizures has been observed.[20]

In 1987 linkage was established between the ABO blood group and the TSC trait, suggesting that a gene for TSC resided on the long arm of chromosome 9.[21] However, evidence for genetic heterogeneity soon emerged, and a second locus was established close to the polycystic kidney disease locus on chromosome 16p13.3.[22] In about 50% of individuals with TSC the disease is attributable to mutations at the chromosome 9 locus known as TSC1 and in the remaining 50% to the chromosome 16 locus, TSC2. The gene at 9q34 remains elusive, but TSC2 was rapidly cloned.[23] TSC2 encodes a protein that has been named tuberin. The function of tuberin has not yet been determined, but it contains an area of sequence homology with the GTPase activating protein rap1GAP, which is consistent with its proposed function as a tumor suppressor gene. TSC1 has been mapped to a 4-cM interval on chromosome 9q34 by the observation of meiotic recombination events and loss of heterozygosity in hamartomas. However, the existence of conflicting data from linkage and haplotype studies has precluded further localization of the disease gene.[24]

At present, accurate genetic counseling requires a full clinical and radiologic workup. Few families are suitable for linkage-based studies given the problems associated with genetic heterogeneity. Mutation analysis of the TSC genes should enable more accurate diagnosis. However, fewer than 10% of mutations in TSC2 are detectable by fluorescent in situ hybridization (FISH), pulsed-field gel electrophoresis (PFGE), or Southern blot analysis, and a wide spectrum of mutations has been observed. The development of alternative methods of analysis should allow the detection of more mutations.

Neurofibromatosis Type I

Neurofibromatosis type I (NF1) is characterized by the presence of café au lait spots, axillary freckling, cutaneous neurofibromas, and Lisch nodules in the iris. Changes in the central nervous system (CNS) include abnormalities of neuronal migration, hamartomas, and gliomas.

The incidence of seizures in NF1 is 3–13%. Seizures occurring in the context of NF1 may be secondary to brain pathologic entities or idiopathic and unrelated to neurofibromatosis. In a retrospective study of 359 individuals with NF1, 22 (6%) had seizures.[25] The age at onset varied from 4 days to 20 years. Generalized tonic-clonic seizures occurred in 11 individuals, in five of whom the seizures were fever-related, and complex partial seizures occurred in nine. Cranial imaging (computed tomography [CT] or MRI scanning) was performed on 21 patients, and the findings appeared normal in 13. Of those with generalized tonic-clonic seizures, two had aqueductal stenosis with consequent dilatation of the third and lateral ventricles. One had cerebral atrophy related to perinatal asphyxia rather than NF1. Three were thought to have primary generalized epilepsy. Pathologic entities seen among those who had complex partial seizures were a Chiari type 1 malformation, a cavum septum pellucidum with culpocephaly, and a small pontomedullary cyst. None had a lesion that corresponded to the site of the epileptic focus. Of the remainder with complex partial seizures and normal imaging findings, only one had normal EEG findings. In an additional patient who presented with infantile spasms, a rapidly growing cervical and mediastinal plexiform neurofibroma and asymmetric cerebral atrophy were noted on an MRI scan. Infantile spasms occurring in individuals with NF1 have been reported elsewhere[26] and appear to correlate with a poor prognosis.

In the majority of patients the seizures were not attributable to NF1. The patients in whom seizures were most likely to be related to NF1 were those with complex partial seizures as well as those with aqueduct stenosis and the one patient with infantile spasms. Most notably, in none of the patients was epilepsy related to the presence of a brain tumor.

The NF1 gene was localized to the long arm of chromosome 17 by linkage analysis in 1987.[27] The gene was cloned in 1990.[28, 29] NF1 is a tumor-suppressor gene encoding neurofibromin, which is a protein homologous to the family of guanosine triphosphatase (GTPase)-activating proteins (GAP proteins). The majority of NF1 patients possess unique mutations, which reduces the usefulness of DNA-based methods of analysis in diagnosis.

Huntington's Disease

Huntington's disease (HD) is an autosomal dominant condition characterized by the degeneration of neurons predominantly in the caudate nucleus and the putamen. The symptoms of HD include a progressive mental disturbance that commences with the characteristic involuntary movements, later accompanied by dementia and psychiatric disturbance. Seizures are not a prominent symptom of HD, occurring in only 10% of men with adult-onset disease. However, seizures occur more frequently in patients with an onset under the age of 10 years. The types of seizure seen include generalized tonic-clonic seizures, atypical absences, and myoclonic seizures. EEG features include spike waves and poly-spike waves.

Linkage between markers on chromosome 4p and the HD trait was established in 1983.[30] No recombination was observed between the marker D4S10 and HD in a large Venezuelan pedigree or in an independent American family with 14 affected members. However, it was not until 1993 that the HD gene was identified.[31] The location of the HD gene was refined to between D4S180 and D4S182.[32] Transcripts from this region were identified using exon trapping, and one, IT15, was found to contain an expanded CAG trinucleotide repeat present in all of the 150 HD families tested. It had been noted that the affected offspring of affected men have a progressively earlier age of onset than their fathers, a phenomenon known as genetic anticipation. Myotonic dystrophy also shows genetic anticipation and is caused by an expanded trinucleotide repeat.

The IT15 messenger ribonucleic acid (mRNA) encodes huntingtin, a novel protein that has no definite homology with any known protein. The trinucleotide repeat lies in the coding region of the gene. In normal individuals the repeat exists in 11–34 copies, whereas in disease alleles the repeat has expanded to contain 42–100 copies. There is an inverse correlation between the length of the trinucleotide repeat and the age of onset of the disease.

Unverricht-Lundborg Disease: Baltic Myoclonus

Progressive myoclonic epilepsy of the Unverricht-Lundborg type (locus symbol, EPM1) is an autosomal recessive disorder that is enriched in the Finnish population with an incidence of 1 in 20,000 births. Stimulus-sensitive myoclonus begins from about age 6 to 15, and with time mild mental retardation, dysarthria, and ataxia develop. Nonspecific histologic changes are found in the brain; Lafora bodies or autofluorescent lipopigment are not found. Present evidence suggests that Unverricht-Lundborg disease (ULD), Baltic myoclonus,[33] and so-called Mediterranean myoclonus[34] are genetically homogenous. The combination of a high degree of consanguinity and a risk rate for siblings of one in four demonstrate that inheritance is autosomal recessive.[35]

ULD was mapped to the long arm of chromosome 21 in a group of 11 nuclear pedigrees from Finland. A genome search was undertaken and linkage found after testing 64 marker loci.[36] A maximum multipoint lod score of 10.08 was obtained with three loci in 21q22.3. The localization has been further refined,[37] most recently through use of the technique of linkage disequilibrium mapping to a region of about 0.3 cM. Linkage studies in non-Finnish families have demonstrated genetic (locus) homogeneity within this phenotype. Candidate genes were isolated from the disease gene region[38] and in 1996 mutations were identified in the gene encoding cystatin B in patients with ULD.[39] Cystatin B is a member of a superfamily of cysteine protease inhibitors.

It is a reversible inhibitor of cathepsins L, H, and B, is present in all tissues, and is thought to inactivate proteases that leak out of the lysosome. It is not yet understood why mutations in the gene encoding cystatin B should be responsible for causing EPM1, which appears to have a tissue-specific phenotype.

Neuronal Ceroid Lipofuscinoses

The neuronal ceroid lipofuscinoses (NCLs) are a group of inherited neurodegenerative disorders characterized by the accumulation of the autofluorescent lipopigments ceroid and lipofuscin in neurones and other cell types.[40] At least five subtypes are recognized on the basis of age of onset, clinicopathologic features, and chromosomal location. The childhood onset varieties are inherited in an autosomal recessive fashion and include infantile NCL (CLN1; Haltia-Santavuori disease, MIM 256730), classical late-infantile NCL (CLN2; Jansky-Bielschowsky disease, MIM 204500), Finnish variant late-infantile NCL (CLN5; MIM 256731), and juvenile NCL (CLN3; Batten or Spielmeyer-Vogt-Sjögren disease, MIM 304200). Until recently the underlying biochemical defects in this group of disorders has been entirely unknown.

Infantile NCL is a Finnish disease with an incidence of one in 20,000 in that population, although occasional patients are found in other populations. Onset occurs in the first 2 years of life with seizures, visual failure, choreoathetosis, and ataxia. The ultrastructural hallmark is so-called granular osmiophilic deposits (GRODS). Initial linkage to a locus on chromosome 1p, D1S57, was established using 26 Finnish families.[41]

The map localization was subsequently refined,[42] and the CLN1 gene was successfully cloned in 1995.[43] The gene encodes palmitoyl protein thioesterase. Prenatal diagnosis has been carried out using linked DNA markers.

Juvenile onset NCL has an incidence of up to 1 in 25,000 births, with an increased prevalence in the northern European population. Onset usually begins with visual failure at age 5–10 years followed by seizures and relentless mental deterioration. The lymphocytes are vacuolated on light microscopic examination, and so-called "finger-print" profiles are the characteristic ultrastructural feature.

The gene locus for Batten disease, CLN3, was assigned to chromosome 16 by demonstration of linkage to the haptoglobin locus.[44] Localization was subsequently refined to the region 16p12 by analysis of additional families and marker loci.[45–48] Strong linkage disequilibrium was identified with four microsatellite loci in the disease gene region: D16S288, D16S299, D16S298, and SPN. Haplotype analysis indicated a strong founder effect with the majority of CLN3 chromosomes having a common origin.[47]

The CLN3 gene was recently cloned. Linkage disequilibrium mapping in the Finnish population suggested that CLN3 was very close to the locus D16S298.[49] Exon amplification of a cosmid containing D16S298 yielded a candidate gene that was disrupted by a 1-kb deletion in all patients carrying the disease chromosome with the common "56" haplotype. Two separate deletions and a point mutation altering a splice site in three unrelated families confirmed that this candidate was CLN3. CLN3 encodes a 438–amino acid protein of unknown function.[50]

Classical late-infantile NCL, CLN2, is characterized by the onset of seizures and progressive dementia at age 2–4 years. The ultrastructural hallmark is so-called "curvilinear profiles." Linkage of CLN2 has been excluded from the CLN3 and CLN1 disease regions on chromosome 16p and 1p.[51] Despite an extensive search, a locus for classical late-infantile NCL has not yet been identified, suggesting that locus heterogeneity exists within this phenotype.[52] A number of variant late-infantile NCL forms exist, including one that is prevalent in Finland. This Finnish variant late-infantile NCL, locus symbol CLN5, has recently been mapped to chromosome 13q.[53]

Lafora's Disease

Progressive myoclonus epilepsy with polyglucosan intracellular inclusion bodies was first described in 1911 by Lafora and has become known as Lafora's disease.[54, 55] It is an autosomal recessive disease characterized by the presence of periodic acid-Schiff–positive cytoplasmic inclusion bodies, known as Lafora's bodies, in neurones, heart, liver, and muscle. The biochemical defect is unknown. During adolescence, affected individuals develop a seizure disorder that may include generalized tonic-clonic seizures, absences, drop attacks, or focal occipital seizures. Soon after presentation, subjects develop asymmetric myoclonic jerks. Dementia rapidly follows accompanied by apraxia and visual loss. Death usually occurs within a decade of presentation. EEG shows high-voltage, bilateral synchronous, spike-wave and polyspike-wave complexes. Diagnosis is based on the presence of Lafora's bodies in the eccrine sweat duct cells, most readily detected on axillary skin biopsy specimens.

In 1991 a gene for progressive myoclonus epilepsy of the ULD type was localized to chromosome 21q22.[36] Subsequent linkage studies demonstrated that Lafora's disease was not allelic to ULD.[37] More recently, linkage analysis performed in nine families with Lafora's disease produced a maximum two-point lod score of 10.54 at $\theta = 0$ at the marker D6S311, localizing the gene to 6q23-25. Homozygosity mapping in four consanguineous families revealed a region of homozygosity extending over a 17-cM interval from D6S292 and D6S420.[56] Candidate genes for Lafora's disease would include enzymes that play a role in carbohydrate metabolism. To date, no genes encoding enzymes involved in the synthesis or degradation of polysaccharides have been mapped to 6q23-25. The disease gene will be amenable to positional cloning techniques, although further families will be required to narrow down the region to which the Lafora's disease gene maps.

Progressive Epilepsy with Mental Retardation

A new autosomal recessive condition, progressive epilepsy with mental retardation (EPMR or northern epilepsy), characterized by epilepsy, dementia, and behavioral disturbances was described in 23 subjects from 11 families from northern Finland in 1994.[57] The onset of epilepsy occurs in the first decade, usually at age 5–10 years. All individuals have generalized tonic-clonic seizures, although some have complex partial seizures in addition. Initially, seizures occur once or twice a month, but the frequency increases through puberty and then declines. Two to 5 years after the onset of epilepsy, mental development starts to decline, especially during the period in which seizures are most frequent. About one-half of the patients have behavioral difficulties during puberty, including irritability, inattentiveness, and disobedience. Neurologic examination findings may be normal, although the majority of subjects have difficulty with fine motor tasks and balance. Of the 23 subjects, four had died, but only one of the deaths was directly related to the condition.

Serial EEG studies have been performed on 14 patients. From childhood onward there is a progressive slowing of background activity, with impaired reactivity to eye opening and the disappearance of sleep patterns. When the condition is fully developed, the wake and sleep recordings are barely distinguishable. The results of metabolic investigations are normal, as are the results of muscle biopsy and karyotype analysis. Cranial imaging shows evidence of brain stem and cerebellar atrophy in young adult patients and signs of cerebral atrophy in adult patients. Necropsy in two cases did not show any specific features in the brain. Of the anticonvulsant drugs administered, clonazepam appeared to give the longest seizure-free period, 1–4 years, even during the period when epilepsy was at its most active.

Further investigation revealed that nine of the 11 families were descended from a common ancestor who originated from northern Finland. The remaining two families were also linked through a common ancestor who originated from the same area of Finland, so that the 11 families formed two pedigrees in which there was a high rate of consanguineous marriage. The disorder has so far not been described outside Finland. Linkage analysis performed in three families using the markers D21S113 and D21S171, which are in strong linkage disequilibrium with EPM1, yielded negative lod scores, demonstrating that EPMR is not allelic to ULD.[56] Subsequently, a genome search was performed and linkage between EPMR and markers on the short arm of chromosome 8 established. A maximum multipoint lod score of 7.03 was observed between the markers AFM185xb2 and D8S264. Eighty-one percent of disease chromosomes shared a haplotype constructed for the five markers studied. This haplotype was not observed in 18 normal chromosomes and supports the hypothesis that the majority of affected individuals derive from a single founding mutation.[58]

Fragile X Syndrome

Fragile X syndrome is the most common form of X-linked mental retardation. It was first described by Martin and Bell in a single family in 1943.[59] Mental retardation is associated with nonspecific facial dysmorphism, including macrocephaly, a prominent jaw, large ears, and a long narrow face. Macro-orchidism is often present after puberty and individuals frequently display behavioral disturbances with autistic features and epilepsy. In 1969, Lubs described the finding of a fragile site at Xq28 in four mentally retarded men with these features, and the condition became known as fragile X syndrome.[60]

In a study of 12 individuals with fragile X syndrome,[61] six (50%) had a history of one or more seizures. All six had generalized tonic or tonic-clonic seizures, two had partial seizures in addition, and one had infantile spasms that evolved into Lennox-Gastaut syndrome. The seizures were usually readily controlled with anticonvulsant monotherapy. EEG studies were performed on all 12 subjects. The waking EEG recording was characterized by 4- to 7-hertz (Hz) background activity spreading to the anterior regions. Five subjects, four of whom had a history of seizures, were found to have similar EEG features during sleep. During slow sleep, focal paroxysmal activity appeared in the form of monophasic or diphasic temporal spikes. The spike amplitude and frequency became lower during rapid eye movement (REM) sleep. Two other groups of fragile X–negative mentally retarded males were also studied. One group had mental retardation and epilepsy, the other had mental retardation only. None of the subjects in these two groups had similar EEG features. The authors suggested that the presence of such characteristic EEG features in individuals with mental retardation indicates a diagnosis of fragile X syndrome. A follow-up study of 18 subjects with fragile X syndrome, eight (44%) of whom had seizures, found that the characteristic EEG features disappeared in three cases during the teenage years.[62] It was not present in any subject older than 17 years nor in any subject younger than 10 years old. The authors concluded that the EEG features were related to brain maturation. Given that individuals with benign childhood epilepsy with centrotemporal spikes (BCECTS) show similar EEG features that are also age-dependent, the authors suggested that the two conditions may be genetically related. However, one study has excluded linkage between the fragile X region and BCECTS in a small group of families.[63]

The genetics of fragile X are not straightforward. Intellectually normal males (so-called normal transmitting males) transmit the fragile X chromosome to their daughters. The daughters are themselves unaffected but will transmit the fragile X chromosome to 50% of their sons, who will all be affected, and 50% of their daughters, of whom 30% will be affected. This unusual pattern of inheritance became known as the Sherman paradox,[64] and the concept of a premutation was put forward.[65] In 1991 the molecular genetics of fragile X was clarified when a CGG triplet repeat was found in the $5'$ untranslated region of a gene now named FMR-1.[66] In unaffected individuals the repeat has 6 and 52 copies but in normal transmitting males and carrier females the repeat expands to up to 230 copies and is known as the premutation. After transmission through a female carrier, the premutation may further expand to greater than 230 copies, up to many thousands of copies, becoming a full mutation. Larger premutations are more likely to expand into the full mutation. The full mutation is accompanied by methylation of the CGG repeat and an adjacent CpG island. This is associated with inactivation of gene transcription, manifestation of the fragile X phenotype, and the appearance of the fragile site on the X chromosome. A reduction in the size of the premutation from parent to child has also been observed; this occurs more commonly when the transmitting parent is an unaffected male.[67] The FMR-1 gene encodes an RNA-binding protein that is widely expressed during fetal life and postnatally in the testis, uterus, and brain. However, the mechanism by which lack of the FMR-1 protein product causes the fragile X syndrome phenotype remains unclear. This and many other aspects of the genetics of fragile X syndrome are the subject of continued investigation.

Neurometabolic Disorders

A vast array of metabolic disorders may present with seizures or include seizures as part of the phenotype. All are rare, but it is important that they be diagnosed correctly so that treatment and genetic counseling may be offered. Certain metabolic disorders may show a characteristic seizure phenotype that will give clues to the diagnosis. These include the neuronal ceroid lipofuscinoses, described elsewhere, the sialidoses, Tay-Sachs and Sandhoff diseases, and disorders of biopterin metabolism. The majority, however, show no specific seizure phenotype. These include amino acid and organic acid disorders, urea cycle disorders, peroxisomal disorders, Menkes' disease, GM1 gangliosidosis, Krabbe's disease, adrenoleukodystrophy, and disorders of vitamin B_{12} metabolism. In this group, the syndrome of pyridoxine dependency is of particular importance. The onset of seizures usually occurs in the first few days of life or even prenatally, although seizure onset may be delayed 12–18 months. Affected individuals typically present with generalized or unilateral status epilepticus, but several seizure types have been described. The seizures respond dramatically to intravenous administration of pyridoxine, which should then be continued orally. Seizures will recur after discontinuation of pyridoxine, although this may not be for weeks or even months. Intravenous pyridoxine should be given for all seizures occurring in the first 18 months of life where the etiology is unclear.[68]

NONMENDELIAN EPILEPSIES

Juvenile Myoclonic Epilepsy

Juvenile myoclonic epilepsy (JME) is a common form of idiopathic generalized epilepsy (IGE) representing 5–10% of epilepsy as a whole. Individuals most commonly present from 8 to 26 years old with early morning myoclonus, symmetric shocklike jerks predominantly of the upper limbs, precipitated by fatigue, alcohol, and menstruation. More than 90% also have generalized tonic-clonic seizures and 30% have absence seizures. The EEG recording characteristically shows bilateral, symmetric, 4- to 6-Hz polyspikes and waves, although it may be normal. JME is usually readily treated with sodium valproate. It is considered to be a benign condition, although susceptibility to seizures remains lifelong.

A genetic contribution to JME has long been established, although the mode of inheritance is unclear. Autosomal dominant,[69] autosomal recessive,[70] two-locus,[71] and multifactorial models[72] have been proposed.

Four studies from two groups have provided evidence for the existence of a locus predisposing individuals to JME on chromosome 6p, and the locus has been designated EJM1. In 1988 Greenberg and colleagues performed linkage analyses in 24 families in which the proband had JME using the classical markers human leukocyte antigen (HLA) and properdin factor B (BF).[73] Eleven families were informative, eight for BF and three for HLA. Asymptomatic relatives with abnormal EEG features were classified as affected. The maximum lod score of 3.04 was obtained when HLA and BF were considered together and under the assumption of autosomal recessive inheritance with full penetrance. When asymptomatic relatives with abnormal EEG features were considered unaffected, the lod score fell to –3.6. By increasing the family resource, the same group later obtained a maximum lod score of 3.78 ($\theta_{m=ff} = 0.01$) with HLA assuming autosomal dominant inheritance and classifying asymptomatic relatives with abnormal EEG features as affected.[74] They suggested that EJM1 lay close to, but not within, the HLA region. In 1991, a study in a separately ascertained group of 33 German families using HLA serologic markers provided further evidence for the existence of a locus on chromosome 6p.[75] A further study of a subset of 20 of these families with one additional family using HLA-DQ restriction fragment length polymorphism markers provided a maximum lod score of 4.1 under the assumption of dominant inheritance with 90% penetrance.[76] More recently, a study in a single large pedigree of Belize origin using microsatellite markers on chromosome 6p obtained a maximum lod score of 3.67 ($\theta_{m=f} = 0$) between the centromeric marker D6S257 and a trait defined as the presence of clinical JME or an EEG study showing diffuse 3.5- to 6-Hz multispike and slow wave complexes.[77]

Two studies from a single group have failed to find evidence for the existence of a locus on chromosome 6p. Linkage analysis was carried out in a third set of 25 families, including a patient with JME and at least one first-degree relative with JME or a related IGE. Pairwise and multipoint linkage analysis was performed using eight loci spanning the HLA region on chromosome 6p and assuming autosomal dominant and autosomal recessive inheritance with age-dependent high and low penetrance.[78] No significant evidence in favor of linkage was obtained. However, because of a lack of suitable markers, the centromeric region of chromosome 6p was not adequately covered. In a more recent study, linkage analysis was performed in 19 families in which the proband and at least one first-degree relative had JME using microsatellite markers spanning a 61-cM region on chromosome 6p and centromeric 6q.[79] Again, no significant evidence in favor of linkage was obtained under any of the models tested. These results suggest that genetic heterogeneity may exist within this epilepsy phenotype. All the studies to date have relied on small groups of families, incapable on their own of demonstrating the presence of heterogeneity. Further work is needed using a large family resource in order to determine whether heterogeneity does exist.

Absence Epilepsies

The human epilepsy syndromes in which absence seizures occur have recently been reviewed,[80] and this review includes a consideration of genetic studies.[81] There is no doubt that there is a genetic contribution to their etiology, but the mode of inheritance and molecular genetic basis remain uncertain, and the field is confounded by some continuing uncertainty about the criteria by which distinct phenotypes should be recognized.[82] There is general agreement that the following discrete syndromes do exist: childhood absence epilepsy (CAE), juvenile absence epilepsy (JAE), myoclonic absence epilepsy, eyelid myoclonia with absences, and JME with absences. JME is considered separately, and the others are considered in turn after some general observations on the genetics of the absence epilepsies.

Earlier "classical" studies included rather broad definitions of the trait under study and are difficult to interpret. Valuable studies have been carried out on the concordance of specific syndromes among relatives of probands with absence epilepsies.[83] It does appear that as more distant relatives are considered, there is substantial heterogeneity of epilepsy types within families—few families have a clinically homogenous form in every affected member.

There is definite evidence for a genetic predisposition to CAE. The concordance rate for monozygotic twins with absence epilepsy is 75%[84] and even higher if

3-Hz spike-waves on EEG studies are included as evidence of affectedness.[85] The mode of inheritance is uncertain, with evidence for autosomal dominant[86] and autosomal recessive[87] models available. Polygenic, multifactorial inheritance is most likely.[88] The comprehensive Italian study of 24 families of probands with CAE demonstrated that the phenotype is concordant (i.e., identical) in first-degree relatives, with more distant relatives showing a variety of epilepsy phenotypes, including febrile seizures, JME, and IGE with generalized tonic-clonic seizures.[83] Results pertaining to whether the putative EJM1 locus on chromosome 6p also confers predisposition to absence epilepsies are controversial, some studies providing evidence in favor[89] and some against.[90]

JAE is distinguished from CAE by a later age of onset (>10 years), less frequent absences, and frequent association with generalized tonic-clonic seizures. Most studies of families of probands with JAE have been undertaken as part of broader analyses of IGE. JAE appears to cluster separately from JME and CAE,[83] but the numbers under study were small. A recent study of 14 families of probands with JAE identified five (36%) first-degree relatives affected with various epilepsy syndromes, including two siblings and an identical twin with JAE.

Epilepsy with myoclonic absences is clearly a distinct syndrome and demonstrates familial clustering, although no extensive genetic studies are available in this comparatively rare syndrome.

Benign Childhood Epilepsy with Centrotemporal Spikes

BCECTS, also known as benign focal epilepsy of childhood and benign rolandic epilepsy, was first described by Nayrae and Beaussart.[91] Seizures occur during awakening and consist of focal facial twitching, speech arrest, and salivation. Consciousness is retained. Interictal EEG abnormalities include spike discharges maximal in or confined to the centrotemporal region.

A family history of seizures or asymptomatic relatives with sharp waves on the EEG recording are found in a high proportion of cases. Genetic analysis is confounded by uncertainty in how best to define the trait that is segregating. Two studies[92, 93] suggested that centrotemporal foci were inherited as an autosomal dominant trait with age-dependent penetrance. A recent study of 43 probands found a positive family history of epilepsy, including individuals with generalized and febrile seizures, in 40%.[94]

Small linkage studies have been carried out in families of probands with benign rolandic epilepsy (BRE) and marker loci from the putative EJM1 region on chromosome 6p and the fragile X region. In each case, negative lod scores were obtained.[63, 95] The latter study was undertaken in view of the observation that seizures occur in a significant proportion of individuals with the fragile X syndrome, in association with EEG abnormalities similar to those found in BRE.[61]

Mitochondrial Disorders

The mitochondrial genome (mtDNA) is a circular DNA molecule, 16,569 bp long, present in up to 10 copies per mitochondrion, and therefore in up to several hundred copies per cell. mtDNA encodes two ribosomal ribonucleic acids

(RNAs), 22 transfer RNAs (tRNAs), and 13 mRNAs encoding components of the inner mitochondrial membrane respiratory chain. The entire mitochondrial genotype of an individual is inherited from the mother.

Human diseases caused by mutations of mtDNA include myopathies, encephalopathies, cardiomyopathies, and various multisystem disorders. Two diseases with CNS involvement manifested in part as epilepsy have been described that are caused by point mutations in mitochondrial transfer RNA genes. These are so-called myoclonic epilepsy with ragged-red fibers (MERRF) and mitochondrial encephalomyopathy, lactic acidosis, and stroke-like episodes (MELAS).

MERRF is characterized by epilepsy, intention myoclonus, muscle weakness, progressive ataxia, and deafness. An A-to-G transition mutation at nucleotide pair 8344 in the pseudouridyl loop of the tRNA^{lys} gene was first described in three unrelated MERRF families.[96] This mutation has now been described in most MERRF families. The patients are heteroplasmic—normal and mutated mtDNA populations are found. Variability of the clinical phenotype appears to depend on the amount and tissue distribution of mutant mtDNA in each individual.

An A-to-G transition at nucleotide 3243 was reported in 26 of 31 unrelated Japanese patients with MELAS. This mutation affects a nucleotide position in the dihydrouridine loop of the transfer RNA for leucine. Again, heteroplasmy was present with 50–92% of mutant mtDNA present.[97] Maternal transmission was documented in one family.

These observations confirm that seizures can be caused by deficiencies in mitochondrial energy production and raise the interesting question of whether mutations in mtDNA could contribute to the unexplained but well-documented maternal influence on the transmission of epilepsy.

CHROMOSOMAL ANOMALIES AND EPILEPSY

Down Syndrome

Down syndrome is the most common cause of mental retardation, with an incidence of about one in 700 live births. In 95% of cases it is caused by trisomy 21, the remainder of cases being caused by a robertsonian translocation, usually between chromosome 21 and one of the D group chromosomes (chromosomes 13–15). The phenotype of Down syndrome is well known, but the prevalence of epilepsy among individuals with Down syndrome is less well recognized. Various studies have estimated the prevalence of seizures in Down syndrome to be between zero and 13%; however, the larger studies place the figure at 5–6%.[98, 99]

Epilepsy occurring in the context of Down syndrome has a number of causes, and the type of epilepsy present is related to the cause and the age of onset. It has been observed that the prevalence of epilepsy increases in subjects with Down syndrome with increasing age. Veall found a prevalence of 1.9% in individuals younger than 20 and 12.2% in individuals older than 55.[99] A more recent but smaller study observed an overall prevalence of 9.4% over the age of 18, increasing to 46% in those 50 years old or older.[100] All the subjects in this study with epilepsy had partial seizures with secondary generalization. Epilepsy in older patients is frequently accompanied by clinical signs of developmental regression as well as an EEG study showing diffuse abnormalities consistent with a diagnosis of dementia. It appears that the onset of epilepsy is related to the neuropathologic changes of Alzheimer's dementia, which is well known to occur in persons with Down syndrome.

A single study of individuals with a seizure onset before the age of 22 found that of 47 individuals with seizures, 29 (62%) had a precipitating cause.[101] The causes fell into three categories: cardiovascular disease, perinatal complications, and infection. The majority in both groups had a seizure onset before the age of 3. The predominant seizure type in both groups was generalized tonic-clonic seizures. Partial seizures were rare in the idiopathic group, although they occurred in four individuals from the known etiology group, all of whom had localized intracerebral pathologic conditions. Infantile spasms occurred in 22% of the idiopathic group compared with 7% in the known etiology group. The EEG recordings showed a spectrum of abnormalities, frequently reflecting the underlying disease process. All patients with infantile spasms had hypsarrhythmia and others showed nonspecific abnormalities, such as a generalized slowing or generalized spikes and slow waves. The prognosis of the two groups was related to etiology. Patients in the idiopathic group largely had a good prognosis, with only 7 of 17 having persistent seizures on anticonvulsants. Reflex seizures have also been reported to be common in individuals with Down syndrome. In a study of 30 Down syndrome patients with epilepsy, six (20%) were found to have reflex seizures.[102] Seizures were precipitated by a variety of stimuli, including photic stimulation, noise, tactile stimulation, and facial contact with water.

Seizures occurring in individuals with Down syndrome should not be assumed to be related to an abnormal brain but should be thoroughly investigated, given that there is frequently an obvious cause.

Angelman Syndrome

Angelman syndrome (AS) is a condition characterized by developmental delay, ataxia, absence of speech, seizures, a happy disposition, and hypopigmentation. It is caused by a lack of a maternal contribution of chromosome 15q11-13, usually arising from de novo deletion or rarely from uniparental disomy. In a minority of families more than one child is affected. In these families no deletion has been found.[103] Recent evidence suggests that a proportion of these may be caused by abnormal methylation patterns in the AS or Prader-Willi syndrome (PWS) region. This suggests that there may be a gene acting in *cis* or *trans* that affects methylation.[104]

Seizures occurring in the context of AS are usually generalized. One study of eight patients with AS and chromosome 15q11-13 deletions found that seizure onset occurred in early childhood. All had atypical absence seizures, and all those that had been through puberty had experienced diminution in clinical seizures.[105] In a study of 19 children with AS aged 11 months to 11 years, one or more of three EEG abnormalities were present in all patients.[106] These were persistent rhythmic 4- to 6-per-second activities reaching more than 200 μV not associated with drowsiness; prolonged runs of rhythmic 2- to 3-per-second activity often more prominent anteriorly; and spikes mixed with 3- to 4-per-second components facilitated by eye closure. The last was seen at some stage in 17 of the 19 patients. These EEG features were thought to be sufficiently characteristic to be useful in diagnosis before the clinical features of AS become obvious.

Extrastructural Abnormal Chromosome 15 Syndrome

An inverted duplication of chromosome 15q (inv dup [15]) was originally described by Shreck et al.[107] The phenotype was further delineated by Wisniewski et al.[108] in a report of five cases and a review of the literature. This report was followed by others in which the inv dup [15] was associated with a normal phenotype, PWS or AS.[109, 110] More recent reports have introduced the term *extrastructural abnormal chromosome 15 syndrome* (ESAC-15 syndrome). In individuals with the phenotype described by Wisniewski et al., generalized tonic-clonic seizures were common and had a variable age of onset. Other consistent abnormalities included hypotonia and developmental retardation in infancy. In childhood the majority develop behavioral problems, including hyperactivity, aggressive behavior, and autism. Abnormal speech and language development is common, and speech may be absent. The dysmorphology is subtle, the only consistent features being strabismus and unusual dermatoglyphics.

Genes on the proximal long arm of chromosome 15 undergo parental imprinting, and it is therefore not surprising that abnormalities of this region usually have a phenotypic consequence. A study of 27 patients attempted to delineate the abnormality at the molecular level.[111] Using FISH with the probes D15Z1 and D15Z, a paracentric probe (pTRA20), and probes in the PWS/AS region, they demonstrated that whereas all patients had two signals on the inv dup [15] chromosome with D15Z1 and pTRA20, only 16 patients had two signals with the PWS/AS probes. They found that the presence of two signals with the PWS/AS probes correlated with the presence of mental retardation, and the authors suggested that it is the presence of additional copies of genes in the PWS/AS region that leads to the abnormal phenotype. However, detailed clinical information was not available from all the patients so that no further genotype/phenotype correlation could be made. An additional study[112] investigated the inverted duplicated chromosome 15 in 11 individuals, of whom seven had severe mental retardation with seizures, three had a normal phenotype, and one had PWS. Using a combination of FISH and quantitative DNA analysis with markers from chromosome 15q11-13, they identified three different sizes of inv dup [15]. The smallest, in which only the centromeric probe D15Z1 was present in two copies, was designated type 1, the largest, in which all probes tested were present in two copies, was designated type 3 and type 2 was intermediate in size. Type 3 was present in all seven patients with mental retardation and seizures and types 1 or 2 in the patients with a normal phenotype or PWS. They found, in addition, that the PWS patient showed maternal uniparental disomy of the normal chromosome 15, which accounted for the presence of PWS. In all the patients with AS or PWS and inv dup [15] in the literature, the syndrome could be ascribed to uniparental disomy or deletion of chromosome 15. It is possible that the presence of the inv dup [15] has an effect on the normal segregation of chromosome 15.

Trisomy 12p

There have been numerous case reports of individuals with trisomy 12p, and it is now recognized as a distinct clinical syndrome.[113] In the majority of cases, one of the parents is found to have a balanced translocation involving chromosome 12, although there have been reports of trisomy 12p arising de novo.[114, 115] The dysmorphic features include a round face with prominent cheeks, hypertelorism, epicanthic folds, a broad and flat nasal bridge, a short nose with anteverted nostrils, a prominent philtrum, and a broad lower lip. Several other features, including spade-shaped fingers, polysyndactyly of the feet, and genu valgum, are also described. Affected individuals have generalized hypotonia in infancy and are severely mentally retarded.

In a study of three patients with trisomy 12p syndrome,[115] two had generalized epilepsy. They both had generalized tonic-clonic seizures and myoclonic seizures. The third case had had a febrile convulsion but no seizures in the absence of fever. EEG studies were performed on all three patients and showed 3-Hz spike and wave discharges. Seizures are not mentioned in other case reports of trisomy 12p, so it is not clear whether they occur commonly in affected individuals. It is possible, however, that there is a gene or genes located on the short arm of chromosome 12 that predispose these individuals and individuals with a normal karyotype and IGE to seizures.

REFERENCES

1. Leppert M, Anderson VE, Quattlebaum T, et al. Benign familial neonatal convulsions linked to genetic markers on chromosome 20. Nature 1989;337:647.
2. Malafosse A, Leboyer M, Dulac O, et al. Confirmation of linkage of benign familial neonatal convulsions to D20S19 and D20S20. Hum Genet 1992;89:54.
3. Ryan SG, Wiznitzer M, Hollman C, et al. Benign familial neonatal convulsions: evidence for clinical and genetic heterogeneity. Ann Neurol 1991;29:469.
4. Lewis TB, Leach RJ, Ward K, et al. Genetic heterogeneity in benign familial neonatal convulsions: identification of a new locus on chromosome 8q. Am J Hum Genet 1993;53:670.
5. Steinlein O, Schuster V, Fischer C, et al. Benign familial neonatal convulsions: confirmation of genetic heterogeneity and further evidence for a second locus on chromosome 8q. Hum Genet 1995;95:411.
6. Steinlein OK, Mullcy JC, Propping P, et al. A missense mutation in the neuronal nicotinic receptor α4 subunit is associated with autosomal dominant nocturnal frontal lobe epilepsy. Nat Genet 1995;11:201.
7. Vigevano F, Fusco L, Di Capua M, et al. Benign infantile familial convulsions. Eur J Pediatr 1992;151:608.
8. Malafosse A, Beck C, Bellet H, et al. Benign infantile familial convulsions are not an allelic form of the benign familial neonatal convulsions gene. Ann Neurol 1994,35.479.
9. Scheffer IE, Bhatia KP, Lopes-Cendes I, et al. Autosomal dominant frontal epilepsy misdiagnosed as sleep disorder. Lancet 1994;343:515.
10. Scheffer IE, Bhatia KP, Lopes-Cendes I, et al. Autosomal dominant nocturnal frontal lobe epilepsy— a distinctive clinical disorder. Brain 1995;118:61.
11. Phillips HA, Scheffer IE, Berkovic SF, et al. Localization of a gene for autosomal dominant nocturnal frontal lobe epilepsy to chromosome 20q13.2. Nat Genet 1995;10:117.
12. Ottman R, Risch N, Hauser WA, et al. Localization of a gene for partial epilepsy to chromosome 10q. Nat Genet 1995;10:56.
13. Bournville DM. Sclérose tubereuse des circonvolutions cérébrales: idiotie et épilepsie hémiplegique. Arch Neurol (Paris) 1880;1:81.

14. Webb DW, Fryer AE, Osborne JP. On the incidence of fits and mental retardation in tuberous sclerosis. J Med Genet 1991;28:395.
15. Shepherd CW, Stephenson JB. Seizures and intellectual disability associated with tuberous sclerosis complex in the west of Scotland. Dev Med Child Neurol 1992;34:766.
16. Pampiglione G, Pugh E. Infantile spasms and subsequent appearance of tuberous sclerosis. Lancet 1975;2:1046.
17. Riikonen R, Simell O. Tuberous sclerosis and infantile spasms. Dev Med Child Neurol 1990;32:203.
18. Shepherd CW, Houser OW, Gomez MR. MR findings in tuberous sclerosis complex and correlation with seizure development and mental impairment. AJNR Am J Neuroradiol 1995;16:149.
19. Tamaki K, Okuno K, Ito M, et al. Magnetic resonance imaging in relation to EEG foci in tuberous sclerosis. Brain Dev 1991;12:316.
20. Bebin EM, Kelly PJ, Gomez MR. Surgical treatment for epilepsy in cerebral tuberous sclerosis. Epilepsia 1993;34:651.
21. Fryer AE, Chalmers A, Connor JM, et al. Evidence that the gene for tuberous sclerosis is on chromosome 9. Lancet 1987;1:659.
22. Kandt RS, Haines JL, Smith M, et al. Linkage of an important gene locus to a chromosome 16 marker for polycystic kidney disease. Nat Genet 1992;2:37.
23. The European Chromosome 16 Tuberous Sclerosis Consortium. Identification and characterization of the tuberous sclerosis gene on chromosome 16. Cell 1993;75:1305.
24. Sampson JR, Harris CP. The molecular genetics of tuberous sclerosis. Hum Mol Genet 1994;3:1477.
25. Korf BR, Carrazana E, Holmes GL. Patterns of seizures observed in association with neurofibromatosis 1. Epilepsia 1993;34:616.
26. Fois A, Tine A, Pavone L. Infantile spasms in patients with neurofibromatosis type 1. Childs Nerv Syst 1994;10:176.
27. Barker D, Wright E, Nguyen K, et al. Gene for von Recklinghausen neurofibromatosis is in the pericentromeric region of chromosome 17. Science 1987;236:1100.
28. Cawthon RM, O'Connell P, Buchberg AM, et al. Identification and characterization of transcripts from the neurofibromatosis 1 region: the sequence and genomic structure of EV12 and mapping of other transcripts. Genomics 1990;7:555.
29. Wallace MR, Marchuk DA, Andersen LB, et al. Type 1 neurofibromatosis gene: identification of a large transcript disrupted in three NF1 patients. Science 1990;249:181.
30. Gusella JF, Wexler NS, Conneally PM, et al. A polymorphic DNA marker genetically linked to Huntington's disease. Nature 1983;306:234.
31. Huntington's Disease Collaborative Research Group. A novel gene containing a trinucleotide repeat that is expanded and unstable on Huntington's disease chromosomes. Cell 1993;72:971.
32. Gusella JF, MacDonald ME. Hunting for Huntington's Disease. In T Friedmann (ed), Molecular Genetic Medicine. London: Academic, 1993;139.
33. Koskiniemi ML. Baltic Myoclonus. In S Fahn, CD Marsden, M van Woert (eds), Myoclonus. New York: Raven, 1986;57.
34. Genton P, Michelucci R, Tassinari CA, et al. The Ramsay-Hunt syndrome revisited: Mediterranean myoclonus versus MERRF and Baltic myoclonus. Acta Neurol Scand 1990;81:8.
35. Norio R, Koskiniemi M. Progressive myoclonus epilepsy: genetic and nosological aspects with special reference to 107 Finnish patients. Clin Genet 1979;15:382.
36. Lehesjoki A-E, Koskiniemi M, Sistonen P, et al. Localization of a gene for progressive myoclonus epilepsy to chromosome 21q22. Proc Natl Acad Sci U S A 1991;88:3696.
37. Lehesjoki A-E, Koskiniemi M, Sistonen P, et al. Linkage studies in progressive myoclonic epilepsy: Unverricht-Lundborg and Lafora disease. Neurology 1992;42:1545.
38. Yamakawa K, Mitchell S, Hubert R, et al. Isolation and characterization of a candidate gene for progressive myoclonus epilepsy on 21q22.3. Hum Mol Genet 1995;4:709.
39. Pennachio LA, Lehesjoki A-E, Stone NE, et al. Mutations in the gene encoding cystatin B in progressive myoclonus epilepsy. Science 1996;271:1731.
40. Vidudala VTS, Pullarkat RK. Report on the fifth annual conference on neuronal ceroid lipofuscinosis. Am J Med Genet 1995;57:125.
41. Jarvela I, Schleutker J, Haataja L, et al. Infantile form of neuronal ceroid lipofuscinosis (CLN1) maps to the short arm of chromosome 1. Genomics 1991;9:170.
42. Hellsten E, Vesa J, Speer MC, et al. Refined assignment of the infantile neuronal ceroid lipofuscinosis (CLN1) locus at 1p32: incorporation of linkage disequilibrium in multipoint analysis. Genomics 1993;16:720.
43. Vesa J, Hellsten E, Verkruyse LA, et al. Mutations in the palmitoyl protein thioesterase gene causing infantile neuronal ceroid lipofuscinosis. Nature 1995;376:584.

44. Eiberg H, Gardiner RM, Mohr J. Batten disease (Spielmeyer-Sjögren disease) and haptoglobins (HP): indication of linkage and assignment to chromosome 16. Clin Genet 1989;36:217.
45. Gardiner RM, Sandford A, Deadman M, et al. Batten disease (Spielmeyer-Vogt disease, juvenile onset neuronal ceroid lipofuscinosis) gene (CLN3) maps to human chromosome 16. Genomics 1990;8:387.
46. Callen DF, Baker E, Lane S, et al. Regional mapping of the Batten disease locus (CLN3) to human chromosome 16p12. Am J Hum Genet 1991;49:1372.
47. Mitchison HM, Thompson AD, Mulley JC, et al. Fine genetic mapping of the Batten disease locus (CLN3) by haplotype analysis and demonstration of allelic association with chromosome 16p microsatellite loci. Genomics 1993;16:455.
48. Lerner TJ, Boustany R-MN, MacCormack K, et al. Linkage disequilibrium between the juvenile neuronal ceroid lipofuscinosis gene and marker loci on chromosome 16p12.1. Am J Hum Genet 1994;54:88.
49. Mitchison HM, O'Rawe AM, Taschner PE, et al. The Batten disease gene, CLN3: linkage disequilibrium mapping in the Finnish population, and analysis of European haplotypes. Am J Hum Genet 1995;56:654.
50. The International Batten Disease Consortium. Isolation of a novel gene underlying Batten disease, CLN3. Cell 1995;82:949.
51. Williams R, Vesa J, Jarvela I, et al. Genetic heterogeneity in neuronal ceroid lipofuscinosis (NCL): evidence that the late-infantile subtype (Jansky-Bielschowsky disease, CLN1) is not an allelic form of the juvenile or infantile subtypes. Am J Hum Genet 1993;53:931.
52. Sharp J, Savukoski M, Wheeler R, et al. Linkage analysis of late-infantile neuronal ceroid lipofuscinosis. Am J Med Genet 1995;57:348.
53. Savukoski M, Kestila M, Williams R, et al. Defined chromosomal assignment of CLN5 demonstrates that at least four genetic loci are involved in the pathogenesis of human ceroid lipofuscinoses. Am J Hum Genet 1994;55:695.
54. Lafora GR. The presence of amyloid bodies in the protoplasm of the ganglion cells: a contribution to the study of the amyloid substance in the nervous system. Bull Gov Hosp Insane 1911;3:83.
55. Lafora GR, Glueck B. Contribution to the histopathology and pathogenesis of myoclonic epilepsy. Bull Gov Hosp Insane 1911;3:96.
56. Serratosa JM, Delgado-Escueta AV, Posada I, et al. The gene for progressive myoclonus epilepsy of the Lafora type maps to chromosome 6q. Hum Mol Genet 1995;5:1657.
57. Hirvasniemi A, Lang H, Lehesjoki A-E, et al. Northern epilepsy syndrome: an inherited childhood onset epilepsy with associated mental deterioration. J Med Genet 1994;31:177.
58. Tahvanainen E, Ranta S, Hirvasniemi A, et al. The gene for a recessively inherited human childhood progressive epilepsy with mental retardation maps to the distal short arm of chromosome 8. Proc Natl Acad Sci U S A 1994;91:7267.
59. Martin JP, Bell J. A pedigree of mental defect showing sex-linkage. J Neurol Neurosurg Psychiatry 1943;6:154.
60. Lubs HA. A marker X chromosome. Am J Hum Genet 1969;21:231.
61. Musumeci SA, Ferri R, Elia M, et al. Epilepsy and fragile X syndrome: a follow-up study. Am J Med Genet 1991;38:511.
62. Musumeci SA, Ferri R, Colognola RM, et al. Prevalence of a novel epileptogenic EEG pattern in the Martin-Bell syndrome. Am J Med Genet 1988;30:207.
63. Rees M, Diebold U, Parker K, et al. Benign childhood epilepsy with centrotemporal spikes and the focal sharp wave trait is not linked to the fragile X region. Neuropediatrics 1993;24:211.
64. Sherman SL, Morton NE, Jacobs PA, et al. The marker (X) syndrome: a cytogenetic and genetic analysis. Ann Hum Genet 1984;48:21.
65. Pembrey ME, Winter RM, Davies KE. A premutation that generates a defect at crossing over explains the inheritance of fragile X mental retardation. Am J Med Genet 1985;21:709.
66. Verkerk AJMH, Pieretti M, Sutcliffe JS, et al. Identification of a gene (FMR-1) containing a CGG repeat coincident with a breakpoint cluster region exhibiting length variation in fragile X syndrome. Cell 1991;65:905.
67. Fisch GS, Snow K, Thibodeau SN, et al. The fragile X premutation in carriers and its effect on mutation size in offspring. Am J Hum Genet 1995;56:1147.
68. Aicardi J. Epilepsy and Inborn Errors of Metabolism. In J Roger, M Bureau, C Dravet, et al. (eds), Epileptic Syndromes in Infancy, Childhood and Adolescence (2nd ed). London: John Libbey, 1992;97.
69. Delgado-Escueta AV, Greenberg D, Weissbecker K. Gene mapping in the idiopathic generalized epilepsies. Epilepsia 1990;31(Suppl 1):519.

70. Panayiotopoulos CP, Obeid T. Juvenile myoclonic epilepsy: an autosomal recessive disease. Ann Neurol 1989;25:440.
71. Greenberg DA, Delgado-Escueta AV, Maldonado HM, Widelitz H. Segregation analysis of juvenile myoclonic epilepsy. Genet Epidemiol 1988;5:81.
72. Andermann E. Multifactorial Inheritance of Generalized and Focal Epilepsies. In VE Anderson, WA Hauser, JK Penry, et al. (eds), Genetic Basis of the Epilepsies. New York: Raven, 1982.
73. Greenberg DA, Delgado-Escueta AV, Widelitz H, et al. Juvenile myoclonic epilepsy may be linked to the BF and HLA loci on human chromosome 6. Am J Med Genet 1988;31:185.
74. Greenberg DA, Delgado-Escueta AV, Widelitz H, et al. Strenghthened evidence for linkage of juvenile myoclonic epilepsy to HLA and BF. Cytogenet Cell Genet 1989;51:1008.
75. Weissbecker KA, Durner M, Janz D, et al. Confirmation of linkage between juvenile myoclonic epilepsy locus and the HLA region on chromosome 6. Am J Med Genet 1991;38:32.
76. Durner M, Sander T, Greenberg DA, et al. Localization of idiopathic generalized epilepsy on chromosome 6p in families of juvenile myoclonic epilepsy patients. Neurology 1991;41:1651.
77. Liu AW, Delgado-Escueta AV, Serratosa JM, et al. Juvenile myoclonic epilepsy locus in chromosome 6p21.2-p11: linkage to convulsions and electroencephalography trait. Am J Hum Genet 1995;57:368.
78. Whitehouse WP, Rees M, Curtis D, et al. Linkage analysis of idiopathic generalized epilepsy and marker loci on chromosome 6p in families of patients with juvenile myoclonic epilepsy: no evidence for an epilepsy locus in the HLA region. Am J Hum Genet 1993;53:652.
79. Elmslie FV, Williamson M, Rees M, et al. Linkage analysis of juvenile myoclonic epilepsy and microsatellite loci spanning 61cM of human chromosome 6p in 19 nuclear pedigrees provides no evidence for a susceptibility locus in this region. Am J Hum Genet 1996;59:653.
80. Duncan JS, Panayiotopoulos CP (eds). Typical Absences and Related Epileptic Syndromes. London: Churchill Communications Europe, 1995.
81. Gardiner RM. Genetics of Human Typical Absence Syndromes. In JS Duncan, CP Panayiotopoulos (eds), Typical Absences and Related Epileptic Syndromes. London: Churchill Communications Europe, 1995.
82. Porter RJ. The absence epilepsies. Epilepsia 1993;34(Suppl 3):542.
83. Bianchi A. Study of Concordance of Symptoms in Families with Absence Epilepsies. In JS Duncan, CP Panayiotopoulos (eds), Typical Absences and Related Epileptic Syndromes. London: Churchill Communications Europe, 1995.
84. Gedda L, Tatarelli R. Essential isochronic epilepsy in MZ twin pairs. Acta Genet Med Gemellol (Roma) 1977;20:380.
85. Lennox WG. Heredity of epilepsy as told by relatives and twins. JAMA 1951;146:529.
86. Metrakos JD, Metrakos K. Genetic Factors in the Epilepsies. In R Alter, WA Hauser (eds), The Epidemiology of Epilepsy: A Workshop. Washington DC: GPO, 1972;97.
87. Serratosa J, Weissbecker K, Delgado-Escueta A. Childhood absence epilepsy: an autosomal recessive disorder? Epilepsia 1990;31:651.
88. Berkovic SF, Andermann F, Andermann E, et al. Concepts of absence epilepsies: discrete syndromes or biological continuum? Neurology 1987;37:993.
89. Sander T, Hildmann BC, Janz D, et al. The phenotypic spectrum related to the human epilepsy susceptibility gene "EJM1." Ann Neurol 1995;38:210.
90. Serratosa JM, Delgado-Escueta AV, Pascual-Castroviejo I, et al. Childhood absence epilepsy: exclusion of genetic linkage to chromosome 6p markers. Abstract presented at International Workshop on Idiopathic Generalized Epilepsies, Alsace, France, April, 1993.
91. Nayrae P, Beaussart M. Les pointes-ondes prerolandique: expression EEG trés particulière. Etude electroclinique de 21 cas. Rev Neurol 1957;99:201.
92. Bray PF, Wiser WC. Hereditary characteristics of familial temporal-central focal epilepsy. Pediatrics 1965;36:207.
93. Heijbel J, Blom S, Rasmuson M. Benign epilepsy of childhood with centrotemporal EEG foci: a genetic study. Epilepsia 1975;16:285.
94. Degen R, Degen H-E, Roth CH. Some genetic aspects of idiopathic and symptomatic absence seizures: waking and sleep EEGs in siblings. Epilepsia 1990;31:784.
95. Whitehouse W, Diebold U, Rees M, et al. Exclusion of linkage of genetic focal sharp waves to the HLA region on chromosome 6p in families with benign partial epilepsy with centrotemporal spikes. Neuropediatrics 1993;24:208.
96. Shoffner JM, Lott MT, Lezza AMS, et al. Myoclonic epilepsy and ragged-red fiber disease (MERRF) is associated with a mitochondrial DNA tRNA^{Lys} mutation. Cell 1990;61:931.
97. Goto Y, Nonaka I, Horai S. A mutation in the tRNA^{Leu} gene associated with the MELAS subgroup of mitochondrial encephalomyelopathies. Nature 1990;348:651.

98. Moore BC. Some characteristics of institutionalized mongols. J Ment Defic Res 1973;17:46.
99. Veall RM. The prevalence of epilepsy among mongols related to age. J Ment Defic Res 1974;18:99.
100. McVicker RW, Shanks OEP, McClelland RJ. Prevalence and associated features of epilepsy in adults with Down's syndrome. Br J Psychiatry 1994;164:528.
101. Stafstrom CE, Patxot OF, Gilmore HE, et al. Seizures in children with Down syndrome: etiology, characteristics and outcome. Dev Med Child Neurol 1991;33:191.
102. Guerrini R, Genton P, Bureau M, et al. Reflex seizures are frequent in patients with Down syndrome and epilepsy. Epilepsia 1990;31:406.
103. Chan CT, Clayton-Smith J, Cheng XJ, et al. Molecular mechanisms in Angelman syndrome: a survey of 93 patients. J Med Genet 1993;30:895.
104. Horsthemke B. Parental imprinting and gene regulation in the Prader Willi syndrome/Angelman syndrome region. Presented at the 27th Annual Meeting of the European Society of Human Genetics (ESHG), Berlin, May, 1995.
105. Matsumoto A, Kumagai T, Miura K, et al. Epilepsy in Angelman syndrome associated with chromosome 15q deletion. Epilepsia 1992;33:1083.
106. Boyd SG, Harden A, Patton MA. The EEG in early diagnosis of the Angelman (happy puppet) syndrome. Eur J Pediatr 1988;147:508.
107. Schreck RR, Breg WR, Erlanger BF, et al. Preferential derivation of abnormal human G-group-like chromosomes from chromosome 15. Hum Genet 1977;36:1.
108. Wisniewski KE, Hassold T, Heffelfinger J, et al. Cytogenetic and clinical studies in five cases of inv dup (15). Hum Genet 1979;50:259.
109. Knight LA, Lipson M, Mann J, et al. Mosaic inversion duplication of chromosome 15 without phenotypic effect: occurrence in a father and daughter. Am J Med Genet 1984;17:649.
110. Robinson WP, Binkert F, Gine R, et al. Clinical and molecular analysis of five inv dup (15) patients. Eur J Hum Genet 1993;1:37.
111. Leana-Cox J, Jenkins L, Palmer CG, et al. Molecular cytogenetic analysis of Inv Dup(15) chromosomes, using probes specific for the Prader-Willi/Angelman syndrome region: clinical implications. Am J Hum Genet 1994;54:748.
112. Cheng S-D, Spinner NB, Zackai EH, et al. Cytogenetic and molecular characterization of inverted duplicated chromosomes 15 from 11 patients. Am J Hum Genet 1994;55:753.
113. Hoo JJ. 12p trisomy: a syndrome? Ann Genet 1976;19:261.
114. Kondo I, Hamaguchi H, Haneda T. Trisomy 12p syndrome: de novo occurrence of mosaic trisomy 12p in a mentally retarded boy. Hum Genet 1979;46:135.
115. Guerrini R, Bureau M, Mattei M-G, et al. Trisomy 12p syndrome: a chromosomal disorder associated with generalized 3-Hz spike and wave discharges. Epilepsia 1990;31:557.

4
Brain Imaging: The Anatomy of Epilepsy

Susan S. Spencer and Dennis D. Spencer

An alteration in brain architecture is widely assumed to underlie the human symptomatic epilepsies, but its consistent demonstration and correlation with the expression of hyperexcitable neuronal activity that defines epilepsy have been slow to evolve. In the last decade, however, computed tomography (CT) and especially magnetic resonance imaging (MRI) have provided increasingly productive means for visualizing the macroscopic anatomic correlates of many symptomatic epilepsies. Furthermore, these changes have been clearly linked to electroencephalographic (EEG) and to clinical variables, prognosis, and pathophysiology. The progress is such that "cryptogenic" symptomatic epilepsy may soon become an anachronism. In this setting, careful analysis of the imaging literature provides a way to study the anatomy of epilepsy.

REVIEW OF PATHOLOGIC SERIES

Before the recent era of sensitive structural imaging techniques, autopsy and surgical series were our windows to epilepsy anatomy.[1–4] These established that epilepsy could arise from lesions of malformative, neoplastic, metabolic, vascular, traumatic, or inflammatory nature. Each category includes a wide variety of specific entities. The distribution within and between these categories could not really be established by autopsy series, being biased toward the patients with the most severe disease, and relied more on pathologic analyses of brain tissue resected from patients who underwent surgery for the treatment of medically uncontrolled epilepsy. As sensitive structural imaging techniques identified other lesions and those lesions were resected with successful seizure control in difficult cases, the spectrum of pathologic features in surgical series also changed. Thus, the available pathology literature represents a spectrum of changing distribution. It is nevertheless illustrative to review the structural abnormalities underlying epilepsy as established by these autopsy and surgical pathology data to understand and contrast current imaging findings and establish their sensitivity and accuracy.

In most reported series on temporal lobe epilepsy surgery, spanning many decades, hippocampal sclerosis is the most common pathologic substrate, accounting for about 70% of abnormalities in resected temporal lobes.[1, 2] The incidence varies somewhat depending on the criteria for patient selection as well as the methods for tissue analysis; hippocampal sclerosis was diagnosed in only 22% of temporal lobe surgery patients in one series.[2] It is reasonable to state, however, based on accumulated literature, that with adequate specimen availability, tissue examination, and criteria for the diagnosis of hippocampal sclerosis that include at least 40–50% neuronal loss in CA1 and other hippocampal subfields, hippocampal sclerosis will remain the most common anatomic correlate of temporal lobe epilepsy.

Only autopsy series could, and did, establish the bilaterality of hippocampal sclerosis in up to 90% of these patients, although it is symmetric in degree in just 10–20%.[5–7] Some patients have multiple abnormalities of structure, but in surgical series, detection of these abnormalities is limited to what is present in the resected specimen. Dual pathologic features in temporal lobe surgical specimens—e.g., the presence of an extrahippocampal temporal lobe pathologic state along with hippocampal sclerosis—is considerably more common with temporal lobe heterotopias (in which it may be observed in up to 50%). With temporal lobe gliomas and other lesions, however, hippocampal cell loss is present to a much lesser degree and does not qualify for a strict pathologic diagnosis of hippocampal sclerosis.[2] In the remaining temporal lobe specimens of surgical series, trauma with meningocerebral cicatrices occurs in very few (3% at the University of California at Los Angeles) as do meningiomas or schwannomas, whereas gliomas (predominantly astrocytomas and oligodendrogliomas) are present in 12–15%.[1–3] Temporal lobe epilepsy surgery series have a disproportionate representation of gangliogliomas as well as the pleomorphic xanthoastrocytomas and dysembryoplastic neuroepithelial tumors (DNT). The latter tumors were initially described specifically in resected tissue of patients with intractable epilepsy. The remaining surgical pathologic findings in temporal lobe epilepsy consist of heterotopias (5–8%) and hamartomas (10–12%). The findings in surgical series of frontal lobe epilepsy also include tumors and developmental abnormalities but consistently there are more traumatic and infectious causes, manifest as meningocerebral cicatrices, neuronal loss with gliosis, and contusion.[4]

In surgical specimens removed from children with refractory epilepsy, a difference in selection criteria creates a bias toward patients with focal lesions demonstrated by neuroimaging. Hippocampal sclerosis is less often identified without a second lesion, making the incidence of dual pathologic states considerably higher in this population.[3] More neuronal migration disorders encompassing dysgenesis, focal cortical dysplasia, tuberous sclerosis, and tumors (low-grade astrocytoma, ganglioglioma, other gliomas, and DNT) are represented in pediatric epilepsy surgery series, with an incidence up to 25–35%. Inflammatory causes are usually Rasmussen's encephalitis. Sturge-Weber syndrome and encephalomalacia secondary to old hypoxic ischemic insults complete the spectrum in childhood surgical epilepsy series.

This brief review of pathology based on autopsy and surgical analyses serves as a point of reference for interpretation of the spectrum of architectural abnormalities encountered by advanced neuroimaging in various groups of epilepsy patients.

COMPUTED TOMOGRAPHY VERSUS MAGNETIC RESONANCE IMAGING

When CT became available 20 years ago, a spate of publications established its use in studying refractory seizure disorders: patients with previously undetected structural lesions were diagnosed and treated by virtue of this new window to the abnormal structural anatomy of the epileptic brain. In 1976, Bachman and colleagues documented structural lesions in 30% of chronic epileptic children, but only 2% of abnormal CTs prompted different treatment.[8] Jabbari et al.[9] and Gilsanz et al.[10] also documented a 2–3% incidence of surgically remediable lesions in their populations of chronic, presumably cryptogenic, epilepsy patients. With the advent of MRI, additional authors reported the superior diagnostic sensitivity of MRI over CT scanning in this clinical setting. Particularly because of its increased sensitivity in the temporal lobes and increased resolution of tissue differences, MRI provides an increased yield of 8–20% over CT scanning in detecting structural lesions associated with epilepsy.[11–19] As early as 1985, Laster et al.[20] found four lesions by MRI in a group of 100 patients with normal CT findings and complex partial seizure disorders that had persisted for more than 5 years. Shortly thereafter, Froment and colleagues[21] found that MRI demonstrated lesions consistent with EEG localization in 17 of 100 epilepsy patients with negative CT findings and refractory complex partial seizures, which is a higher yield in the patient population with refractory epilepsy. However, contrast enhancement with gadopentetate dimeglumine was not found to enhance the yield.[22] In the singular situation of cerebral calcification, exemplified by patients with tuberous sclerosis,[23] CT scanning was reported to be complimentary to MRI. Caution has been advised in interpreting the MRI findings in refractory epilepsy because of repeated documentation of "disappearing lesions" associated with epilepsy, which are only sometimes a result of metabolic alterations in and around the area of epileptogenesis (Figure 4.1).[24–26] With these caveats, however, there is little disagreement that a discussion of advanced neuroimaging in epilepsy and its ability to demonstrate the "anatomy of epilepsy" is equivalent to a discussion of MRI in epilepsy and that CT scanning is not necessary when MRI is available. The discussion below will address MRI almost exclusively, since information obtained from MRI series in epilepsy is likely to be more comprehensive and therefore more reflective of the spectrum of architectural alterations in the epileptic brain.

CAVEATS ON MAGNETIC RESONANCE IMAGING IN EPILEPSY

Certain microscopic abnormalities cannot be visualized by currently available MRI techniques. Cortical dysgenesis is likely to represent the most frequently undetected anatomic correlate of the epileptogenic process, although vigilance and development of newer quantitative techniques are improving this yield above its current level of 50% or less. Nevertheless, some of these developmental abnormalities may also remain undetected in pathologic or surgical series, since microscopic analysis in those groups depends on a sufficient degree of suspicion concerning the involved cortical region. In patients with epilepsy not severe enough to warrant a surgical approach and in patients with medically refractory

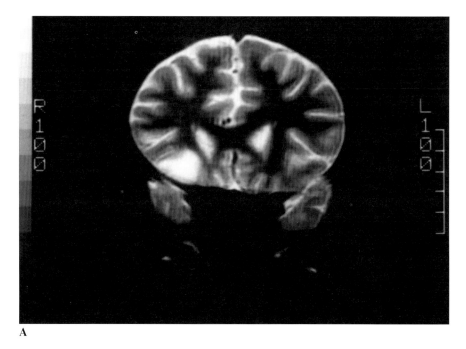

Figure 4.1   Coronal spin-spin magnetic resonance imaging sequences performed 1 month apart in a patient with Rasmussen's encephalitis. An area of increased signal (A) associated with partial status epilepticus resolves 1 month later (B) with improved seizure control.

epilepsy whose surgery fails to resect the appropriate portion of involved brain and therefore does not improve the seizures, only neuroimaging can provide a window to the anatomic correlate. The anatomic changes underlying *controlled* epilepsy and the structural correlates of epilepsy in various groups of patients, such as those with new onset, late onset, or neonatal onset seizures, are only just becoming "visible" through MRI. Furthermore, the presence of more than one separate anatomic abnormality in a patient can be accurately defined only with neuroimaging, because surgical series depend on the second pathologic entity being contiguous with the first (so that it is included in the specimen). For these reasons, our concepts of what underlies the epileptic process are under revision thanks to modern neuroimaging.

MAGNETIC RESONANCE IMAGING FINDINGS IN EPILEPSY

Newly Diagnosed Epilepsy

The only systematic analysis of structural imaging in patients with newly diagnosed epilepsy was done with CT scans and 0.02-tesla MRI studies in Sweden and was restricted to adult-onset seizure disorders (after age 17).[26] Of 44 individuals, 20 had normal findings on neuroimaging studies, whereas five had ischemic lesions, four had contusions, five had neoplasms, two had hamartomas, one had hydrocephalus, one had an aneurysm, one had heterotopia, and four had encephalomalacia from various causes. These authors noted four patients with lesions detected only by CT scanning, whereas a single patient had a lesion detected by MRI scanning alone. The 10- to 15-mm slice thickness on a low-strength magnet makes comparison with later series difficult. What is remarkable, however, is the high overall incidence of structural abnormalities *even at initial presentation*, with a spectrum that parallels that of the population with refractory epilepsy (see below).

Late-Onset Epilepsy

A more focused evaluation of MRI in 50 patients with late-onset seizures (after age 25) was performed in Australia but restricted to patients whose CT findings were negative or nondiagnostic.[27] The series therefore does not provide a comprehensive survey of structural abnormalities accompanying late-onset epilepsy. Nonetheless, four patients had positive findings on MRI studies with negative findings on CT scans. The final diagnoses included 10 cortical infarctions, five tumors, two arteriovenous malformations, one mesial temporal sclerosis (MTS), and one multiple sclerosis. The authors observed that small, deep, white-matter lesions were no more common in this group than in a control, nonepileptic population and concluded that such lesions bear no relationship to the epilepsy. The higher incidence of ischemic lesions is consistent with the older population (mean age 51) as is the absence of developmental lesions, but these scans were performed at 0.3 tesla and are thus not comparable with later studies.

Nonrefractory Epilepsy

An issue of great interest is the incidence of demonstrable structural abnormality in *unselected* patients with *controlled* epilepsy. Indeed, combining these with the refractory series might provide a true estimate of the distribution of anatomic abnormalities in epilepsy. Two reports from the same center included such a population but restricted patients to those with "moderately severe, controlled" temporal lobe epilepsy.[28, 29] A 1.5-tesla magnet was used, all patients had negative findings on CT scans within 3 months of the MRI studies, and individuals with post-traumatic epilepsy were excluded. Since the reports were overlapping, only the latter (on 40 patients) will be described.[29] Twenty-one patients had normal findings, while nine had findings consistent with MTS. Four patients had signal changes in temporal/basal locations, of which one was a ganglioglioma and three were presumed (but not proven) to be vascular anomalies. Finally, six patients had small focal abnormal signals in the frontoparietal white matter, of which five were multiple. Even assuming the lack of significance of the frontoparietal white matter lesions in the epileptic process (as suggested by previous authors and by their lack of correlation with EEG findings), one-third of these patients with controlled temporal lobe epilepsy had structural abnormalities on high-resolution MRI scans and most of these abnormalities were consistent with MTS.

Refractory Epilepsy

For obvious reasons, the group of patients with refractory epilepsy is the group about which we have the most structural imaging data. In two separate reports of MRI in unselected patients with refractory epilepsy who underwent surgery, foreign tissue lesions (including gliomas and vascular lesions) were detected by MRI at an incidence of 12–25%, and developmental lesions (including cortical dysplasia, polymicrogyria, and tuberous sclerosis) were detected in 10–12%; these were all confirmed by pathologic analysis after surgery.[18, 30] The detection of MTS, on the other hand, was variable despite similar magnet strengths and protocols. Nevertheless, a pathologic diagnosis of MTS in these surgical groups was made in 60–70% of the patients. Dowd et al.[30] and Brooks et al.[18] reported findings in patients with refractory complex partial seizures on 1.5-tesla MRI. Dowd et al. found MRI abnormalities in 16 of 20 patients who had pathologic findings after surgery; 7 of 11 patients with MTS had positive findings on MRI scans in a medial temporal lobe region, and MRI demonstrated all other abnormalities, including two neoplasms, two vascular malformations, one hamartoma, one case of polymicrogyria, one arachnoid cyst, one case of tuberous sclerosis, and one case of hemiatrophy. In contrast, Brooks et al. found that MRI detected lesions in 28% of patients with epilepsy refractory to surgery with only 8% sensitivity to MTS but 93% sensitivity in diagnosing 11 of 12 tumors and all three vascular malformations in this population.

The distribution of anatomic pathologic features as demonstrated by MRI in specific locations differs only slightly based on these reports. In 135 patients with refractory *temporal* lobe complex partial seizures who underwent surgery, 85 had hippocampal sclerosis (63%), 20 had foreign tissue lesions, and two had cortical dysplasia based on the findings of preoperative MRI scans; MRI had a sensitivity of 97% for MTS and 100% for foreign tissue lesions.[31] Among another series of 34 temporal lobe epilepsy surgery patients, MRI documented all five foreign tissue lesions and had a sensitivity of 52% for the medial temporal changes associated with MTS in 20 patients.[32] Overall, the underlying substrate in refractory temporal lobe epilepsy was 14–15% foreign tissue lesions and 60–63% MTS, which is a remarkable concordance in two studies performed on opposite sides of the world. In the single report of 48 patients with refractory *frontal* lobe epilepsy, 33% had a focal lesion, including 12 foreign tissue lesions (10 neoplasms, two vascular lesions).[33] Considering the likely bias in a group of patients with frontal lobe epilepsy selected for surgery, these are not substantial differences in the incidence of the anatomic changes underlying refractory partial epilepsy in frontal and temporal lobes.

Remarkably, the anatomic findings in refractory epilepsy populations appear to approximate the incidence of abnormalities in new-onset, late-onset, and controlled epilepsy series, confirming the impression that, notwithstanding differences in patient populations, magnets, technique, and interpretation criteria, the anatomic basis of epilepsy is demonstrated by MRI in 50% or more of patients. MTS accounts for the largest group, and foreign tissue lesions represent the underlying cause in 10–20% of remaining cases. Furthermore, and most remarkably, the distribution of structural abnormalities in refractory epilepsy parallels its distribution in controlled epilepsy, suggesting that all these pathologic structural lesions have a spectrum of associated seizure severity.

Children

Reports on the utility of MRI in evaluating the structural basis of the epileptic process in children have been restricted to those addressing refractory epilepsy of childhood. In that population as well, MRI has proven to be a remarkably sensitive tool. Twenty-seven of 37 children with refractory epilepsy had MRI-demonstrated abnormalities that corresponded to the EEG-documented epileptogenic focus according to Otsubo et al.[34] These authors documented positive findings in eight of nine children with focal cortical dysplasia, 11 of 11 children with hemimegalencephaly, and five of six children with tumors. MRI was also sensitive to MTS in this population, which was, however, more often associated with an additional structural lesion in the temporal lobe (7 of 12). Although CT scanning has been found to be more sensitive to the calcification of Sturge-Weber syndrome, MRI is more sensitive to the angiomatous enhancement in this disease, making it an equally sensitive tool for diagnosis.[35] Dietrich et al. reported 29 children who underwent hemispherectomy in whom MRI studies, CT scans, or both detected lesions in 19.[35] More recently, Kuzniecky et al. found abnormalities concordant with the EEG findings in 84% of children with refractory epilepsy who were surgically treated, with developmental abnormalities in 25%, hippocampal sclerosis in 50% (almost all over the age of 12 years), and gliomas in 25% (but with a tendency for gangliogliomas to be more prevalent than astrocytomas under the age of 12 years).[36] In a group of 30 refractory epileptic children who did not undergo surgery, Cross and colleagues found abnormalities of the hippocampus or temporal lobe in 25, of whom 16 had hippocampal abnormalities of various sorts, six had temporal neocortical abnormalities, and three had temporal lobe foreign tissue lesions.[37] These discrepant results emphasize the selection bias in the prior reports of surgically treated children who were probably selected for resective surgery in part because of the focally abnormal MRI findings consistent with the EEG localization. In four infants with West syndrome, MRI detected focal abnormalities of cortical development despite negative findings on CT studies.[38] Finally, among 15 term infants with seizures, MRI detected focal ischemic injury in five, diffuse cerebral edema in six, and superior sagittal thrombosis in one. The findings in this group were not predicted by the clinical history.[39] MRI is as sensitive to the abnormal structure associated with epilepsy in childhood as it is in adulthood, although with a slightly different distribution of findings.

ISSUES IN THE INTERPRETATION OF MAGNETIC RESONANCE IMAGING FINDINGS IN EPILEPSY

That the lesion detected with MRI was usually consistent with the localization of the EEG abnormality and that its resection most often cured the epilepsy underline the relevance of these images of structure to the epileptic process, regardless of its severity.

In refractory frontal lobe epilepsy, the presence of a single MRI-identified lesion was associated with the best surgical prognosis, whereas patients with normal MRI findings or multiple lesions fared less well with respect to surgical response after resection.[33] Similarly, in refractory temporal lobe epilepsy, the finding of a foreign tissue lesion on the MRI study predicted seizure freedom after temporal lobe resection, and hippocampal atrophy or spin-spin MRI (T2) signal abnormality in the hippocampus was also associated with surgical success in seizure control after removal of the MRI-identified abnormality.[31, 32]

Furthermore, despite the tendency to assume that electrical demonstration of the epileptogenic zone is necessary even when a structural lesion is seen on neuroimaging, several authors have emphasized the proximity of the lesion to the brain area causing seizures regardless of what other means are used to define the epileptogenic zone and what they show—at least with respect to foreign tissue lesions. Thus, Awad et al. observed 47 patients with tumors, vascular lesions, or developmental lesions, of whom four of six had excellent seizure control after resection of the epileptogenic zone alone (defined by chronic extraoperative EEG recordings), nine of ten with resection of the lesion alone, and six of eight with resection of the lesion plus the epileptogenic zone.[40] The authors concluded that resection of the lesions offers the best chance of seizure control. Similarly, Fish et al. found only five of 20 patients with lesional epilepsy had seizure control when resection was confined to the epileptogenic zone and did not resect the lesion identified with neuroimaging.[41] Some others have documented the need to resect the lesion and the surrounding structurally abnormal or electrically abnormal area in proximity to the lesion for seizure control,[42, 43] but Britton et al. found equal and excellent results in seizure control with resection of the lesion with or without the "epileptogenic zone."[44] Postoperative electrocorticography may be especially valuable in deciding the extent of resection in patients with developmental lesions, where MRI definition of anatomic abnormalities may not be complete because of more microscopic intraparenchymal cerebral involvement.[45] The distillation of this literature suggests that the anatomic abnormalities seen on MRI scans in patients with refractory epilepsy at least define the primary region of epileptogenesis, although more or less surrounding, microscopically involved cortical tissue may also play a role in the process of seizure generation.

DUAL ANATOMIC PATHOLOGIC PROCESSES

The above considerations do not solve the problem of multiple anatomic lesions seen on MRI scans in patients with epilepsy and the distinction between these lesions with respect to their potential epileptogenicity. One specific instance of dual pathologic entities is the patient with hippocampal atrophy and a foreign tissue lesion. Fried and colleagues found that patients with temporal lobe tumors in more medial locations or of longer duration, and patients with developmental abnormalities or arteriovenous malformations, had more hippocampal cell loss; the authors, however, did not address the epileptogenic potential of the hippocampal sclerosis.[46] Watson and Williamson did not document hippocampal atrophy in any of 30 patients with foreign tissue lesions outside of the temporal lobe, regardless of their character,[47] and Cascino et al. found only one such example in 18 patients.[48] Cendes et al. and others emphasized the more frequent existence of dual pathologic processes in the form of hippocampal sclerosis and developmental lesions in the temporal lobe,[49] and Rush and Morrell documented independent epileptogenesis in those two areas in four patients with this type of dual lesions.[50] The coexistence of developmental abnormalities with hippocampal sclerosis is even more common in children with refractory epilepsy.[51] In these situations, then, a possible structural basis of epilepsy is indeed dual and can also be documented by MRI, whereas in some others (for example, adults with temporal lobe gliomas) the dual anatomic abnormalities may not always represent dual epileptogenicity.

Cendes et al. recently published the most extensive study thus far to address these issues.[49] Dual pathologic processes in the form of hippocampal sclerosis and a lesion were found in 25 of 167 patients with refractory epilepsy and included individuals with temporal and extratemporal lesions. The incidence of hippocampal atrophy was highest in patients with developmental lesions in any lobe, vascular abnormalities close to the hippocampus, and a history of febrile seizures, but was low in patients with gliomas, which confirms many of the prior findings. Although they speculated about possible dual epileptogenicity, the authors did not provide information to assess the epileptogenic potential of the hippocampal atrophy in these dual pathology patients, which remains unknown in most such situations. Still, this quandary is present in a minority of epilepsy patients with structural lesions.

MAGNETIC RESONANCE IMAGING: TECHNICAL ISSUES IN EPILEPSY

If any differences emerge from the above overview of the distribution of structural abnormalities in epilepsy, it is the discrepancy between the ability to detect medial temporal lobe changes that is most striking. Most MRI protocols detect nearly 100% of the foreign tissue lesions associated with epilepsy (of any severity, location, type, or duration). To maximize results in the temporal lobe, the usual protocol consists of sagittal spin-lattice MRI (T1) images; axial and coronal T2; and inversion recovery sequences with overlapping 3- to 5-mm sections.[52, 53] Features that are most consistent include an increased hippocampal T2 signal and decreased gray/white demarcation on T1 signals, but other findings may include decreased size of the hippocampus or temporal lobe and increased size of the temporal horn.[54] It has been demonstrated that gadolinium does not enhance the yield of MRI studies in epilepsy, but it can serve to define the nature of a demonstrated structural abnormality.[55]

Volumetric analysis of the hippocampus has been used in the management of epilepsy since 1989, with various centers employing somewhat different techniques and methods of normalization and with control values generated by individual centers showing considerable variability.[56] The technique has found its greatest utility in the demonstration of lateralized hippocampal atrophy. Significant correlations between the presence of hippocampal atrophy and hippocampal cell loss and between hippocampal atrophy and surgical outcome have been shown.[57–59] The technique of hippocampal volumetric analysis has a sensitivity of 60–90% for the presence of MTS, which is, as noted above, the most common structural substrate associated with temporal lobe epilepsy.[60] Not all MTS is detected, however, and some patients with hippocampal atrophy have seizure onset elsewhere, so hippocampal atrophy is not an independent indicator of medial temporal lobe epilepsy.[61] Nevertheless, it remains a highly accurate and sensitive noninvasive diagnostic study, the results of which should be confirmed by electrical evidence of epileptogenicity. MTS is also associated with increased T2 signal in the hippocampus, and quantitation of T2 signal by relaxometry is being used as a more objective and sensitive measure of this change.[62] However, increased T2 signal and decreased hippocampal size can usually be appreciated by qualitative analysis.

Volumetric techniques are being extended to extrahippocampal regions. Barkovich and colleagues used high resolution, three-dimensional, Fourier transform volumetric MRI with 1.5 mm partition size in 15 patients with simple partial epilepsy and found cortical abnormalities in eight.[63]

SPECIFIC GROUPS

With an understanding of the distribution of structural abnormalities in various epilepsy groups and an appreciation of the spectrum of pathologic findings, we consider below the most common substrates in terms of MRI and the additional insights into pathophysiology that this structural demonstration provides.

Gliosis

Although many epilepsy patients demonstrate some gliosis on pathologic examination of resected tissue from various cerebral locations, it is the gliosis of

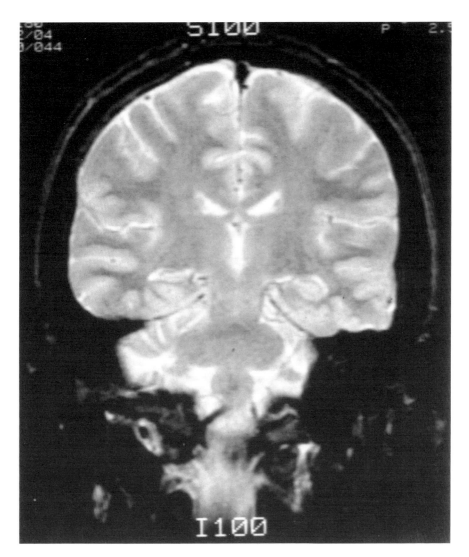

Figure 4.2 Coronal spin-spin magnetic resonance image demonstrates atrophy and increased signal in the right hippocampus associated with refractory medial temporal lobe epilepsy.

medial temporal lobe structures that is most commonly found and has therefore been most extensively studied (Figure 4.2). As documented above, volumetric assessment of the hippocampus has become common in documenting the reduction in the size of the hippocampus associated with neuronal loss in medial temporal lobe epilepsy,[56, 61] but this atrophy is visualized on qualitative examination with appropriate sequences and sections.[64, 65] The side of hippocampal atrophy correlates with the side of the EEG abnormality in 90% or more of patients,[57, 59, 66–68] but rare individuals with medial temporal lobe epilepsy do not have hippocampal atrophy.[69] Some have hippocampal atrophy without medial temporal lobe epilepsy,[61] and others have bilateral hippocampal atrophy most prominent contralateral to the predominant side of seizure onset.[70, 71] Nevertheless, comparative investigations in the most difficult group of epileptic patients, those undergoing intracranial EEG studies, found that hippocampal volume loss had higher sensitivity and specificity than any other noninvasive technique, including scalp electroencephalography, in predicting the epileptogenic region.[60] In conjunction with electroencephalography, MRI has reduced the need for intracranial EEG studies by 50% in this group of patients.[72]

Quantitative volumetric analysis or qualitative analysis of the hippocampus can be performed in regions or in toto.[64, 65] The presence of regional hippocampal atrophy, as well as its relationship to the epileptogenic process, is not well defined. Although segmental hippocampal atrophy can exist even in isolation, most often the atrophy involves the hippocampus throughout, or at least the body.[65] However, the implications for the localization of seizure onset within the hippocampus or for surgical outcome of these variations are essentially unknown, with the single exception that isolated amygdala atrophy has been shown to be a poor prognostic sign for surgery.[73]

Hippocampal atrophy correlates with neuronal density in the hippocampus.[57, 67] Cell loss of less than 30% usually cannot be detected by current techniques. This degree of cell loss is more commonly seen in association with foreign tissue lesions in patients who apparently do not have independent hippocampal seizure onset.[46, 57, 74] In patients with sufficient neuronal loss to demonstrate hippocampal atrophy (qualitatively or quantitatively), the finding correlates with surgical outcome.[58, 59] Hippocampal atrophy is identified in 90% of patients with hippocampal seizure onset associated with MTS.[57, 59, 66–68]

Foreign Tissue Lesions

Within the category of foreign tissue lesions, representing 10–20% of the structural substrates of epilepsy, fall neoplastic and vascular lesions. They are all convincingly, accurately, and uniformly demonstrated by MRI. Recently, Bronen et al. discussed the MRI characteristics of these lesions.[75] Among 33 neoplasms and eight vascular lesions in patients with refractory epilepsy confirmed by subsequent surgical resection and pathologic analysis, MRI detected 100% and predicted the pathologic entity in 95%. Lesions were predominantly temporal (70% of the neoplasms and 63% of the vascular lesions), usually peripheral (within or adjacent to the cortex or hippocampus), and often remodeled the overlying calvarium. Sixty-one percent of the tumors produced mass effect, whereas vascular lesions usually did not. Tumors were usually heterogeneous, while vascular lesions were most frequently cavernous angiomas and had the characteristic appearance of a central high signal surrounded by a zone of signal void.

Boon et al. described the neuropsychological, EEG, and clinical seizure characteristics of this group of patients.[76] Of 250 patients with intractable epilepsy who underwent surgery, 50 had foreign tissue lesions. Most (>90%) were seizure free or markedly improved after resection of the lesion, but localization of the site of the lesions by neuropsychological assessment (26%) and interictal EEG recording (30%) was poor.

Some authors have discussed vascular or neoplastic lesions specifically. Of 67 patients with cerebral vascular malformations, including 35 AVMs, 29 cryptic malformations, and 11 venous angiomas, 25 patients had epilepsy and 42 did not.[77] The epileptic cerebral vascular malformations were more peripheral and more often associated with a perilesional increase in T2 on MRI. Surgery with resection of the lesion and the surrounding hemosiderin-stained cortex in 20 patients with epilepsy and with vascular malformations was reported to produce good or excellent seizure control in all but two patients at the Mayo Clinic.[78] Of interest was the presence of more than one vascular lesion in five of these vascular malformation patients. Concordance of the EEG findings with the site of the lesion resected was the most important factor in predicting good surgical outcome. Seventeen of the resected lesions were cavernomas.

In another report restricted entirely to cavernous angiomas, MRI detected the lesion in all 18 patients.[79] Some of these patients had multiple cavernomas, a finding that sometimes occurred as part of a familial syndrome with additional hepatic and retinal cavernous hemangiomas.[80]

With respect to venous malformations in epilepsy, no agreement exists on their epileptic potential. Rigamonti et al. noted seizures in only two of 30 patients with such malformations,[81] whereas Crecco et al. found that of 17 patients with venous angiomas, four had associated cavernomas and 50% had epilepsy.[82] Authors agree that other lesions may coexist with venous angiomas and may be responsible for symptoms or signs of neurologic illness and that MRI is the most valuable technique for demonstrating the other lesions and the venous angiomas.

Most neoplasms associated with epilepsy are slow-growing intraparenchymal tumors; in one study, seizures occurred in 70% of patients with astrocytomas (Figure 4.3), 92% of patients with oligodendrogliomas (Figure 4.4), and 37% of patients with glioblastomas.[83] Most neoplastic determinants of epilepsy are astrocytomas, oligodendrogliomas, oligoastrocytomas, gangliogliomas, or DNT. MRI is the procedure of choice for demonstrating these lesions and nearly always does so; in some series it is 50–100% more sensitive than CT scanning.[84] A constant proportion, about 10–25%, of patients with refractory epilepsy undergoing surgery have neoplasms; although neoplasms are more common among adult-onset epilepsies, they remain an important cause of seizures in children as well. In one report, 46% of children undergoing epilepsy surgery had primary brain neoplasms; all were gliomas.[85]

The pleomorphic xanthoastrocytoma is a glioma, first recognized in 1979, arising from subpial astrocytes and characteristic of younger patients with epilepsy; almost all of these patients have seizures. Despite its pleomorphic and bizarre appearing cells, the prognosis is good.[86] DNT is a newly recognized lesion with a high degree of cellular polymorphism, a multinodular architecture, and associated cortical dysplasia. The lesion presents with seizures at a young age, is almost always in the temporal lobe, often medial, and responds well to resection, which results in seizure control and lack of recurrence in most patients.[87] Younger patients with refractory epilepsy also tend to have gangliogliomas; again, these tumors are most common in the temporal lobe (more than 60%), and patients have an excellent response to resection with respect to seizures and cure of the lesion.[88] This latter tumor, like DNT, may be associated with developmental abnormalities in 5–25% of patients and is considered hamartomatous by some authors. In one report of 51 such patients, 92% had

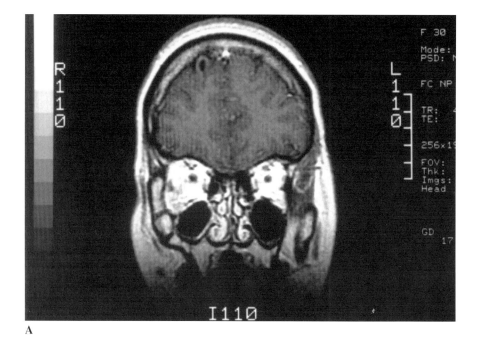

A

B

Figure 4.3   Coronal spin-lattice magnetic resonance (A) and sagittal spin-spin magnetic resonance (B) images of an astrocytoma associated with refractory frontal lobe epilepsy.

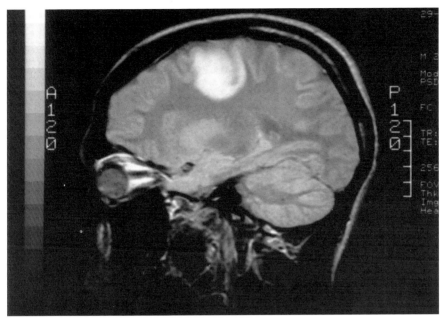

A

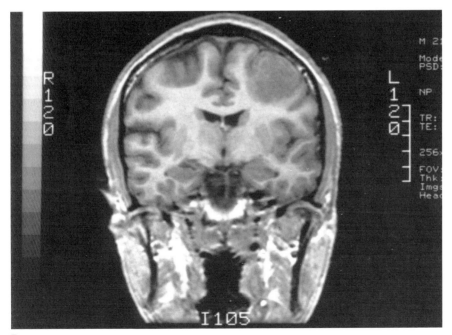

B

Figure 4.4 Sagittal (A) and coronal (B) spin-lattice magnetic resonance images illustrating a cortical oligodendroglioma associated with intractable epilepsy.

seizures, 84% of the neoplasms were temporal, and 50% were cystic; the operation cured the seizures in all patients.[89]

Developmental Abnormalities

Abnormalities of cortical development are an important cause of epilepsy of
various severities and have been demonstrated with increasing sensitivity by
MRI. These lesions, however, because of their variable nature and degree,
remain the structural causes of epilepsy in which our imaging techniques are
least sensitive. Even pathologic descriptions have been continuously modified
by virtue of increasing recognition and pathologic analysis. We still do not have
complete agreement in some of these as to their epileptogenic or even their
pathologic nature.

These developmental abnormalities can be severe, as manifested by
lissencephaly or agyria with failed cerebral gyration and lamination, but gyral
abnormalities can also be more restricted (hemimegalencephaly, pachygyria,
polymicrogyria, schizencephaly, focal cortical dysplasia) (Figure 4.5).[90]
Developmental abnormalities can also be manifested by scattered or clustered
ectopic neurons (band or nodular heterotopia). By virtue of the sensitivity of
MRI to most of these abnormalities, more frequent diagnoses of developmental abnormalities are being made, and a classification scheme based on MRI has
been devised.[91]

The distribution of developmental abnormalities in epilepsy patients has been
reported in a variety of publications. Of 100 patients with developmental abnormalities and epilepsy collected from two centers in London, 39 had abnormalities of gyration, 28 had heterotopias, five had tuberous sclerosis, seven had focal
cortical dysplasia, and 21 had cortical dysgenesis associated with neoplasms
(DNT).[90] Of interest, CT scans appeared normal in 69% of these patients, and
MRI findings had been negative on a previous occasion in 19 of the 36 patients
who were studied before. Although MRI scans with 1.5-mm continuous coronal
slices did demonstrate the developmental abnormalities in all but one of the
reported patients, subsequent surgery with histologic analysis confirmed additional areas of cortical dysplasia in six others that were not demonstrated by the
MRI scan. Raymond et al.[51] emphasized the importance of obtaining thin MRI
slices through the entire brain and multiple planes to enhance the yield of MRI-
based diagnosis of cortical dysplasia.

MRI findings in developmental abnormalities may include broad sulci, thick-
ened cortex, blurring of the gray/white interface, increased T2 signals, and
clefts.[92] Several distinct syndromes have been defined, mostly by MRI, including the congenital bilateral perisylvian syndrome[93] (characterized by bilateral
opercular polymicrogyria, developmental delay, pseudobulbar palsy, and variable
pyramidal signs) and subependymal heterotopia (which affects predominantly
females and presents with epilepsy in the second decade or later in individuals
with normal intelligence).[94] Band or laminar heterotopia, also known as double
cortex syndrome, may be associated with mental retardation, epilepsy, and thick-
ening of the overlying cortex; the severity is variable.[95, 96] A syndrome of posterior agyria and pachygyria with polymicrogyria was reported in two brothers with
mental retardation and refractory epilepsy.[97]

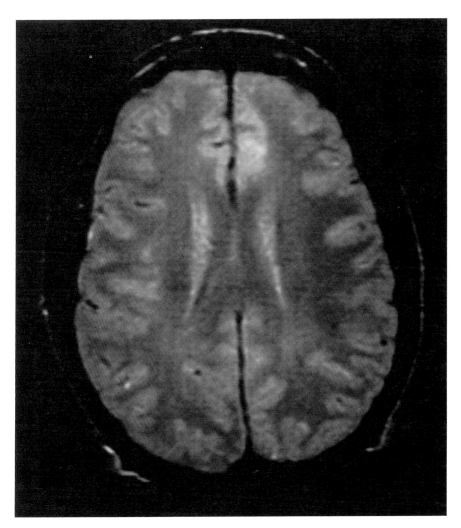

Figure 4.5 Axial spin-spin magnetic resonance image shows left medial frontal area of increased signal, which was proven by pathologic analysis to represent focal cortical dysplasia.

In tuberous sclerosis, the cortical tubers (hamartomas) are well demonstrated on MRI scans by virtue of an increased T2 signal and can be distinguished from those of subependymal heterotopia by their gadolinium enhancement, isointensity with white matter, and elongated shape.[98] This is another syndrome of developmental abnormality with a spectrum of neurologic and genetic manifestations. In 34 children with tuberous sclerosis, topographic correlation of the MRI and EEG findings was found for at least one tuber per patient. A more obscure developmental abnormality is the hypothalamic hamartoma; these lesions are associated with cortical abnormalities, ictal laughter, multiple seizure types, and cognitive deterioration. These are also ideally demonstrated by MRI.[99]

Microdysgenesis is the form of developmental abnormality that is not visualized by MRI. It is a phenomenon of scattered heterotopic neurons of insufficient density to be detected by current imaging techniques. Its significance also remains unresolved with respect to epilepsy, although it has been reported in patients with temporal lobe epilepsy and generalized epilepsy.

The incidence of epilepsy in patients with developmental abnormalities has also been studied. In 53 patients with developmental abnormalities treated at the Montreal Neurological Institute, 32 had localized cortical dysplasias, 10 had bilateral perisylvian dysplasia, six had diffuse migration abnormalities, four had hemimegalencephaly, and one had nodular gray matter heterotopia. Of those with focal cortical dysplasia, all had epilepsy. Of the 10 patients with bilateral perisylvian dysplasia, two did not have epilepsy, although all had significant neurologic compromise.[92] In most patients who underwent surgery for seizure control, success correlated with the extent of resection of the abnormality demonstrated on the MRI scan but remained at 50% or less. The cytoarchitectonic abnormalities may exceed our ability to detect them.

With respect to the incidence of developmental abnormalities in epilepsy patients, in a group of 303 epileptic patients in Norway studied with variable MRI technique, 13 had developmental abnormalities (four schizencephaly, one hemimegalencephaly, two heterotopias, six localized pachygyria or polymicrogyria).[100] This study suggests an incidence of 5% for developmental abnormalities in epilepsy; this figure is probably lower than that usually reported for the refractory epilepsy population and may also be falsely low because of suboptimal MRI techniques. In a single study evaluating developmental abnormalities specifically in temporal lobe epilepsy patients, 16 of 222 patients with temporal lobe epilepsy were found to have developmental abnormalities.[101] These included one heterotopia, six focal cortical dysplasias, five hippocampal malformations, and four patients with a combination of the above. These patients did not differ clinically from the remainder of the temporal lobe epilepsy population. MRI can thus be critical in defining the underlying substrate, which can affect the approach to medical or surgical treatment and the prognosis.

Although not a cortical dysplasia per se, abnormal development leading to occult encephalocele of the temporal lobe has also been reported to result in epilepsy. These lesions are rare and have been diagnosed at surgery but not by MRI.[102]

CONCLUSION

MRI applied to general and specific populations of epilepsy patients has clarified, defined, discovered, and documented the living anatomy of epilepsy. A systematic synthesis of available information shows that the distribution from more common to less common anatomic accompaniments of epilepsy includes gliosis (particularly medial temporal), neoplasms (particularly gliomas), vascular lesions (especially cavernous angiomas), and developmental abnormalities (especially focal cortical dysplasias). This distribution varies minimally in patients with refractory, newly diagnosed, late- and early-onset, and controlled epilepsy. Available data also provide considerable evidence to support the contention that the anatomic abnormalities seen by MRI are indeed related to the cause of the epilepsy, although multiple structural abnormalities may confuse the final determination of the epileptogenic zone as defined by EEG.

All patients with epilepsy should have an MRI study, since symptomatic generalized and unsuspected partial epilepsies can masquerade as primary epilepsy and structural abnormalities of importance for treatment or prognosis may be detected in epilepsy of any age or duration. High-resolution studies with fine cuts in multiple planes and volumetric analysis hold promise for further definition of some elusive developmental abnormalities. Already, MTS and foreign tissue lesions can be defined with nearly 100% sensitivity. The continued scrutiny of anatomic abnormalities associated with epilepsy will help define additional syndromes, which may open doors to genetic definition and treatment as well as modify surgical and medical approaches.

REFERENCES

1. Vinters HV, Armstrong DL, Babb TL, et al. The Neuropathology of Human Symptomatic Epilepsy. In J Engel Jr (ed), Surgical Treatment of the Epilepsies. New York: Raven, 1993;593.
2. Babb TL, Brown WJ. Pathological Findings in Epilepsy. In J Engel Jr (ed), Surgical Treatment of the Epilepsies (2nd ed). New York: Raven, 1987;511.
3. Jay V, Becker L. Surgical pathology of epilepsy: a review. Pediatr Pathol 1994;14:731.
4. Robitaille Y, Rasmussen T, Dubeau F, et al. Histopathology of nonneoplastic lesions in frontal lobe epilepsy. Adv Neurol 1992;57:499.
5. Sano K, Malamud N. Clinical significance of sclerosis of the cornu ammonis. Arch Neurol Psychiatry 1953;70:40.
6. Mouritzen-Dam A. Hippocampal neuron loss in epilepsy and after experimental seizures. Acta Neurol Scand 1982;66:601.
7. Margerison JH, Corsellis JAN. Epilepsy and the temporal lobes. Brain 1966;89:499.
8. Bachman DS, Hodges FJ III, Freeman JM. Computerized axial tomography in chronic seizure disorders of childhood. Pediatrics 1976;58:828.
9. Jabbari B, Huott AD, Di Chiro G, et al. Surgically correctable lesions detected by CT in 143 patients with chronic epilepsy. Surg Neurol 1978;10:319.
10. Gilsanz V, Strand R, Barnes P, Nealis J. Results of presumed cryptogenic epilepsy in childhood by CT scanning. Ann Radiol (Paris) 1979;22:184.
11. Latack JT, Abou-Khalil BW, Siegel GJ, et al. Patients with partial seizures: evaluation by MR, CT, and PET imaging. Radiology 1986;159:159.
12. Conlon P, Trimble MR, Rogers D, Callicott C. Magnetic resonance imaging in epilepsy: a controlled study. Epilepsy Res 1988;2:37.
13. Theodore WH, Dorwart R, Holmes M, et al. Neuroimaging in refractory partial seizures: comparison of PET, CT, and MRI. Neurology 1986;36:750.
14. Sperling MR, Wilson G, Engel J Jr, et al. Magnetic resonance imaging in intractable partial epilepsy: correlative studies. Ann Neurol 1986;20:57.
15. Kuzniecky R, De La Sayette V, Ethier R, et al. Magnetic resonance imaging in temporal lobe epilepsy: pathologic correlations. Ann Neurol 1987;22:341.
16. Lesser RP, Modic MT, Weinstein MA, et al. Magnetic resonance imaging (1.5 tesla) in patients with intractable focal seizures. Arch Neurol 1986;43:367.
17. Gerard G, Shabas D, Rossi D. MRI in epilepsy. Comput Radiol 1987;11:223.
18. Brooks BS, King DW, El Gammal T, et al. MR imaging in patients with intractable complex partial epileptic seizures. AJNR Am J Neuroradiol 1990;11:93.
19. Heinz ER, Heinz TR, Radtke R, et al. Efficacy of MR vs CT in epilepsy. AJNR Am J Neuroradiol 1988;9:1123.
20. Laster DW, Perry JK, Moody DM, et al. Chronic seizure disorders: contribution of MR imaging when CT is normal. AJNR Am J Neuroradiol 1985;6:177.
21. Froment JC, Mauguiere F, Fischer C, et al. Magnetic resonance imaging in refractory focal epilepsy with normal CT scans. J Neuroradiol 1989;16:285.

22. Elster AD, Mirza W. MR imaging in chronic partial epilepsy: role of contrast enhancement. AJNR Am J Neuroradiol 1991;12:165.
23. Shepherd CW, Houser OW, Gomez MR. MR findings in tuberous sclerosis complex and correlation with seizure development and mental impairment. AJNR Am J Neuroradiol 1995;16:149.
24. Rao TH, Libman RB, Patel M. Seizures and disappearing brain lesions. Seizure 1995;4:61.
25. Fujikawa Y, Kubota H, Matsuda K, et al. Reversal of MRI lesion with relapse and remission of partial motor seizures in epilepsia partialis continua. Jpn J Psychiatr Neurol 1991;45:410.
26. Forsgren L, Fagerlund M, Zetterlund B. Electroencephalographic and neuroradiological findings in adults with newly diagnosed unprovoked seizures. Eur Neurol 1991;31:61.
27. Kilpatrick CJ, Tress BM, O'Donnell C, et al. Magnetic resonance imaging and late-onset epilepsy. Epilepsia 1991;32:358.
28. Triulzi F, Franceschi M, Fazio F, Del Maschio A. Non-refractory temporal lobe epilepsy: 1.5-T MR imaging. Radiology 1988;166:181.
29. Franceschi M, Triulzi F, Ferini-Srambi L, et al. Focal cerebral lesions found by magnetic resonance imaging in cryptogenic nonrefractory temporal lobe epilepsy patients. Epilepsia 1989;30:540.
30. Dowd CF, Dillon WP, Barbaro NM, Laxer KD. Magnetic resonance imaging of intractable complex partial seizures: pathologic and electroencephalographic correlation. Epilepsia 1991;32:454.
31. Berkovic SF, McIntosh AM, Kalnins RM, et al. Preoperative MRI predicts outcome of temporal lobectomy: an actuarial analysis. Neurology 1995;45:1359.
32. Kuzniecky R, Burgard S, Faught E, et al. Predictive value of magnetic resonance imaging in temporal lobe epilepsy surgery. Arch Neurol 1993;50:65.
33. Lorenzo NY, Parisi JE, Cascino GD, et al. Intractable frontal lobe epilepsy: pathological and MRI features. Epilepsy Res 1995;20:171.
34. Otsubo H, Chuang SH, Hwang PA, et al. Neuroimaging for investigation of seizures in children. Pediatr Neurosurg 1992;18:105.
35. Dietrich RB, Saden SE, Chugani HT, et al. Resective surgery for intractable epilepsy in children: radiologic evaluation. AJNR Am J Neuroradiol 1991;12:1149.
36. Kuzniecky R, Murro A, King D, et al. Magnetic resonance imaging in childhood intractable partial epilepsies: pathologic correlations. Neurology 1993;43:681.
37. Cross JH, Jackson GD, Neville BGR, et al. Early detection of abnormalities in partial epilepsy using magnetic resonance. Arch Dis Child 1993;69:104.
38. Van Bogaert P, Chiron C, Adamsbaum C, et al. Value of magnetic resonance in West syndrome of unknown etiology. Epilepsia 1993;34:701.
39. Rollins NK, Morris MC, Evans D, Perlman JM. The role of early MR in the evaluation of the term infant with seizures. AJNR Am J Neuroradiol 1994;15:239.
40. Awad IA, Rosenfeld J, Ahl F, et al. Intractable epilepsy and structural lesions of the brain: mapping, resection strategies, and seizure outcome. Epilepsia 1991;32:179.
41. Fish D, Andermann F, Olivier A. Complex partial seizures and small posterior temporal or extratemporal structural lesions: surgical management. Neurology 1991;41:1781.
42. Pilcher WH, Silbergeld DL, Berger MS, Ojemann GA. Intraoperative electrocorticography during tumor resection: impact on seizure outcome in patients with gangliogliomas. J Neurosurg 1993;78:891.
43. Spencer DD, Spencer SS, Mattson RH, Williamson PD. Intracerebral masses in patients with intractable partial epilepsy. Neurology 1984;34:432.
44. Britton JW, Cascino GD, Sharbrough FW, Kelly PJ. Low-grade glial neoplasms and intractable partial epilepsy: efficacy of surgical treatment. Epilepsia 1994;35:1130.
45. Palmini A, Gambardella A, Andermann F, et al. Intrinsic epileptogenicity of human dysplastic cortex as suggested by corticography and surgical results. Ann Neurol 1995;37:476.
46. Fried I, Kim JH, Spencer DD. Hippocampal pathology in patients with intractable seizures and temporal lobe masses. J Neurosurg 1992;76:735.
47. Watson C, Williamson B. Volumetric magnetic resonance imaging in patients with epilepsy and extratemporal structural lesions. J Epilepsy 1994;7:80.
48. Cascino GD, Jack CR Jr, Sharbrough FW, et al. MRI assessments of hippocampal pathology in extratemporal lesional epilepsy. Neurology 1993;43:2380.
49. Cendes F, Cook MJ, Watson E, et al. Frequency and characteristics of dual pathology in patients with lesional epilepsy. Neurology 1995;45:2058.
50. Rush E, Morrell MJ. Cortical dysplasia with mesiotemporal sclerosis: evidence for kindling in humans [abstract]. Epilepsia 1993;34(Suppl 6):15.
51. Raymond AA, Fish DR, Stevens JM, et al. Association of hippocampal sclerosis with cortical dysgenesis in patients with epilepsy. Neurology 1994;44:1841.

52. Kuzniecky RI, Cascino GD, Palmini A, et al. Structural Neuroimaging. In J Engel Jr (ed), Surgical Treatment of the Epilepsies (2nd ed). New York: Raven, 1993;197.
53. Cascino GD, Jack CR Jr, Hirschorn KA, Sharbrough FW. Identification of the Epileptic Focus: Magnetic Resonance Imaging. In WH Theodore (ed), Surgical Treatment of Epilepsy. Epilepsy Research Supplement 5. Amsterdam: Elsevier, 1992;95.
54. Meiners LC, Van Gils A, Jansen GH, et al. Temporal lobe epilepsy: the various MR appearances of histologically proven mesial temporal sclerosis. AJNR Am J Neuroradiol 1994;15:1547.
55. Cascino GD, Hirschom KA, Jack CR, Sharbrough FW. Gadolinium-DTPA-enhanced magnetic resonance imaging in intractable partial epilepsy. Neurology 1989;39:1115.
56. McCarthy G, Luby M. Imaging the structural changes associated with human epilepsy. Clin Neurosci 1994;2:82.
57. Lencz T, McCarthy G, Bronen RA, et al. Quantitative magnetic resonance imaging in temporal lobe epilepsy: relationship to neuropathology and neuropsychological function. Ann Neurol 1992;31:629.
58. Garcia PA, Laxer KD, Barbaro NM, Dillon WP. Prognostic value of qualitative magnetic resonance imaging hippocampal abnormalities in patients undergoing temporal lobectomy for medically refractory seizures. Epilepsia 1994;35:520.
59. Jack CR Jr, Sharbrough FW, Cascino GD, et al. Magnetic resonance image-based hippocampal volumetry: correlation with outcome after temporal lobectomy. Ann Neurol 1992;31:138.
60. Spencer SS, McCarthy G, Spencer DD. Diagnosis of medial temporal lobe seizure onset: relative specificity and sensitivity of quantitative MRI. Neurology 1993;43:2117.
61. Spencer SS. MRI and epilepsy surgery [editorial]. Neurology 1995;45:1248.
62. Jackson GD, Connelly A, Duncan JS, et al. Detection of hippocampal pathology in intractable partial epilepsy: increased sensitivity with quantitative magnetic resonance T2 relaxometry. Neurology 1993;43:1793.
63. Barkovich AJ, Rowley HA, Andermann F. MR in partial epilepsy: value of high-resolution volumetric techniques. AJNR Am J Neuroradiol 1995;16:339.
64. Kim JH, Tien RD, Felsberg GJ, et al. MR measurements of the hippocampus for lateralization of temporal lobe epilepsy: value of measurements of the body versus the whole structure. AJR Am J Roentgenol 1994;163:1453.
65. Bronen RA, Fulbright RK, Kim JH, et al. Regional distribution of MR findings in hippocampal sclerosis. AJNR Am J Neuroradiol 1995;16:1193.
66. Berkovic SF, Andermann F, Olivier A, et al. Hippocampal sclerosis in temporal lobe epilepsy demonstrated by magnetic resonance imaging. Ann Neurol 1991;29:175.
67. Cascino GD, Jack CR Jr, Parisi JE, et al. Magnetic resonance imaging-based volume studies in temporal lobe epilepsy: pathological correlations. Ann Neurol 1991;30:31.
68. Cook MJ, Fish DR, Shorvon SD, et al. Hippocampal volumetric studies in frontal and temporal lobe epilepsy. Brain 1992;115:1001.
69. Jackson GD, Kuzniecky RI, Cascino GD. Hippocampal sclerosis without detectable hippocampal atrophy. Neurology 1994;44:42.
70. King D, Spencer SS, McCarthy G, et al. Bilateral hippocampal atrophy in medial temporal lobe epilepsy. Epilepsia 1995;36:905.
71. Jack CR Jr, Trenerry MR, Cascino GD, et al. Bilaterally symmetric hippocampi and surgical outcome. Neurology 1995;45:1353.
72. Spencer SS. Selection of Candidates for Invasive Monitoring. In GD Cascino, CR Jack Jr (eds), Neuroimaging in Epilepsy: Principles and Practice. Boston: Butterworth–Heinemann, 1996;219.
73. Miller LA, McLachlan RS, Bouwer MS, et al. Amygdalar sclerosis: preoperative indicators and outcome after temporal lobectomy. J Neurol Neurosurg Psychiatry 1994;57:1099.
74. Spencer DD, Spencer SS. Clinical perspectives: hippocampal resection and the use of human tissue in defining temporal lobe epilepsy syndromes. Hippocampus 1994;4:243.
75. Bronen RA, Fulbright RK, Spencer DD, et al. MR characteristics of neoplasms and vascular malformations associated with epilepsy. Magn Reson Imaging 1995;13:1153.
76. Boon P, Calliauw L, DeReuck J, et al. Clinical and neurophysiological correlations in patients with refractory partial epilepsy and intracranial structural lesions. Acta Neurochir (Wien) 1994;128:68.
77. Trussart V, Berry I, Manelfe C, et al. Epileptogenic cerebral vascular malformations and MRI. J Neuroradiol 1989;16:273.
78. Dodick DW, Cascino GD, Meyer FB. Vascular malformations and intractable epilepsy: outcome after surgical treatment. Mayo Clin Proc 1994;69:741.
79. Requena I, Arias M, Lopez-Ibor L, et al. Cavernomas of the central nervous system: clinical and neuroimaging manifestations in 47 patients. J Neurol Neurosurg Psychiatry 1991;54:590.

80. Drigo P, Mammi I, Battistella PA, et al. Familial cerebral, hepatic and retinal cavernous angiomas: a new syndrome. Childs Nerv Sys 1994;10:205.
81. Rigamonti D, Spetzler RF, Medina M, et al. Cerebral venous malformations. J Neurosurg 1990;73:560.
82. Crecco M, Floris R, Vidiri A, et al. Venous angiomas: plain and contrast-enhanced MRI and MR angiography. Neuroradiology 1995;37:20.
83. Cascino GD. Epilepsy and brain tumors: implications for treatment. Epilepsia 1990;31(Suppl 3):S37.
84. Bergen D, Blech T, Ramsey R, et al. Magnetic resonance imaging as a sensitive and specific predictor of neoplasms removed for intractable epilepsy. Epilepsia 1989;30:318.
85. Sato Y. Pediatric primary brain tumors. Top Magn Reson Imaging 1992;4:64.
86. Davies KG, Maxwell RE, Seljeskog E, Sung JH. Pleomorphic xanthoastrocytoma—report of four cases with MRI scan appearances and literature review. Br J Neurosurg 1994;8:681.
87. Raymond AA, Halpin SFS, Alsanjari N, et al. Dysembryoplastic neuroepithelial tumor: features in 16 patients. Brain 1994;117:461.
88. Celli P, Scarpinati B, Cervoni L, Cantore GP. Gangliogliomas of the cerebral hemispheres. Report of 14 cases with long-term follow-up and review of the literature. Acta Neurochir 1993;125:52.
89. Zentner J, Wolf HK, Ostertun B, et al. Gangliogliomas: clinical, radiological and histopathological findings in 51 patients. J Neurol Neurosurg Psychiatry 1994;57:1497.
90. Raymond AA, Fish DR, Sisodiya SM, et al. Abnormalities of gyration, heterotopias, tuberous sclerosis, focal cortical dysplasia, microdysgenesis, dysembryoplastic neuroepithelial tumor and dysgenesis of the archicortex in epilepsy. Brain 1995;118:629.
91. Kuzniecky RI. MRI in cerebral developmental malformations and epilepsy. Magn Reson Imaging 1995;13:1137.
92. Palmini A, Andermann F, Tampieri D, et al. Epilepsy and Cortical Cytoarchitectonic Abnormalities: An Attempt at Correlating Basic Mechanisms with Anatomo-Clinical Syndromes. In J Engel Jr, C Wasterlain, EA Cavalheiro, et al. (eds), Molecular Neurobiology of Epilepsy. Epilepsy Research Supplement 9. Amsterdam: Elsevier, 1992;19.
93. Kuzniecky R, Andermann F, Tampieri D, et al. Bilateral central macrogyria: epilepsy, pseudobulbar palsy, and mental retardation—a recognizable neuronal migration disorder. Ann Neurol 1989;25:547.
94. Raymond AA, Fish DR, Stevens JM, et al. Subependymal heterotopia: a distinct neuronal migration disorder associated with epilepsy. J Neurol Neurosurg Psychiatry 1994;57:1195.
95. Palmini A, Andermann F, Aicardi J, et al. Diffuse cortical dysplasia, or the "double cortex" syndrome: the clinical and epileptic spectrum in 10 patients. Neurology 1991;41:1656.
96. Barkovich AJ, Guerrini R, Battaglia G, et al. Band heterotopia: correlation of outcome with magnetic resonance imaging parameters. Ann Neurol 1994;36:609.
97. Ferrie CD, Jackson GD, Giannakodimos S, Panayiotopoulos CP. Posterior agyria-pachygyria with polymicrogyria: evidence for an inherited neuronal migration disorder. Neurology 1995;45:150.
98. Cusmai R, Chiron C, Curatolo P, et al. Topographic comparative study of magnetic resonance imaging and electroencephalography in 34 children with tuberous sclerosis. Epilepsia 1990;31:747.
99. Berkovic SF, Andermann F, Melanson D, et al. Hypothalamic hamartomas and ictal laughter: evolution of a characteristic epileptic syndrome and diagnostic value of magnetic resonance imaging. Ann Neurol 1988;23:429.
100. Brodtkorb E, Nilsen G, Smevik O, Rinck PA. Epilepsy and anomalies of neuronal migration: MRI and clinical aspects. Acta Neurol Scand 1992;86:24.
101. Lehericy S, Dormont D, Semah F, et al. Developmental abnormalities of the medial temporal lobe in patients with temporal lobe epilepsy. AJNR Am J Neuroradiol 1995;16:617.
102. Hyson M, Andermann F, Olivier A, Melanson D. Occult encephaloceles and temporal lobe epilepsy: developmental and acquired lesions in the middle fossa. Neurology 1984;34:363.

5
Brain Imaging: Physiology of Epilepsy

William H. Theodore

Electroencephalography was the first "functional imaging" method for the management of epilepsy. It still has advantages that other imaging methods do not share (Table 5.1). However, newer techniques, including positron emission tomography (PET), single photon emission computed tomography (SPECT), magnetic resonance spectroscopy (MRS), and "functional" magnetic resonance imaging (fMRI), are having an increasing effect on the evaluation of patients with epilepsy. They offer new approaches to localization of epileptic foci and preoperative cognitive mapping as well as to understanding the pathophysiology of seizure disorders and the effect of seizures on behavior, language, and memory. A wide variety of physiologic processes, including cerebral blood flow (CBF), glucose metabolism (CMRglc), high-energy phosphate stores, and neuroreceptor distribution, can now be studied.

The complexity of these techniques and the amount of quantitative information they contain preclude a routine "radiologic" approach to their interpretation. Delineation of clear clinical questions or research hypotheses before investigations are begun is essential. Clinical observation and, if possible, electroencephalographic (EEG) recording, are important adjuncts to functional imaging studies, particularly SPECT and PET. Recently, techniques have been developed for performing EEG monitoring during magnetic resonance imaging (MRI).[1] To improve anatomic specificity, functional images can be coregistered with structural MRI scans.

SINGLE PHOTON EMISSION COMPUTED TOMOGRAPHY, POSITRON EMISSION TOMOGRAPHY, MAGNETIC RESONANCE SPECTROSCOPY/FUNCTIONAL MAGNETIC RESONANCE IMAGING: ADVANTAGES AND DISADVANTAGES

SPECT uses commercially available isotopes labeled with iodine 128 or technetium 99m. Specially designed multiheaded SPECT head scanners have improved resolution compared with standard gamma cameras, but resolution,

Table 5.1   Characteristics of an ideal imaging method for epilepsy

---

Good time resolution
   Sensitivity to seizure spread
Millimeter spatial resolution
Wide availability
Safety
Low cost
Reliability
   Standardization
   Replicability

---

about 8 mm in plane, is less than that of PET. SPECT can measure CBF as well as distribution of ligands for muscarinic, cholinergic, and benzodiazepine receptors. Until recently, most SPECT CBF scans were performed with technetium 99m hexamethylene propylene amine oxime (^{99m}Tc-HMPAO), which was chemically unstable and had to be mixed immediately before injection. A new, more stable tracer, ^{99m}Tc-ethyl cysteinate dimer (Neurolyte) will probably replace HMPAO.[2]

SPECT has two major advantages over PET: It is cheaper, and it uses longer-lived isotopes. Ictal SPECT scans are a practical possibility, particularly with ^{99m}Tc-ethyl cysteinate dimer, since the tracer can be kept premixed on a monitoring unit to be injected as soon as a seizure is detected. Since ^{99m}Tc has a 6-hour half-life, the actual scan can be performed at a delay after tracer injection. An EEG recording should be obtained when the isotope is administered. The major disadvantages of SPECT are lower resolution than PET and its lack of clinical value for interictal CBF studies. SPECT is only a relatively quantitative technique, which is a particular disadvantage for research purposes. Values can be expressed in ratio to the cerebellum, for example, but comparison of serial scans where global changes may have occurred is difficult.

PET is more expensive than SPECT. However, it is far more versatile and is capable of measuring a wide variety of physiologic processes. Inhaled oxygen-15–labeled molecular oxygen (^{15}O), carbon dioxide ($C^{15}O_2$), and carbon-11–labeled carbon monoxide (^{11}CO), can be used to measure cerebral blood flow, cerebral metabolic rate for oxygen consumption, and cerebral blood volume. More frequently, oxygen-15–labeled water ($H_2{}^{15}O$) is injected to estimate CBF alone. Ligands are available for benzodiazepine receptors and several opiate and dopamine receptor subtypes. Since the tracers have short half-lives (^{15}O, 2 minutes; ^{11}C, 20 minutes; ^{18}F-deoxyglucose, 110 minutes), an on-site cyclotron should be part of the scanning facility. State-of-the-art PET scanners can produce sets of 30–50 images that can be reconstructed in coronal, sagittal, and transverse planes with true three-dimensional resolution. The spatial resolution of the best PET scanners, 3–4 mm, is still slightly inferior to that of MRI. If an arterial line is used to obtain a tracer input curve, absolute quantitative data can be derived from PET.

Although MRS and fMRI can be performed on standard 1.5-T clinical scanners, higher field strength improves the signal-to-noise ratio.[3, 4] Customized hardware, such as surface coils, and special software for data acquisition and analysis are necessary. PET and MRS/fMRI require specialized personnel, including cyclotron operators, radiochemists, imaging physicists, and computer programmers, which increases operational costs. For a PET center, the initial investment for the scanner, cyclotron, and laboratories would be approximately $4 million. Yearly running costs could range from $500,000 to several million dollars depending on the complexity of the procedures performed. Initial costs for MRS/fMRI are similar, but the center may be somewhat cheaper to run.

PARTIAL SEIZURES: CLINICAL AND PHYSIOLOGIC INSIGHTS

Interictal Cerebral Blood Flow and Energy Metabolism

Functional imaging detects focal dysfunction in patients with partial seizures. At the site of the focus, interictal fluorodeoxyglucose–PET (FDG-PET) detects hypometabolism and ictal SPECT detects increased CBF in 70–90% of patients who have well-localized temporal lobe foci on surface EEG recordings; a slightly lower percentage is found when the surface EEG recording is nonlocalizing[5–12] (Figure 5.1). False lateralization is unusual.[7, 12, 13] Inaccurate patient positioning, unrecognized ictal activity, or, in the case of PET, failure to perform quantitative analysis, are possible pitfalls.

For PET, scanner resolution has proved to be an important factor in sensitivity: Only 56% of patients with a localized seizure focus had hypometabolism on a single-slice scanner with 17-mm resolution, compared with 86% on a multislice scanner with 5-mm resolution.[5] FDG-PET shows focal hypometabolism in children with uncontrolled temporal lobe epilepsy nearly as frequently as it does in adults, reflecting the similar underlying pathologic states.[14] Children with new-onset partial seizures, however, may be less likely to have hypometabolism, suggesting that persistent seizures can lead to progressive neuronal dysfunction.[15]

FDG-PET can localize seizure onset to, but not within, the temporal lobe. In many studies, patients with temporal lobe foci had greater lateral than mesial hypometabolism, even when mesial temporal seizure onset was demonstrated electrophysiologically and when mesial temporal sclerosis was found at surgery.[16–19] More recent reports using higher resolution scanners suggest that mesial and lateral hypometabolism are equal, although variability is greater in the former region, probably because of partial volume effects in the smaller structure.[7, 20, 21] In a study using foramen ovale electrodes to define mesial temporal onset, patients had equal mesial and lateral temporal hypometabolism, although a small group of patients with apparently lateral neocortical foci had only lateral temporal hypometabolism.[22]

Patients with temporal lobe seizures can have associated hypometabolism in the frontal, thalamic, basal ganglia, and parietal areas.[20, 23, 24] Bilateral cerebellar hypometabolism has been reported, caused by a combination of the effects of phenytoin and the seizures themselves.[25] In some patients it may be possible to lateralize the hypometabolism but not to localize it to the temporal or frontal lobe. In patients with frontal lobe seizure onset, initial studies suggested that PET was less likely to detect focal hypometabolism.[20, 26, 27] However, recent investigations

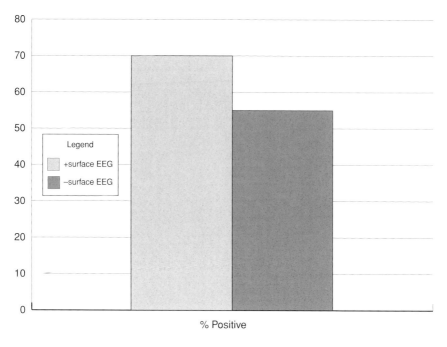

Figure 5.1   Percentage of patients with seizures of temporal lobe origin lateralized by interictal fluorodeoxyglucose–positron emission tomography. (EEG = electroencephalogram.)

using a rigorous quantitative technique showed that FDG-PET has good sensitivity and specificity for frontal lobe foci.[28]

Interictal CBF studies using PET or SPECT have been less sensitive to temporal lobe foci than ictal SPECT or FDG-PET,[9, 12, 29–35] and false lateralization may occur in 15–20% of patients. Because of the energy of the emitted positrons, ^{15}O-labeled PET scans, using inhaled gases or injected water, have lower intrinsic spatial resolution than FDG-PET. Also, several lines of evidence suggest that mesial temporal sclerosis may lead to a greater reduction in metabolism than in perfusion.[32] When a structural lesion is present, however, hypoperfusion is detected more frequently.[35, 36]

Lateral neocortical and mesial temporal FDG-PET hypometabolism are related to the degree of hippocampal volume loss measured by volumetric MRI.[37, 38] However, there may be only a weak relationship between FDG-PET hypometabolism and hippocampal neuron loss in resected specimens.[39] Hypometabolism could in part be caused by amygdalar, thalamic, or neocortical as well as hippocampal neuronal loss. Alterations in synaptic organization, which have been demonstrated in kindled animals and may be related to a prolonged postictal effect of intermittent seizures, might lead to metabolic dysfunction independent of pathologic changes.[40] Metabolism is depressed to a greater degree than CBF in epileptic foci, which could be due to a greater reduction in substrate utilization than supply or impaired glucose transport at the blood–brain barrier level.[32, 41]

Initial reports suggested that the rate-limiting transporter GlutR1 is upregulated in epileptic foci, but subsequent studies may not corroborate this finding.[42] After surgery, extratemporal and contralateral hypometabolism tend to normalize, also suggesting that synaptic mechanisms rather than cell loss could, in part, be responsible for hypometabolism.[43]

MRS can measure relative changes in the levels of high energy phosphates as well as N-acetyl-aspartate (NAA), which is a compound found in high levels in neurons and which serves as a marker for neuronal numbers. One advantage of MRS is its excellent time resolution; spatial resolution, however, is inferior to that of PET or SPECT.[3] In temporal lobe foci, decreased ratios of NAA to creatinine have been reported by several groups; such ratios probably reflect neuronal loss.[44–48] In addition to reduced NAA levels, some but not all investigators noted increased hydrogen ion concentration (pH), decreased phosphomonoester levels, and increased postictal lactate levels.[45, 46, 49, 50] The reduction in interictal high-energy phosphate stores also may reflect neuronal loss. Reduced ratios of NAA to creatinine have been detected in frontal lobe foci.[51] Animal seizure models investigated with MRS have shown many of the same features, such as reduced NAA levels in regions of neuronal loss.[52] The evidence suggests that MRS can be used to localize epileptic foci.

Functional Imaging and Neuropsychological Studies

FDG-PET hypometabolism predicts cognitive deficits in affected brain regions.[53] Depression, for example, is associated with bilateral inferior frontal or left temporal hypometabolism. Relative left lateral temporal hypometabolism predicts lower verbal intelligence quotient (IQ) and memory scores.[54, 55] In one study, patients with psychosis and epilepsy had relatively greater depression of oxygen metabolism than blood flow compared with normal controls and patients with epilepsy who did not have psychosis.[56] Antipsychotic treatment partially reversed these deficits.

Ictal Studies: Blood Flow

Early measurements of ictal blood flow used various techniques, including thermocouples, direct cortical stimulation, and inhaled or injected ^{133}Xe, and demonstrated global or hemispheric flow increases during partial seizures.[57–60] More recently, ictal SPECT studies have proven to be useful clinically, but PET has provided more detailed physiologic data. Quantitative measurements of ictal CBF increases vary considerably. Focal CBF, measured by ^{13}NH$_3$-PET, increased 25–40% during partial seizures of temporal onset. Flow increases measured with bolus H$_2$^{15}O ranged from 70% to 80% for complex partial seizure (CPS) and from 60% to 133% for generalized tonic-clonic seizure (GTCS).[61] A child with intrauterine asphyxia and hypoxic ischemic encephalopathy had focal seizures with clonic jerking of the right arm and deviation of the eyes to the right; peak CBF of 80 ml per minute per 100 g in the left temporoparietofrontal region compared with 57 ml per minute per 100 g on the right.[62] PET methods, although more accurate than previous techniques, still underestimate CBF at high flows; true ictal increases may be 150–200%.[63, 64]

Ictal SPECT CBF studies using various tracers have shown areas of increased CBF (often multilobar) that correlated well with EEG lateralization.[9–12, 33] Injections that are immediately postictal demonstrate mesial temporal hyperperfusion with relative neocortical hypoperfusion.[9] Based on studies of patients at different time intervals after seizure onset, mesial hyperperfusion appeared to decline in 5–10 minutes for most patients.[65] A similar time course was seen in a patient who had multiple $H_2^{15}O$ injections during PET after a CPS.[62]

Ictal SPECT may be particularly sensitive to extratemporal foci; it shows localized activation that correlates with EEG foci and in particular with structural lesions.[10, 12, 66–69]

Recently, echo planar fMRI has been used for ictal studies; increased signal was observed in several patients with simple partial seizures even when no clinical manifestations were present. Both patients had ictal SPECT scans that showed hyperperfusion in the same region.[70, 71] Although fMRI cannot provide quantitative data, its excellent time resolution may allow more detailed investigation of seizure spread.

Ictal Metabolism

Ictal FDG-PET studies in human partial or secondarily generalized seizures have shown variable patterns, with focal and generalized increases in CMRglc of 80–120%[17, 30, 64, 72] (Figure 5.2). The extent of metabolic alteration is related to clinical ictal manifestations and seizure spread. Because of the long FDG uptake period, "ictal" scans may reflect postictal depression and thus show only hypometabolism.[17, 72]

In animal studies, heterogeneous patterns of activation during seizures also occur and are related to clinical manifestations as well as to the species of animal and convulsant used. Some structures may show decreased metabolism, whereas others are still active.[73] Experimental epileptic foci in the motor cortex are associated with increased CMRglc in ipsilateral as well as contralateral homotopic regions; patterns of subcortical activation appear to follow glutaminergic pathways.[74–76] Progressive recruitment of subcortical structures may be crucial for mechanisms of seizure spread and secondary generalization. Hypometabolism lateral to the focus has also been reported in somatosensory cortex but not in motor, perirhinal, or occipital cortex, and may be the result of widespread inhibition via activation of thalamic nuclei.[77]

It is uncertain whether increased CMRglc, measured by human FDG-PET, is present during "interictal" spiking, but data from animal studies suggest that the metabolic distinction between interictal and ictal states may be less certain than previously thought. In rats, bicuculline-induced EEG spiking—without clinical manifestations—caused an increase in "interictal" glucose utilization and in c-fos immunoreactivity in superficial and middle cortical layers at spiking sites. Seizures themselves led to a more widespread increase in CMRglc.[78] In humans, repetitive paroxysmal lateralizing epileptiform discharges are also associated with increased CMRglc.[79] Focal hypermetabolism has been reported during continuous spike-wave discharges of sleep in children.[80]

With FDG scans, relative increases in CMRglc can persist 24–48 hours after partial seizures.[81] Although blood flow studies suggest a more rapid return to base-

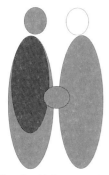

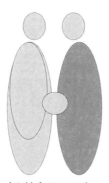

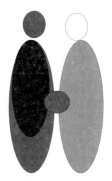

Interictal left temporal hypometabolism. More extensive than mesial pathology. May have frontal, thalamic hypometabolism.

Ictal left temporal hypermetabolism. Variable spread to extratemporal, contralateral cortex.

Postictal exaggerated left temporal hypome-tabolism persists.

Time: 0

Figure 5.2   Fluorodeoxyglucose-positron emission tomography in patients with complex partial seizures of temporal lobe origin.

line values, blood flow and metabolism may be uncoupled in epileptic foci. Metabolism and CBF increases during focal seizures may extend to the contralateral temporal lobe, frontal regions, and subcortical structures, such as the thalamus and basal ganglia, reflecting pathways of seizure spread.[82] Preliminary evidence suggests aerobic glycolysis may occur in the actively spiking tissue in humans as well as in epileptic tissue in animal models. However, possible seizure-induced alterations in the lumped constant, which describes the relationship between tracer (fluorodeoxyglucose) uptake and the use of physiologic substrate (glucose), makes it difficult to interpret quantitative ictal metabolic data.[83]

Unusual conditions, such as epilepsia partialis continua, show complex patterns of physiologic derangement on functional imaging studies. In contrast to patients with a shorter disease duration, patients who have had focal seizures for many years may not show increased glucose metabolism or lactate production, suggesting a compensated steady state.[84, 85]

POSITRON EMISSION TOMOGRAPHY AND SINGLE PHOTON EMISSION COMPUTED TOMOGRAPHY RECEPTOR STUDIES IN PATIENTS WITH PARTIAL SEIZURES

In patients with CPS, mu-opiate receptors are increased in number or binding potential ipsilateral to the focus.[86] The upregulation is more marked in lateral than mesial temporal cortex. This intriguing observation could be related to lateral temporal hypometabolism in patients with mesial temporal foci, as well as to the

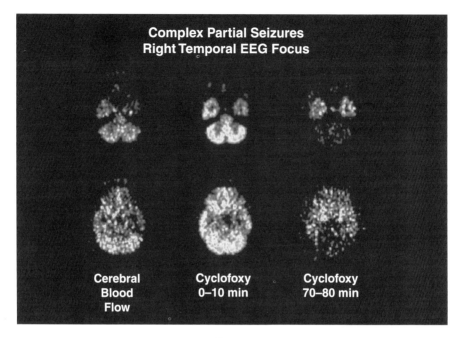

Figure 5.3   Cerebral blood flow and ^{18}F-Cyclofoxy scans in a patient with a right temporal focus. There is interictal hypoperfusion. The initial Cyclofoxy scan shows a distribution similar to that of blood flow. The late scan shows absent binding in the cerebellum and occipital cortex but increased binding ipsilateral to the epileptic focus in the right temporal lobe.

presurgical and postsurgical depression experienced by many patients with temporal lobe epilepsy.[87] Studies with a kappa-opiate ligand gave mixed results, in which increased activity, which could be mesial as well as lateral, was seen in some patients but not others (Figure 5-3).[88] Delta receptors do not appear to be altered.[89] Mixed ligands were used in the latter two studies, and it is possible that depressed kappa or delta binding could have been masked by increased mu binding. The difference in results with mu and kappa ligands may be the result of greater prominence of the latter in the hippocampus and amygdala.

Reduced benzodiazepine-binding or receptor number has been shown using iodine-123 labeled 3-(5-cyclopropyl-1,2,4-oxadiazo-3-yl)- 7-iodo-5, 6-dihydro-5-methyl-6-oxo-4H-imidazo[1,5-a][1,4]-benzodiazepine (NNC 13-8241), a SPECT ligand, and ^{11}C-RO-15-1788, a PET ligand.[90–92] The benzodiazepine receptor abnormalities are localized to mesial temporal cortex even when hypometabolism is widespread and reliably localizes epileptic foci.[92, 93] They appear to reflect neuronal loss rather than altered function in intact receptors.[91, 94] Reduced benzodiazepine receptor ligand binding may occur in frontal lobe epileptic foci as well.[95] Increased H1 histamine and MAO-B receptor binding and decreased muscarinic acetylcholine binding probably represent focal gliosis and neuronal loss.[96–98]

PRIMARY GENERALIZED EPILEPSY

In patients with primary generalized absence seizures, there are no regions of interictal hypometabolism.[99, 100] During seizures, marked increases in CMRglc are usually found, although one study in adults reported no consistent activation, possibly because of a paucity of spike-wave discharges during FDG uptake.[101] Although localized activation was not found on studies of ictal glucose metabolism, CBF, measured with $H_2^{15}O$, increased to a greater degree in the thalamus than in cortical regions during absence seizures.[102] Decreased ictal binding of a nonspecific ligand that measures mu, delta, and kappa receptors may be evidence for increased ictal release of endogenous opiates during absence seizures.[103] No ictal or interictal abnormalities in benzodiazepine receptors have been found.[104]

SECONDARY GENERALIZED EPILEPSY

In patients with Lennox-Gastaut syndrome (LGS), initial FDG-PET studies showed variable patterns of global or multifocal hypometabolism that were related to the presence or absence or structural lesions as well as the underlying cause.[105, 106] SPECT studies in patients with LGS have shown regions of multiple CBF deficits.[107]

Many patients with neuronal migration disorders also have secondary generalized seizures associated with multiple hypometabolic regions on PET scans; these regions usually correspond to abnormalities noted on MRI scans.[108] FDG-PET is useful in predicting surgical outcome in patients with hemimegalencephaly. Hypometabolism contralateral to the hemimegalencephalic side is a contraindication to surgery.[109] FDG-PET is more sensitive than structural imaging to the presence of an epileptic focus in children with severe developmental deficits and secondary generalized epilepsy but may not provide the precise structural information necessary for detailed surgical planning.[110] In children being considered for hemispherectomy, unilateral hypoperfusion detected with SPECT may predict a good outcome irrespective of EEG findings.[111]

Ictal scans in children with secondary generalized epilepsy have shown varying patterns of asymmetric or symmetric hypermetabolism of the striatum and thalamus; hypermetabolism of unilateral cortical, contralateral cerebellar, hippocampal, or insular regions; or cortical hypermetabolism alone.[112] Focal hypermetabolism has been reported in patients with active "interictal" spiking but without clinical signs of seizure activity.[113] In some children with LGS, ictal discharges may be associated with reduced metabolism.[105]

Distinguishing ictal from interictal states in many of these children may be difficult, particularly when infantile spasms are present. Symmetric increases in lenticular nuclei metabolism were found, as was focal cortical hypometabolism, in patients with infantile spasms, which perhaps explains why focal abnormalities could lead to generalized seizure patterns.[114] Focal hypoperfusion was found on SPECT scans in children with electrical status epilepticus of sleep, usually in a widespread frontotemporoparietal region, particularly in children who had had the syndrome for a year or more.[115]

Differences between metabolic patterns in children and adults with seemingly similar epilepsy syndromes may be due to developmental factors. In animal models, metabolic features of seizures may evolve with age. Kindling, which is a model for "development" or "progression" of epilepsy, may affect ictal and interictal metabolic features of seizures. Stage 1 and stage 2 electrically kindled seizures in rats showed increases in CMRglc only in the amygdala and its direct projection fields ipsilateral to the focus; stages 3–5 showed less limbic activation but recruitment of substantia nigra bilaterally, specific and nonspecific thalamic nuclei, globus pallidus, and neocortex.[116] Audiogenic seizure–sensitive rats showed lower increases in metabolism after kindling, particularly in brain stem regions. Interestingly, the amygdala was the only region where the increase was greater in kindled rats than naive rats.[117] In newborn rats, relative lack of activation of some structures during pentylenetetrazol-induced status epilepticus may help to explain resistance to neuronal damage.[118]

Imaging findings in children with infantile spasms are particularly exciting. Unilateral posterior quadrant hypometabolism was found on FDG-PET in patients with normal findings on MRI scans; most of these patients had had focal EEG findings at some point in the course of their disease,[119] and microscopic cortical dysplasia was found at surgery. At a mean of 28 months of follow-up (4–67 months), 18 of 23 children who had surgery based on imaging findings were seizure-free or significantly improved.[120] SPECT scans in children with a history of infantile spasms showed patterns of abnormal CBF reflecting clinical deficits: Children with visual impairment alone showed only parieto-occipital perfusion defects (unilateral or bilateral), whereas globally impaired patients had multiple deficits.[121]

IMAGING AND ANTIEPILEPTIC DRUGS

Imaging of drug distribution and effect may provide clues to drug mechanism of action as well as toxicity. PET imaging of ^{11}C-labeled phenytoin showed uniform distribution throughout the cerebral cortex without increased accumulation in epileptic foci.[122] Occipital gamma-aminobutyric acid (GABA) levels, measured by MRS, were higher in patients taking vigabatrin, a GABA-transaminase inhibitor, than in controls.[123]

Neuropsychological side effects of antiepileptic drugs may be related to their reduction of CMRglc and CBF. Phenobarbital reduces CMRglc by 37%, phenytoin (PHT) by 13%, carbamazepine (CBZ) by 12%, and valproic acid (VPA) by 12–20% depending on whether the drug was given to normal volunteers or patients taking CBZ.[124, 125] The effect of VPA on CBF was particularly marked in the thalamus, which is interesting in view of its importance in the treatment of primary generalized absence seizures.[126] On acute administration, diazepam reduced CMRglc by 20%.[127] These results suggest that the GABA-agonist effects of drugs such as barbiturates and benzodiazepines, which are often associated with cognitive impairment, reduce cerebral glucose metabolism. Drugs such as PHT and CBZ, without clinically important GABA-agonist effects, have less effect on metabolism.

SEIZURES AND NEURONAL INJURY

The concept of epilepsy as a "progressive" disease is controversial. Data from clinical and pathologic studies are disputed, but many investigators believe that persistent seizures can lead to neurologic dysfunction, neuropsychologic deficits, and neuronal loss. It is well established that metabolic dysfunction, possibly related to alterations in neurotransmitter binding, extends beyond the pathologic focus. Preliminary evidence from FDG studies also suggests that temporal hypometabolism may not be present at the onset of epilepsy and can develop over time if seizures continue.

Studies in animal seizure models have attempted to elucidate possible mechanisms of neuronal injury during seizures, including physiologic compromise, neuronal substrate depletion (with mismatch between supply and demand), and repetitive neuronal firing itself ("excitotoxic injury"). In animal models, focal epileptic activity may influence distant brain areas via far-reaching connections.[128] Sustained focal discharges in the motor cortex, for example, may lead to thalamic damage.[129] Regions showing neuronal damage are usually those exhibiting the greatest increases in activity during prolonged seizures.[130, 131] Although decreases in CBF may contribute at a late stage to damage in structures with persistent hypermetabolism, energy failure appears only to make a late and lesser contribution to the damage caused by oxidative mechanisms in cells with excessive neuronal activity.[132–134] Injury can occur during prolonged seizures even when physiologic variables, such as oxygen, glucose, and blood pressure, are maintained at control levels. MRS during prolonged seizures shows persistently high lactate levels, despite recovery of pH level and EEG features, suggesting possible damage resulting from enhanced neuronal activity itself.[135] Prolonged lactate levels can persist despite the return of high-energy phosphate stores to normal levels.[136, 137] Limited data on humans parallel these results. During prolonged neonatal seizures studied with MRS, high-energy phosphate stores may become depleted, while oxidative metabolism increases.[138] Although the ratio of phosphocreatine to inorganic phosphate (Pcr/Pi), which is a measure of cerebral energy reserve, returned to normal when seizures stopped, the children who developed neurologic sequelae had the lowest ratios. Increased ictal neuronal activity itself, rather than exhaustion of substrate supply, leads to neuronal damage. It is uncertain, however, whether prolonged seizures are necessary or whether the cumulative effect of repeated, short episodes—especially if frequent—could have a similar effect.

CLINICAL USE OF IMAGING TECHNIQUES

Surgical Localization

Functional imaging is a reliable means of localization for planning surgery. Hypometabolism on FDG-PET, hyperperfusion on ictal SPECT scans, but no hypoperfusion on PET or interictal SPECT studies, predict successful temporal lobectomy.[7, 11, 12, 139–141] It is likely that MRS may be equally as accurate, particularly as spatial resolution is improved, although fewer data have been collected.

Direct comparison of the various techniques is difficult, since few investigators possess optimal hardware, software, and experience for all of these techniques.

FDG-PET and ictal SPECT scans are often obtained to provide "confirmatory" evidence for ictal video-EEG localization of the epileptic focus. In this context, imaging may add little of clinical value. One might argue, however, presuming that the diagnosis of localization-related epilepsy has been confirmed, that it would be safer and more convenient for patients (as well as cheaper) to undergo one or two brain scans (particularly FDG-PET and MRI, which can be done on an outpatient basis), than to admit the patient for antiepileptic drug withdrawal and ictal monitoring.

Initial reports of the role of FDG-PET in detecting epileptic foci in children with infantile spasms are very encouraging. If future studies confirm the imaging findings and surgical success, children with infantile spasms should undergo an FDG-PET scan even if there is no reason to suspect focal seizure onset based on MRI, EEG, or clinical data.

Functional Mapping

One of the most exciting potential applications for functional imaging is its use for preoperative cognitive mapping and prediction of neuropsychological deficits.

PET and fMRI studies in normal volunteers have shown a good correlation between functional imaging results and traditional ideas of cortical language representation.[142] The ability to perform multiple activation tasks during the same PET session makes the short-lived $H_2^{15}O$ very useful for cognitive studies. fMRI and $H_2^{15}O$ PET activation have been compared with the intracarotid amobarbital (Amytal) test for language lateralization in adults and children, with good agreement for speech lateralization.[143–147] Surgical results in 11 patients suggested PET was at least as accurate as the intracarotid amobarbital test for prediction of postoperative deficits.[146] SPECT studies with ^{99m}Tc injection performed immediately after amobarbital administration for Wada testing showed CBF reductions of 10–50%; the contralateral hemisphere was not affected.[148, 149]

Patients with seizures may have functional reorganization. Studies using FDG-PET showed an accentuation of left temporal hypometabolism in patients with left temporal foci during a speech discrimination task.[150] In a patient with a large left-sided heterotopia, a verbal fluency task led to increased right frontotemporal glucose metabolism.[151] Patients with primary generalized epilepsy may have altered activation patterns detected by FDG-PET, particularly in the dorsolateral prefrontal cortex.[152]

In addition to replacing the intracarotid amobarbital test for speech and memory lateralization, PET and fMRI may be able to provide more precise localizing data and may replace direct cortical mapping. In studies using digital image coregistration, patients who were candidates for temporal lobectomy performed the same task during $H_2^{15}O$ PET and subdural stimulation mapping. Increased CBF was found only at electrode points where naming errors occurred during electrical stimulation; CBF did not increase at electrodes where stimulation did not produce errors.[153] fMRI language lateralization matches Wada results; future refinements of this technique may provide more precise language localizing data.[154]

SUMMARY

Neuroimaging will have an increasingly important role in the evaluation of epilepsy and may replace traditional techniques. Although technical difficulties, particularly visualization of inferior temporal regions, still must be overcome to take full advantage of these approaches, integration of structural, metabolic, and electrophysiologic data in common anatomic reference frames is already possible. Data integration may help to explain the complex interaction of physiologic factors leading to the clinical manifestations of seizure disorders. In vivo imaging of neurochemical and metabolic processes using PET and MRS should provide new insights into the pathophysiology of epilepsy.

REFERENCES

1. Ives JR, Warash S, Schmidt F, et al. Monitoring the patients' EEG during echo planar MRI. Electroencepahlogr Clin Neurophysiol 1993;87:417.
2. Holman BL, Hellman, RS, Goldsmith SJ, et al. Biodistribution, dosimetry, and clinical evaluation of technetium-99m-ethyl cysteinate dimer in normal subjects and in patients with chronic cerebral infarction. J Nucl Med 1989;30:1018.
3. Pritchard JW. Nuclear magnetic resonance spectroscopy of seizure states. Epilepsia 1994;35(Suppl 6):S14.
4. Cuenod C, Bookheimer S, Hertz-Pannier L, et al. Functional MRI during word generation using conventional equipment: a potential tool for language localization in a clinical environment. Neurology 1995;45:1841.
5. Engel J, Henry T, Risinger MW, et al. Presurgical evaluation for epilepsy: relative contributions of chronic depth electrode recordings versus FDG-PET and scalp-sphenoidal EEG. Neurology 1990;40:1670.
6. Debets RM, van Veelen CWM, Maquet P, et al. Quantitative analysis of 18FDG-PET in the presurgical evaluation of patients suffering from refractory partial epilepsy. Acta Neurochir (Wien) 1990;(Suppl 50):88.
7. Theodore WH, Sato S, Kufta C, et al. Temporal lobectomy for uncontrolled seizures: the role of positron emission tomography. Ann Neurol 1992;32:789.
8. Benbadis SR, So NK, Antar MA, et al. The value of PET scan (and MRI and Wada test) in patients with bitemporal epileptiform abnormalities. Arch Neurol 1995;52:1062.
9. Rowe CC, Berkovic SF, Sia STB, et al. Localization of epileptic foci with postictal single photon emission computed tomography. Ann Neurol 1989;26:660.
10. Stefan H, Bauer J, Feistel H, et al. Regional cerebral blood flow during focal seizures of temporal and frontocentral onset. Ann Neurol 1990;27:162.
11. Newton MR, Austin MC, Chan JG, et al. Ictal SPECT using technetium-99m-HMPAO: methods for rapid preparation and optimal deployment of tracer during spontaneous seizures. J Nucl Med 1993;34:666.
12. Ho SS, Berkovic SF, Berlangieri SU, et al. Comparison of ictal SPECT and interictal PET in the presurgical evaluation of temporal lobe epilepsy. Ann Neurol 1995;37:738.
13. Sperling MR, Alavi A, Reivich M, et al. False lateralization of temporal lobe epilepsy with FDG positron emission tomography. Epilepsia 1995;36:722.
14. Gaillard WD, White S, Malow B, et al. FDG–PET in children and adolescents with epilepsy: role in epilepsy surgery evaluation. Epilepsy Res 1995;20:77.
15. Gaillard WD, Conry J, Weinstein S, et al. FDG-PET in children with new-onset partial seizures [abstract]. Epilepsia 1995;36(Suppl 4):S163.
16. Engel J Jr, Kuhl DE, Phelps ME, Mazziotta JC. Interictal cerebral glucose metabolism in partial epilepsy and its relation to EEG changes. Ann Neurol 1982;12:510.
17. Theodore WH, Newmark ME, Sato S, et al. 18-F-Fluorodeoxyglucose positron emission tomography in refractory complex partial seizures. Ann Neurol 1983;14:429.
18. Sackellares JC, Siegel GJ, Abou-Khalil BW, et al. Differences between lateral and mesial temporal hypometabolism interictally in epilepsy of mesial temporal origin. Neurology 1990;40:1420.

19. Abou-Khalil BW, Siegel GJ, Sackellares JC, et al. Positron emission tomography studies of cerebral glucose metabolism in chronic partial epilepsy. Ann Neurol 1987;22:480.
20. Henry TR, Mazziotta JC, Engel JP, et al. Quantifying interictal metabolic anatomy in human temporal lobe epilepsy. J Cereb Blood Flow Metab 1990;10:748.
21. Theodore WH, Fishbein D, Dubinsky R. Patterns of cerebral glucose metabolism in patients with partial seizures. Neurology 1988;38:1201.
22. Hajek M, Antonini A, Leenders KL, Wieser WG. Mesiobasal versus lateral temporal lobe epilepsy: metabolic differences in the temporal lobe shown by interictal; 18F-FDG positron emission tomography. Neurology 1993;43:79.
23. Holmes MD, Kelly K, Theodore WH. Complex partial seizures: correlation of clinical and metabolic features. Arch Neurol 1988;45:1191.
24. Henry TR, Mazziotta JC, Engel JP. Interictal metabolic anatomy of mesial temporal lobe epilepsy. Arch Neurol 1993;50:582.
25. Theodore WH, Fishbein D, Deitz M, Baldwin P. Complex partial seizures: cerebellar metabolism. Epilepsia 1987;28:319.
26. Swartz BE, Halgren E, Delgado-Escueta AV, et al. Neuroimaging in patients with seizures of probable frontal origin. Epilepsia 1989;30:547.
27. Radtke RA, Hanson MW, Hoffman JM, et al. Positron emission tomography: comparison of clinical utility in temporal lobe and extratemporal epilepsy. J Epilepsy 1994;7:27.
28. Swartz BE, Khonsari A, Brown C, et al. Improved sensitivity of 18FDG-positron emission tomography scans in frontal and "frontal plus" epilepsy. Epilepsia 1995;36:388.
29. Bernardi S, Trimble MR, Frackowiak RS, et al. An interictal study of partial epilepsy using positron emission tomography and the oxygen-15 inhalation technique. J Neurol Neurosurg Psychiatry 1983;46:473.
30. Franck G, Sadzot B, Salmon E, et al. Regional Cerebral Blood Flow and Metabolic Rates in Human Focal Epilepsy and Status Epilepticus. In AV Delgado-Escueta, AA Ward, DM Woodbury, RJ Porter (eds), Basic Mechanisms of the Epilepsies: Molecular and Cellular Approaches. Advances in Neurology 44. New York: Raven, 1986;935.
31. Leiderman DB, Balish M, Sato S, et al. Comparison of PET measurements of cerebral blood flow and glucose metabolism for the localization of human epileptic foci. Epilepsy Res 1992;13:153.
32. Gaillard WD, Fazilat S, White S, et al. Interictal metabolism and blood flow are uncoupled in temporal lobe cortex of patients with partial epilepsy. Neurology 1995;45:1841.
33. Lee BI, Markand ON, Wellman HN, et al. HIPDM–SPECT in patients with medically intractable complex partial seizures: ictal study. Arch Neurol 1988;45:397.
34. Stefan H, Pawlik G, Bocher-Schwarz HG, et al. Functional and morphological abnormalities in temporal lobe epilepsy: a comparison of interictal and ictal EEG, CT, MRI, SPECT, and PET. J Neurol 1987;234:377.
35. Ryvlin P, Philippon B, Cinotti L, et al. Functional neuroimaging strategy in temporal lobe epilepsy: a comparative study of 18FDG-PET and 99mTc-HMPAO SPECT. Ann Neurol 1992;31:650.
36. Duncan R, Patterson J, Hadley DM, MacPherson P. CT, MR, and SPECT imaging in temporal lobe epilepsy. J Neurol Neurosurg Psychiatry 1990;53:11.
37. Gaillard WD, Bhatia S, Bookheimer SY, et al. FDG-PET and MRI volumetry in partial seizure focus localization. Neurology 1995;45:123.
38. Semah F, Baulac M, Hasboun D, et al. Is interictal temporal hypometabolism related to mesial temporal sclerosis? A positron emission tomography/magnetic resonance imaging confrontation. Epilepsia 1995;36:447.
39. Henry TR, Babb TL, Engel J, et al. Hippocampal neuron loss and hypometabolism in temporal lobe epilepsy. Ann Neurol 1994;36:925.
40. Sloviter RS. The functional organization of the hippocampal dentate gyrus and its relevance to the pathogenesis of temporal lobe epilepsy. Ann Neurol 1994;35:640.
41. Pardridge WM. Glucose transport and phosphorylation: which is rate limiting for brain glucose utilization? Ann Neurol 1994;35:511.
42. Cornford EM, Hyman S, Swartz BE. The human brain glut1 glucose transporter: ultrastructural localization to the blood-brain barrier endothelia. J Cereb Blood Flow Metab 1994;14:106.
43. Hajek M, Wieser HG, Khan N, et al. Preoperative and postoperative glucose consumption in mesiobasal and lateral temporal lobe epilepsy. Neurology 1994;44:2125.
44. Connelly A, Jackson GD, Duncan JS, et al. Magnetic resonance spectroscopy in temporal lobe epilepsy. Neurology 1994;44:1411.
45. Hugg J, Laxer K, Matson G, et al. Lateralization of human focal epilepsy by ^{31}P magnetic resonance spectroscopic imaging. Neurology 1992;42:2011.

46. Hugg JW, Laxer KD, Matson GB, et al. Neuron loss localizes human temporal lobe epilepsy by in vivo proton magnetic resonance spectroscopic imaging. Ann Neurol 1993;34:788.

47. Cendes F, Andermann F, Pruel MC, Arnold DL. Lateralization of temporal lobe epilepsy based on regional metabolic abnormalities in proton magnetic resonance spectroscopic images. Ann Neurol 1994;35:211.

48. Breiter SN, Arroyo S, Matthews VP, et al. Proton MR spectroscopy in patients with seizure disorders. AJNR Am J Neuroradiol 1994;15:373.

49. Garcia PA, Laxer KD, van der Grond J, et al. Phosphorous magnetic resonance spectroscopic imaging in patients with frontal lobe epilepsy. Ann Neurol 1994;35:217.

50. Kuzniecky R, Elgavish GA, Hetherington HP, et al. In vivo ^{31}P nuclear magnetic resonance spectroscopy of human temporal lobe epilepsy. Neurology 1992;42:1586.

51. Garcia PA, Laxer KD, van der Grond J, et al. Proton magnetic resonance spectroscopic imaging in patients with frontal lobe epilepsy. Ann Neurol 1995;279:281.

52. Young R, Petroff O. Neonatal seizures: magnetic resonance spectroscopic findings. Semin Perinatol 1990;14:238.

53. Rausch R, Henry TR, Ary C, et al. Asymmetric interictal glucose hypometabolism and cognitive performance in epileptic patients. Arch Neurol 1994;51:139.

54. Victoreff JI, Benson DF, Grafton ST, et al. Depression in complex partial seizures: electroencephalography and cerebral metabolic correlates. Arch Neurol 1994;51:155.

55. Bromfield EB, Altshuler L, Leiderman DB, et al. Cerebral metabolism and depression in patients with complex partial seizures. Arch Neurol 1992;49:617.

56. Gallhofer B, Trimble MR, Frackowiack R, et al. A study of cerebral blood flow and metabolism in epileptic psychosis using positron emission tomography and oxygen. J Neurol Neurosurg Psychiatry 1985;48:201.

57. Gibbs FA, Lennox WG, Gibbs EL. Cerebral blood flow preceding and accompanying epileptic seizures in man. Arch Neurol Psychiatry 1934;32:257.

58. Penfield W, von Kalman S, Cipriani A. Cerebral blood flow during induced epileptiform seizures in animals and man. J Neurophysiol 1939;2:257.

59. Hougaard K, Oikawa T, Sveinsdottir E, et al. Regional cerebral blood flow in focal cortical epilepsy. Arch Neurol 1976;33:527.

60. Sakai F, Meyer JS, Naritomi H, Hsu M. Regional cerebral blood flow and EEG in patients with epilepsy. Arch Neurol 1978;35:648.

61. Theodore WH, Balish MB, Leiderman DB, et al. The effect of seizures on cerebral blood flow measured with ^{15}O-H$_2$O and positron emission tomography. Epilepsia 1996;37:796.

62. Perlman JM, Herscovitch P, Kreusser KL, et al. Positron emission tomography in the newborn: effect of seizure on regional cerebral blood flow in an asphyxiated infant. Neurology 1985;35:244.

63. Brodersen P, Paulson OB, Bolwig TG, et al. Cerebral hyperemia in electrically induced epileptic seizures. Arch Neurol 1973;28:334.

64. Engel J Jr, Kuhl DE, Phelps ME. Patterns of human local cerebral glucose metabolism during epileptic seizures. Science 1982;218:64.

65. Rowe CC, Berkovic SF, Austin MC, et al. Patterns of postictal cerebral blood flow in temporal lobe epilepsy. Neurology 1991;41:1096.

66. Kuzniecky R, Mountz J, Wheatley G, Morawetz R. Ictal single photon emission computed tomography demonstrates localized epileptogenesis in cortical dysplasia. Ann Neurol 1993;34:627.

67. Marks DA, Katz A, Hoffer P, Spencer SS. Localization of extratemporal epileptic foci during ictal single photon emission computed tomography. Ann Neurol 1992;31:250.

68. Harvey AS, Hopkins IJ, Bowe JM, et al. Frontal lobe epilepsy: clinical seizure characteristics and localization with ictal ^{99m}Tc HMPAO SPECT. Neurology 1993;43:1966.

69. Ho SS, Berkovic SF, Newton MR, et al. Parietal lobe epilepsy: clinical features and seizure localization by ictal SPECT. Neurology 1995;44:2277.

70. Jackson GD, Connelly A, Cross JH, et al. Functional magnetic resonance imaging of focal seizures. Neurology 1994;44:850.

71. Detre JA, Sirven JI, Alsop DC, et al. Localization of subclinical ictal activity by functional magnetic resonance imaging: correlation with invasive monitoring. Ann Neurol 1995;38:618.

72. Engel J Jr, Kuhl DE, Phelps ME, et al. Local cerebral metabolism during partial seizures. Neurology 1983;33:400.

73. Ben-Ari Y, Tremblay E, Riche E, et al. Electrographical, clinical, and pathological alterations following systemic administration of kainic acid, bicuculline, or pentetrazole: metabolic mapping using the deoxyglucose method with special reference to the pathology of epilepsy. Neuroscience 1981;6:1361.

74. Collins RC, Kennedy C, Sokoloff L, Plum F. Metabolic anatomy of focal motor seizures. Arch Neurol 1976;33:536.
75. Caveness WF, Kato M, Malamut BL, et al. Propagation of focal motor seizures in the pubescent monkey. Ann Neurol 1980;7:213.
76. Meldrum BS, Brierley JB. Prolonged epileptic seizures in primates: ischemic cell change and its relation to ictal physiologic events. Arch Neurol 1973;28:10.
77. Bruehl C, Kloiber O, Hossman KA, et al. Regional hypometabolism in an acute model of focal epileptic activity in the rat. Eur J Neurosci 1995;7:192.
78. Handforth A, Finch DM, Peteres R, et al. Interictal spiking increases 2-deoxy ^{14}C glucose uptake and c-fos–like reactivity. Ann Neurol 1994;35:724.
79. Handforth A, Cheng JT, Mandelkern MA, Treiman DA. Markedly increased mesiotemporal lobe metabolism in a case with PLEDs: further evidence that PLEDs are a manifestation of partial status epilepticus. Epilepsia 1994;35:876.
80. Park YD, Hoffman JM, Radtke RA, DeLong GR. Focal cerebral metabolic abnormality in a patient with continuous spike-waves during slow-wave sleep. J Child Neurol 1994;9:139.
81. Leiderman DB, Albert P, Balish M, et al. The dynamics of metabolic change following seizures as measured by positron emission tomography with 18-fluoro-2-deoxyglucose. Arch Neurol 1994;51:932.
82. Theodore WH, Porter RJ, Albert P, et al. The secondary generalized tonic-clonic seizure: a videotape analysis. Neurology 1994;44:1403.
83. Cowan JMA, Rothwell JC, Wise RJS, Marsden CD. Electrophysiological and positron emission studies in a patient with cortical myoclonus, epilepsia partialis continua, and motor epilepsy. J Neurol Neurosurg Psychiatry 1986;49:796.
84. Matthews PM, Andermann F, Arnold DL. A proton magnetic resonance study of focal epilepsy in humans. Neurology 1990;40:985.
85. DeCarli C, Gaillard WD, Ko D, Theodore WH. Cerebral metabolism in epilepsia partialis continua [abstract]. Epilepsia 1994;35(Suppl 8):147.
86. Frost JJ, Mayberg HS, Fisher RS, et al. Mu–opiate receptors measured by positron emission tomography are increased in temporal lobe epilepsy. Ann Neurol 1988;23:231.
87. Altshuler LL, Devinsky O, Post RM, Theodore WH. Depression, anxiety, and temporal lobe epilepsy: laterality of focus and symptomatology. Arch Neurol 1990;47:284.
88. Theodore WH, Carson RE, Andreasen P, et al. PET imaging of opiate receptor binding in human epilepsy using (^{18}F) Cyclofoxy. Epilepsy Res 1992;13:129.
89. Mayberg HS, Sadzot B, Meltzer CC, et al. Quantification of mu and non-mu opiate receptors in temporal lobe epilepsy using positron emission tomography. Ann Neurol 1991;30:3.
90. Savic I, Roland P, Sedvall G, et al. In vivo demonstration of reduced benzodiazepine receptor binding in human epileptic foci. Lancet 1988;2:863.
91. Johnson EW, de Lanerolle NC, Kim JH, et al. Central and peripheral benzodiazepine receptors: opposite changes in human epileptogenic tissue. Neurology 1992;42:811.
92. Henry TR, Frey KA, Sackellares JC, et al. In vivo cerebral metabolism and central benzodiazepine-receptor binding in temporal lobe epilepsy. Neurology 1993;43:1998.
93. Savic I, Ingvar M, Stone-Elander S. Comparison of [^{11}C]flumazenil and [^{18}F]FDG as PET markers of epileptic foci. J Neurol Neurosurg Psychiatry 1993;56:615.
94. Burdette DE, Sakuri SY, Henry TR, et al. Temporal lobe central benzodiazepine binding in unilateral mesial temporal lobe epilepsy. Neurology 1995;45:934.
95. Savic I, Thorell JO, Roland P. ^{11}C-flumazenil positron emission tomography visualizes frontal epileptogenic regions. Epilepsia 1995;36:1225.
96. Iinuma K, Yokoyama H, Otsuki T, et al. Histamine H1 receptors in complex partial seizures [abstract]. Lancet 1993;341:238.
97. Kumlien E, Bergstrom M, Lilja A, et al. Positron emission tomography with ^{11}C-deuterium-deprenyl in temporal lobe epilepsy. Epilepsia 1995;36:712.
98. Muller-Gartner HW, Mayberg HS, Fisher RS, et al. Decreased hippocampal muscarinic cholinergic receptor binding measured by ^{123}I-iododexetimide and single-photon emission computed tomography in epilepsy. Ann Neurol 1993;34:235.
99. Theodore WH, Brooks R, Sato S, et al. Positron emission tomography in generalized seizures. Neurology 1985;35:684.
100. Engel J Jr, Lubens P, Kuhl DE, Phelps ME. Local cerebral metabolic rate for glucose during petit mal absences. Ann Neurol 1985;17:121.
101. Ochs RF, Gloor P, Tyler JL, et al. Effect of generalized spike-and-wave discharge on glucose metabolism measured by positron emission tomography. Ann Neurol 1987;21:458.

102. Prevett MC, Duncan JS, Jones T, et al. Demonstration of thalamic activation during typical absence seizures using $H_2^{15}O$ and PET. Neurology 1995;45:1396.

103. Prevett MC, Cunningham VJ, Brooks DJ, et al. Opiate receptors in idiopathic generalized epilepsy measured with ^{11}C-diprenorphine and positron emission tomography. Epilepsy Res 1994;19:71.

104. Prevett MC, Lammertsma AA, Brooks DJ, et al. Benzodiazepine GABA—a receptor binding during absence seizures. Epilepsia 1995;36:592.

105. Theodore WH, Rose D, Patronas N, et al. Cerebral glucose metabolism in the Lennox-Gastaut syndrome Ann Neurol 1987;21:14.

106. Chugani HT, Engel J Jr, Mazziotta JC, Phelps ME. The Lennox-Gastaut syndrome: metabolic subtypes determined by 2-deoxy-2-[^{18}F]-fluoro-D-glucose positron emission tomography. Ann Neurol 1987;21:4.

107. Heiskala H, Launes J, Pihko H, et al. Brain perfusion SPECT in children with frequent fits. Brain Dev 1993;15:214.

108. Lee N, Radtke RA, Gray L, et al. Neuronal migration disorders: positron emission tomography correlations. Ann Neurol 1994;35:290.

109. Rintahaka PJ, Chugani HT, Messa C, Phelps ME. Hemimegalencephaly: evaluation with positron emission tomography. Pediatr Neurol 1993;9:21.

110. Dietrich RB, el Saden S, Chugani HT, et al. Resective surgery for intractable epilepsy in children: radiologic evaluation. AJNR Am J Neuroradiol 1991;12:1149.

111. Carmant L, Otuama LA, Roach PJ, et al. Technetium-99m HMPAO brain SPECT and outcome of hemispherectomy for intractable seizures. Pediatr Neurol 1994;11:203.

112. Chugani HT, Rintahaka PJ, Shewmon DA. Ictal patterns of cerebral glucose utilization in children with epilepsy. Epilepsia 1994;35:813.

113. Chugani HT, Shewmon DA, Khanna S, Phelps ME. Interictal and postictal focal hypometabolism on positron emission tomography. Pediatr Neurol 1993;9:10.

114. Chugani HT, Shewmon DA, Sankar R, et al. Infantile spasms: 2. Lenticular nuclei and brain stem activation on positron emission tomography. Ann Neurol 1992;32:212.

115. Gaggero R, Caputo M, Fiorio P, et al. SPECT and epilepsy with continuous spike waves during slow wave sleep. Childs Nerv Syst 1995;11:154.

116. Engel J, Wolfson L, Brown L. Anatomical correlates of electrical and behavioral events related to amygdaloid kindling. Ann Neurol 1978;3:538.

117. Nehlig A, Vergnes M, Hirsch E, et al. Mapping of cerebral blood flow changes during audiogenic seizures in Wistar rats: effect of kindling. J Cereb Blood Flow Metab 1995;15:259.

118. Pereira de Vasconcelos A, Boyet S, Koziel V, Nehlig A. Effects of pentylenetetrazole-induced status epilepticus on local cerebral flow in the developing rat. J Cereb Blood Flow Metab 1995;15:270.

119. Chugani HT, Shields WD, Shewmon DA, et al. Infantile spasms: 1. PET identifies focal cortical dysgenesis in cryptogenic cases for surgical treatment. Ann Neurol 1990;27:406.

120. Chugani HT, Shewmon DA, Shields WD, et al. Surgery for intractable infantile spasms: imaging perspectives. Epilepsia 1993;34:764.

121. Jambaque I, Chiron C, Dulac O, et al. Visual inattention in West syndrome: a neuropsychological and neurofunctional imaging study. Epilepsia 1993;34:692.

122. Baron JC, Roeda D, Munari C, et al. Brain regional pharmacokinetics of ^{11}C-labeled diphenylhydantoin: positron emission tomography in humans. Neurology 1983;33:580.

123. Petroff OAC, Rothman DL, Behar KL, Mattson RH. Initial observations on effect of vigabatrin on in vivo ^1H spectroscopic measurements of γ-aminobutyric acid, glutamate, and glutamine in human brain. Epilepsia 1995;36:457.

124. Theodore WH. Antiepileptic drugs and cerebral glucose metabolism. Epilepsia 1988;29(Suppl 2):48.

125. Leiderman, DB, Balish MB, Bromfield EB, Theodore WH. The effect of valproic acid on human cerebral glucose metabolism. Epilepsia 1991;32:417.

126. Gaillard WD, White S, Fazilat S, et al. Effect of valproate on cerebral glucose metabolism and cerebral blood flow as determined by ^{18}FDG and ^{15}O water PET [abstract]. Epilepsia 1992;33(Suppl 3):55.

127. Foster NL, VanDerSpek AFL, Aldrich MS, et al. The effect of diazepam sedation on cerebral glucose metabolism in Alzheimer's disease as measured using positron emission tomography. J Cereb Blood Flow Metab 1987;7:415.

128. Sloviter RS, Damiano BP. Sustained electrical stimulation of the perforant path duplicates kainate-induced electrophysiological effects and hippocampal damage in rats. Neurosci Lett 1981;24:279.

129. Collins RC, Olney JW. Focal cortical seizures cause distant thalamic lesions. Science 1982;218:177.

130. Siesjo BK, Abdul-Rahman A. A metabolic basis for the selective vulnerability of neurons in status epilepticus. Acta Physiol Scand 1979;106:377.

131. Horton RW, Meldrum BS, Pedley TA, McWilliam JR. Regional cerebral blood flow in the rat during prolonged seizure activity. Brain Res 1980;192:399.

132. Ingvar M, Siesjo BK. Local blood flow and glucose consumption in the rat brain during sustained bicuculline-induced seizures. Acta Neurol Scand 1983;68:129.

133. Blennow G, Folbergrova J, Nilsson B, Siesjo BK. Effects of bicuculline-induced seizures on cerebral metabolism and circulation of rats rendered hypoglycemic by starvation. Ann Neurol 1979;5:139.

134. Blennow G, Brierly JB, Meldrum BS, Siesjo BK. Epileptic brain damage: the role of systemic factors that modify cerebral energy metabolism. Brain 1978;101:687.

135. Petroff OAC, Prichard JW, Ogino T, et al. Combined ^{1}H and ^{31}P nuclear magnetic resonance spectroscopic studies of bicuculline-induced seizures in vivo. Ann Neurol 1986;20:185.

136. Meric P, Barrere B, Peres M, et al. Effects of kainate-induced seizures on cerebral metabolism: a combined ^{1}H and ^{31}P NMR study in rat. Brain Res 1994;638:53.

137. Young RSK, Chen B, Petroff, OAC, et al. The effect of diazepam on neonatal seizures: in vivo ^{31}P and ^{1}H NMR study. Pediatr Res 1989;25:27.

138. Younkin DP, Delivoria-Papadopoulos M, Maris J, et al. Cerebral metabolic effects of neonatal seizures measured with in vivo ^{31}P NMR spectroscopy. Ann Neurol 1986;20:513.

139. Theodore WH, Gaillard WD, Sato S, et al. Measurement of cerebral blood flow and temporal lobectomy. Ann Neurol 1994;36:241.

140. Radke RA, Hanson MW, Hoffman JM, et al. Temporal lobe hypometabolism on PET: predictor of seizure control after temporal lobectomy. Neurology 1993;43:1088.

141. Manno EM, Sperling MR, Ding X, et al. Predictors of outcome after temporal lobectomy: positron emission tomography. Neurology 1994;44:2331.

142. Demonet IF, Wise R, Frackowiack RSJ. Language functions explored in normal subjects by positron emission tomography: a critical review. Hum Brain Map 1993;1:39.

143. Mueller R-A, Chugani HT, Muzik O, et al. Presurgical functional brain mapping in children by means of ^{15}O–water positron emission tomography. Neurology 1995;45(Suppl 4):A295.

144. Gaillard WD, Hertz-Pannier L, Mott S, et al. Identification of cortical language areas using 1.5T functional magnetic resonance imaging in children with epilepsy. Ann Neurol 1994;36:504.

145. Morris GL, Mueller WM, Yetkin FZ, et al. Functional magnetic resonance imaging in partial epilepsy. Epilepsia 1994;35:1194.

146. Pardo JV, Fox PT. Preoperative assessment of the cerebral hemispheric dominance for language with CBF PET. Hum Brain Map 1993;1:57.

147. Mendius JR, Sum JM, Desmond JE, et al. Localization of language using functional MRI in patients with complex partial seizures. Epilepsia 1994;35(Suppl 8):87.

148. Ryding E, Sjoholm H, Skeidsvoll H, Elmqvist D. Delayed decrease in hemispheric cerebral blood flow during Wada test demonstrated by ^{99m}Tc-HMPAO single photon emission computed tomography. Acta Neurol Scand 1989;80:248.

149. Biersack HJ, Linke D, Brossel F, et al. Technetium-99m HMPAO brain SPECT in epileptic patients before and during unilateral hemispheric anesthesia (Wada test): report of 3 cases. J Nucl Med 1987;28:1763.

150. Bromfield EB, Ludlow CL, Sedory S, et al. Cerebral activation during speech perception in temporal lobe epilepsy. Epilepsy Res 1991;9:49.

151. Calabrese P, Fink GR, Markowitsch HJ, et al. Left hemisphere neuronal heterotopia: a PET, MRI, EEG, and neuropsychological investigation. Neurology 1995;44:302.

152. Swartz B, Simpkins F, Halgren E, et al. Cortical activation by an abstract visual memory task in frontal and primary generalized epilepsy. Neurology 1995;45(Suppl 4):A264.

153. Bookheimer SY, Zeffiro TA, Theodore W, et al. Multimodality functional imaging for language localization in epilepsy. Neurology 1993;43(Suppl):A193.

154. Desmond JE, Sum JM, Wagner AD, et al. Functional MRI measurement of language lateralization in Wada-tested patients. Brain 1995;118:1411.

6
Electroencephalogram: Advances and Pitfalls

Colin D. Binnie

ABNORMAL ELECTROENCEPHALOGRAPHIC DISCHARGES

The electroencephalogram (EEG) is a spatiotemporal average of electrical activity from cortical neurons, reflecting the activity that occurs synchronously in substantial populations of neurons, orientated parallel to one another. Cerebral activity in epilepsy, during and between seizures, is characterized by neuronal discharges that may be excessive and abnormally synchronous. Because the electroencephalogram detects synchronous cortical activity, it should be particularly suitable for the study of epilepsy.

Synchronous postsynaptic potentials and possibly paroxysmal depolarization shifts recorded with microelectrodes in human and experimental epilepsies (see Chapter 2) appear in the EEG as abrupt potential changes, designated as "spikes" if they last less than 80 ms, or as "sharp waves" if they last 80–120 ms (Figure 6.1). Such transients are usually electronegative over the area of cortex where they arise, as one would expect if they were caused by depolarization in the dendrites of radially oriented pyramidal cells. They are usually followed by slower waves, which in the case of the "spike-wave [SW] epilepsies" (see Chapter 2) can be shown to be associated with neuronal hyperpolarization and reduced firing. These phenomena may be isolated or continuous and rhythmic; the more sustained discharges being more likely to be ictal—i.e., accompanied by clinical manifestations. The occurrence of overt clinical events depends on the duration and extent of the discharge and possibly on involvement of specific neuronal populations. The distinction between ictal and nonictal discharges is somewhat artificial, because with suitable methods of assessment, such as continuous psychological testing (e.g., see reference 1), changes can be detected during apparently subclinical discharges, even when these are brief and focal.

EEG phenomenology supports the conventional division of seizures into two basic types: generalized and partial. Generalized seizures are characterized by a sudden, widespread disturbance of the EEG, typically bilaterally synchronous and fairly symmetrical spikes or SW discharges. The discharges also cease abrup-

112

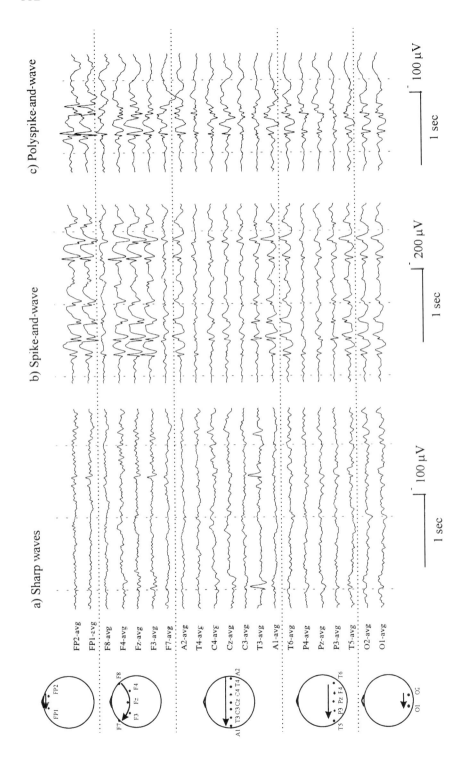

tly but may be followed by postictal slowing of the EEG and continued impairment of consciousness. Partial seizures begin with discharges confined to a restricted brain region. These may remain focal, spread locally, or become generalized. The clinical manifestations are determined by the site and extent of discharge. Again, postictal electrographic and clinical dysfunction may persist after the seizure.

Seizures

Generalized

The sudden appearance of bilaterally synchronous discharges invited the explanation of a pacemaker, involving deep midline structures, that triggered and synchronized the activity. Past and current theories concerning mechanisms of generalized SW activity are discussed in Chapter 2. The current "corticoreticular" theory assigns the cortex a primary role in generalized epileptogenesis but leaves important issues unresolved. A localized discharge may spread, eventually giving rise to "secondarily generalized" SW activity, and, similarly, a seizure may commence with symptoms of local dysfunction and then evolve to a generalized convulsion. Gloor[2] accommodated such "secondary bilateral synchrony" due to a focal cortical pacemaker within the corticoreticular model. This may seem to undermine the concept of primarily generalized epileptogenesis: Even in generalized seizures without evidence of a focus, local epileptogenesis in a discrete neuronal aggregate may appear more plausible than simultaneous activation of the entire cortex. It may then be argued that the distinction between generalized and focal seizures is simply a question of the rate and extent of spread of a physiologic disturbance of local onset. There is clinical evidence, admittedly somewhat arcane, to support this disquieting view:

1.   The phenomenology of the archetypical generalized seizure, the absence, may include features indicating that cerebral dysfunction is asymmetrical or focal. Versive movements can occur in otherwise clinically and electrographically typical absences, which respond selectively to valproate therapy. Detailed video-EEG studies[3] reveal an asymmetric craniocaudal march of motor phenomena in some absences.

◀ *Figure 6.1*   Epileptiform discharges. In this and following figures the electrode positions are shown on a stylized head outline. In this particular case, each channel records the potential between a single electrode and the average of the entire array ("average reference derivation"). In some subsequent figures, voltages between pairs of adjacent electrodes are shown ("bipolar derivation"). There are technical reasons for choosing one or the other of these recording methods, which serve to highlight different electroencephalographic features, but these considerations are outside the scope of the present text. To assist in the reading of electroencephalograms, the channels are arranged such that electrode sequences run from right to left and front to back, as indicated by the dotted lines and arrows. (a) Focal sharp waves arising at the left temporal electrode, designated T3. (b) Generalized spike-and-wave discharges in runs repeating at about 3.5 per second. (c) Generalized spike-and-wave with a more complex waveform, including multiple spikes, as seen in juvenile myoclonic epilepsy.

2.   Pattern sensitivity provides a means of studying localized cortical epileptogenesis: Hemifield pattern stimulation in some 50% of susceptible subjects with idiopathic generalized epilepsy demonstrates an asymmetrical threshold for initiating discharges.[4]

3.   Reflex seizures with specific cognitive triggers, such as reading, which presumably involve particular brain regions or neuronal systems, occur mainly in the context of idiopathic generalized epilepsy.

4.   Callosotomy in patients with generalized discharges and seizures may unmask focal discharges and partial seizures.

Present classifications of seizures and epilepsies provide practical aids to communication and prognosis but necessarily involve oversimplification. A neurobiologic description of the etiology and pathophysiology of the seizure disorder in a particular patient, taking account of the various contributions of local pathology and corticoreticular mechanisms, allows a more individualized approach.[5, 6]

Most generalized seizures are accompanied by generalized spikes or SW activity of sudden, symmetrical onset and termination. Other types of ictal change include an electrodecremental event, a sudden reduction in amplitude of ongoing activity typical of atonic seizures, and fast activity in tonic seizures.

Interictal EEG recordings in patients with generalized seizures commonly show essentially similar discharge types but these are briefer than those accompanied by overt clinical events.

Absences   Typical absences are characterized by generalized SW activity at about 3 per second that begins and terminates abruptly without postictal EEG disturbance (Figure 6.2). The paradox of a dramatic EEG change with minimal clinical symptoms may be explained by the inhibitory origin of the slow wave component, which is accompanied by hyperpolarization due to recurrent inhibition. The spike and the slow wave are topographically distinct, although there remains some disagreement about the details of their distribution.[7] The discharges usually show bifrontal maxima, and a single midline maximum is reported to be associated with an atypical clinical picture and poor response to medication.[8]

Clinical seizures are not necessarily observed during every SW discharge but, it is claimed, can always be detected given sufficiently close observation; thus, "in absence seizures inter-ictal discharges probably do not occur."[9] The interictal EEG is usually normal, but ongoing rhythms may be slightly slowed. Some patients exhibit striking, rhythmic posterior slow activity at about 3 per second, which builds up to a generalized SW discharge on overbreathing. This feature is reported to be a favorable prognostic sign and is more common in the childhood form of absence epilepsy. Overbreathing elicits SW activity in patients with absence seizures so consistently that the lack of this finding in an untreated patient who hyperventilates efficiently must cast doubt on the diagnosis.

The main differential diagnosis of absences is brief complex partial seizures, and if focal ictal discharges rapidly generalize, their origin may not be apparent. Minor asymmetries of SW activity are common in absences, and it is uncertain what degree of asymmetry should raise the suspicion of a focal onset. It has been argued that absences and brief complex partial seizures with SW activity are

115

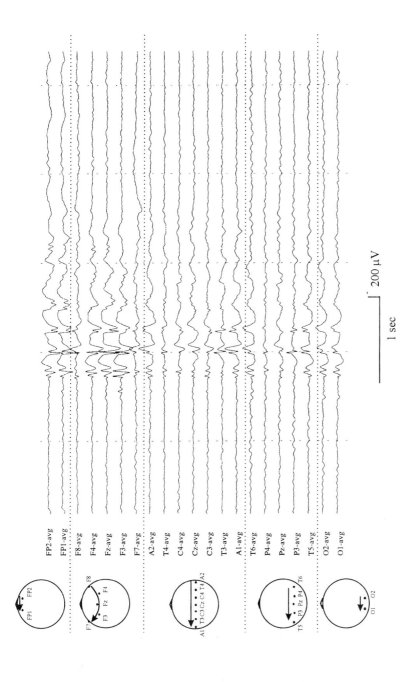

Figure 6.2 Absence seizure in a 14-year-old boy. The patient was observed to stare and flutter his eyelids during the generalized spike-and-wave discharge. This episode occurred spontaneously, but more frequent and longer discharges occurred on overbreathing.

argued that absences and brief complex partial seizures with SW activity are physiologically similar.[6]

"Atypical absences" are accompanied by more irregular, slower discharges in which the spikes are often multiple. Specifically, Lennox-Gastaut syndrome is associated with SW activity at not more than 2 per second.

Myoclonic Seizures   In juvenile myoclonic epilepsy, ictal and interictal discharges consist of multiple spikes and slow waves. Fifty percent of patients are photosensitive (see the section on photosensitivity). Similar findings may be present in other epilepsies associated with myoclonus, although many of these syndromes are associated with diffuse cerebral disease, the effects of which may dominate the EEG picture.

Tonic Seizures   Tonic seizures are accompanied by fast low-voltage activity, starting in the beta or mid-alpha range, slowing and increasing in amplitude during the attack. These too occur often in the context of the various syndromes of symptomatic generalized epilepsy with other associated EEG abnormalities.

Tonic-Clonic Seizures   EEGs recorded during tonic-clonic seizures are generally obscured by large amounts of muscle artifact. However, characteristically the tonic phase is accompanied by generalized spikes and the clonic phase by SW activity that is synchronous with the jerks and slows and becomes irregular as they do. In the postictal state, a generalized reduction in amplitude of EEG activity may be seen, followed by the gradual appearance of slow activity, which may at first be episodic but becomes continuous and faster as the normal interictal pattern is restored. Interictal recordings from patients who suffer only tonic-clonic seizures may appear normal or may be characterized by occasional bursts of generalized, multiple spikes and slow waves, particularly during sleep.

Atonic Seizures   Atonic seizures occur mainly in the context of syndromes of symptomatic, generalized epilepsy, which are characterized by a variety of interictal EEG abnormalities. In pure atonic seizures, without other clinical features, the ictal EEG often shows only an electrodecremental event.

Partial

In recordings from extracellular electrodes at the site of origin of a partial seizure, the onset is typically characterized by the appearance of a sharply localized, fast activity at frequencies of 50 hertz (Hz) or more (see Figure 6.9). Individual neurons may or may not show any change in activity; some fire rapidly for up to 2 seconds but do not continue throughout the discharge. Only a small proportion, some 7–14%, of neurons contribute at any time to the population discharge.[10] Typically, after a few seconds or sometimes as long as a minute, the discharge spreads to involve a larger volume of tissue and changes in character, producing SW activity or, more commonly, rhythmic sharp wave forms that gradually increase in amplitude and diminish in frequency—"rhythmic ictal transformation."[11]

This activity typically becomes slower and irregular and may give way to SW discharges, which in their turn slow to about 1 per second, become irregular, and abruptly cease. Sometimes SW activity is seen from the start of the seizure; however, this is less sharply localized than the fast activity described above, suggesting that onset is "regional" or possibly that there is no electrode positioned at the causal focus.

After the seizure, there may be a postictal disturbance characterized by a reduction in amplitude of all activity and the appearance of slow waves, which gradually increase in frequency until the normal rhythms are restored. This sequence of events may be confined to a small part of the brain, but the discharges may spread to a localized, usually homotopic, area of the opposite hemisphere or, indeed, become generalized.

Partial seizures are often preceded by an electrodecremental event, from less than 1 second to 10 seconds in duration, which may be localized or generalized. When focal, it does not necessarily correspond to the site of seizure onset.[12] The occurrence of an event that may be generalized or falsely localizing at the start of a partial seizure is perplexing. One explanation is that it reflects an afferent event in the reticular activating system that triggers the seizure; another is that the cortical desynchronization is caused by activity propagated from an earlier focal ictal discharge that is undetectable.

Frequent interictal discharges are usually seen in intracranial recordings from patients with partial seizures. They usually consist of spikes, sharp waves, or isolated SW complexes, but may include runs of fast activity similar to those seen at seizure onset. Rhythmic ictal transformation is not a usual finding. However, a prolonged evolving sequence of epileptiform activities may be interpreted as an electrographic seizure, again calling into question the distinction between ictal and interictal events, particularly if subtle cognitive changes occur.

In experimental epilepsy, focal discharges may spread to the homotopic area of the contralateral hemisphere. Eventually, the "mirror focus" becomes autonomous and fires independently. Ascending the evolutionary scale, mirror foci develop more slowly, and it is uncertain whether they occur in humans. Many patients with temporal lobe epilepsy have bilateral foci, but such pathologic entities as mesial temporal sclerosis may also be bilateral. Falconer and Kennedy[13] and Morrel and Whisler[14] found contralateral foci that disappeared after removal of the epileptogenic lesion, and Hughes[15] reported that 40% of foci become bilateral. Others argue that the occurrence of mirror foci in humans has not been established.[16, 17]

The scalp EEG in patients with partial seizures fails to demonstrate the rich phenomenology seen in intracranial recordings. The interictal discharges usually consist of isolated spikes or sharp waves, usually with a succeeding slow component, and are less frequent than at intracranial electrodes. Their topography corresponds approximately to that of the intracranial focus, but if this is deeply located they are more likely to arise from physiologic propagation to overlying neocortex than by volume conduction of the electrical field arising at the focus.[18] Their reliability for purposes of localization is therefore limited and unlikely to be enhanced by complex computational techniques intended to display their topography (see Topographic Displays: Uses and Abuses below).

Ictal EEG recordings rarely show the initial fast events of partial seizures. Indeed, ictal changes may not be detected on the scalp, particularly in brief, simple partial seizures, presumably involving small areas of the brain. Often the seizure pattern does not consist of spikes but rather of rhythmic activity in the theta or alpha range; this activity may be localized, lateralized, or more widespread. When a secondarily generalized tonic-clonic seizure occurs, widespread spikes followed by SW activity are seen.

Seizures Arising in the Temporal Lobes   Temporal lobe epilepsy is typically associated with interictal temporal spikes, sharp waves, or SW complexes, bilateral in some 20–50% of patients.[19–21] A 4 to 1 preponderance on one side may be regarded as evidence of lateralization.[22] Where the seizures arise in mesial temporal structures, the interictal spikes are usually of greatest amplitude on the scalp at a site about 1 cm behind the external canthus (Figure 6.3). They are generally about 30% larger at a sphenoidal electrode, but because they are adequately recorded at an anterior temporal scalp placement, the value of sphenoidal recording is questionable.[23]

In patients with mesial temporal epilepsy, the discharges typically exhibit a bipolar field, with a sharply localized negative spike in the anterior temporal region and a more diffuse low-amplitude positivity in the contralateral central area. This characteristic topography is not seen in patients with seizures arising in the lateral temporal neocortex[24] (Figure 6.4).

Nonepileptiform abnormalities are often found—reduction of fast activity ipsilateral to the focus and possibly localized theta or delta activity, occurring at the site of the spike focus or more widely. These abnormalities may reflect underlying pathologic states, but often the slowing appears to be more closely related to seizure activity, increasing in or confined to postictal recordings.

The initial ictal EEG change may consist of clear temporal spikes but often only theta or slower activity is seen, which may be bitemporal or generalized. Ictal scalp EEGs are lateralizing in only 50% of patients and even then indicate the side of origin of temporal lobe seizures with only 80% reliability.[25, 26] Some seizures of temporal lobe origin are preceded by a generalized electrodecremental event, and sometimes this is the only EEG change. Others, notably simple partial seizures with viscerosensory or psychic symptoms, may produce no visible alteration of the scalp EEG (see Intracranial Recording). In view of the postulated bilateral limbic involvement in complex partial seizures, it might be expected that these would always produce bilateral changes in the EEG. Although this is generally the case, complex partial seizures can occur with unilateral discharges and with no apparent change in the scalp EEG (Figure 6.5).

Seizures of Frontal Origin   In patients with partial seizures of frontal origin, localized interictal or ictal foci in the scalp EEG are uncommon.[27] A frontal interictal focus may be found in as few as 9% of patients, and some 59% exhibit regional discharges over the frontocentral or frontotemporal areas.[28] The poor EEG localization may reflect the inaccessibility of medial or orbital foci, rapid spread of discharges within and beyond the frontal lobes, and sometimes an extensive epileptogenic zone.[29, 30]

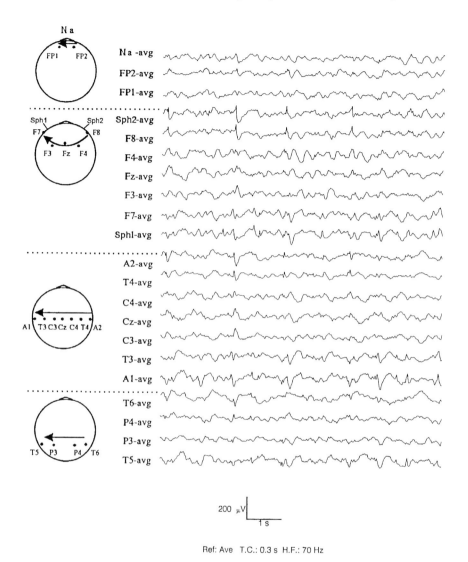

Figure 6.3   Sphenoidal recording of anterior temporal spikes in a 14-year-old boy with right mesial temporal sclerosis. Note that the spikes are largest at the right sphenoidal electrode (Sph2) but are well seen at F8, located on the scalp in the anterior temporal region. Contrast Figure 6.4, a sylvian temporal focus caused by epilepsy of lateral neocortical origin, and Figure 6.5, an intracranial recording from this patient obtained 4 years later.

In patients with seizures of mesial or orbital frontal origin, ictal and interictal records may show secondarily generalized slow waves or SW discharges.[31-33] An irregular waveform and possible asymmetry distinguish these from the typical 3-per-second SW activity of idiopathic generalized epilepsy. Ictal discharges consisting only of frontal slow waves are easily overlooked or mistaken for artifact.

120

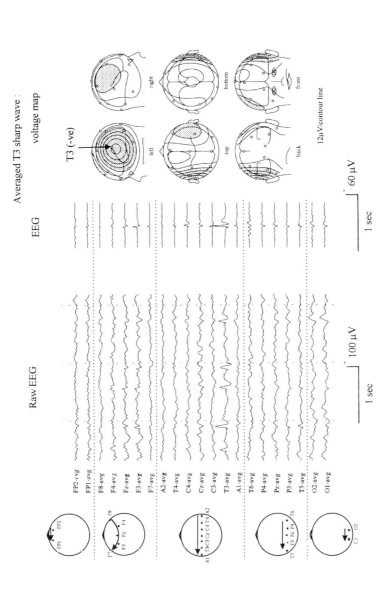

Figure 6.4 Interictal temporal sharp waves in the sylvian temporal region from an 11-year-old boy with seizures of lateral temporal neocortical origin (caused by cortical dysgenesis). A brain map plotted from an average of 50 discharges shows the type II pattern of Ebersole.[24] The shaded areas are negative with respect to the average; thus the discharge is widespread over the left centrotemporal region and there is no contralateral positivity.

Because seizures of mesiobasal frontal origin are often bizarre and readily supposed to be psychogenic, the EEG findings if not carefully interpreted may serve only to compound the diagnostic confusion (see Intracranial Recording). Seizures arising from the cingulate gyrus may resemble absences clinically and electrographically. Those from the supplementary motor area typically produce characteristic ictal posturing and are often associated with ictal and interictal sharp waves at the vertex.

Simple partial seizures with motor symptoms may be associated with central foci of ictal and interictal discharges (most strikingly in the syndrome of benign epilepsy of childhood with rolandic spikes). Interictal temporal spikes or generalized spikes and slow waves may be present. However, a lack of interictal abnormalities is more usual in symptomatic perirolandic epilepsies, and even ictal records may show no epileptiform activity if the motor phenomena are brief and of restricted extent.

Seizures of Parieto-Occipital Origin   Occipital foci are uncommon and do not necessarily reflect the site of origin of seizures. Symptomatic epilepsies arising from the occipital lobes are yet rarer. Ictal and interictal discharges may be appropriately localized,[34] temporal, or generalized.[35] Posterior temporal and occipital epileptogenic lesions commonly produce abnormalities of ongoing EEG activity, particularly alpha asymmetry. In the nonlesional "benign epilepsy of childhood with occipital paroxysms," discharges are usually biooccipital but may be focal in one or other posterotemporo-occipital region.

Localizing EEG signs of parietal epileptogenic lesions are rare, beyond a possible local reduction in amplitude of ongoing activity. Interictal discharges tend to be located in the middle to posterior temporal region. Ictal spikes are often generalized but may be lateralized to the side of seizure origin.[36]

Partial Seizures Evolving to Secondarily Generalized   During partial seizures that become secondarily generalized, a corresponding EEG evolution is seen with the focal or bilateral discharges, as described above, giving way to generalized spikes and later to SW activity. Late ictal activity and postictal disturbances may be more apparent contralateral to the site of onset and are therefore of little localizing value.

STANDARD ELECTROENCEPHALOGRAPHIC RECORDINGS

Epileptiform Abnormalities and Common Causes of Confusion

Artifacts

A basic principle of reading EEGs is to identify first those features that are artifactual, and then those that are normal, before considering findings that may be pathologic.

Spiky artifacts do not often present an interpretative problem. Difficulties may arise from electromyographic (EMG) potentials, or sudden, brief electrode artifacts

122

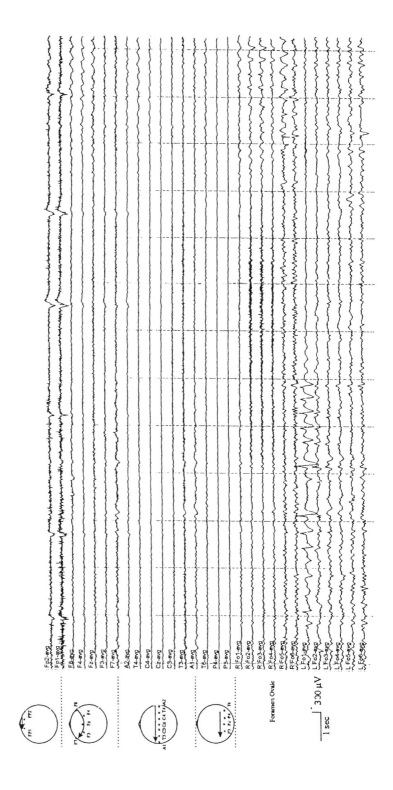

accompanying apparent myoclonic jerks, but usually these are distinguishable, being of shorter duration than spikes of cerebral origin seen in the scalp EEG. Rhythmic movements, as in tonic-clonic seizures, often produce generalized synchronous artifacts with spike and slow components mimicking SW activity. The identifying feature is usually the topography, which is often different on the right and left, and characterized by multiple potential maxima, producing double phase reversals on bipolar recording, which is a distribution very rarely shown by genuine EEG phenomena and clearly different from the bifrontal maxima of true generalized SW discharges. Greater problems are presented by ictal EEG changes in seizures of medial frontal origin, which are often inconspicuous and may consist of frontal slow activity. This can readily be mistaken for oculographic artifact unless careful attention is directed to the topography, with a high frontal maximum and often marked asymmetry, which exclude an ocular origin.

Normal Spiky Waveforms

Various sharp or frankly spiky waveforms, which commonly occur in normal subjects, are of little or no significance in relation to the diagnosis of epilepsy (see references 37 and 38 for reviews).

Six- and 14-Per-Second Positive Spikes Epileptiform discharges are usually of negative polarity. A distinctive normal waveform consists of positive spikes in runs at 6 or 14 per second. Positive spikes occur in some 20–30% of adolescents and young adults during drowsiness and light sleep. A statistical association has been claimed with various conditions, ranging from behavior disorders to allergies, but is in any event too weak for positive spikes to be of practical diagnostic significance.

◀ *Figure 6.5* Onset of a complex partial seizure of right temporal lobe origin recorded with foramen ovale electrodes (multipolar wire electrodes inserted through the foramen ovale to lie along the medial aspect of the temporal lobe). The patient, an 18-year-old youth, became seizure-free after right temporal resection. The pathologic entity was mesial temporal sclerosis. The interictal record showed spikes and slow waves at the *left* foramen ovale contacts (L Fo 1–2), seen here for 3 seconds before the seizure; these cease shortly after seizure onset. At clinical and electrographic onset of the attack, the patient immediately becomes inaccessible and high-frequency discharges are recorded at the right foramen ovale contacts (R Fo 2–4), but no change can be seen in the scalp electroencephalogram (EEG) recording. Later, diffuse frontotemporal theta activity at 4.5 per second appears, which is more prominent on the right. This example demonstrates that (1) gross focal ictal discharges recorded with intracranial electrodes may not be visible in the scalp EEG recording, (2) impairment of consciousness in complex partial seizures can occur without apparent bilateral spread of the discharges, (3) ictal changes in the scalp EEG recording during temporal lobe seizure often consist only of poorly localized slow activity without overtly spiky discharges, and (4) interictal discharges may have a very different morphology and topography from ictal phenomena.

Benign Epileptiform Transients of Sleep   Benign epileptiform transients of sleep (BETS), or "short sharp spikes," are spiky transients of brief duration, usually polyphasic and followed by a slow wave, often in the theta range, seen in the temporal regions during sleep. They occur in many normal subjects but show a very weak association with epilepsy. Depth recording in patients with partial epilepsies shows that BETS arise at sites different from the seizures and therefore probably play no part in the epileptic mechanism in these patients.[39] They do not materially support a diagnosis of epilepsy.

Rhythmic Mid-Temporal Discharge   Rhythmic mid-temporal discharge (RMTD) is a rare, unilateral or bilateral temporal rhythmic activity at about 6 per second found in repeated records of some normal subjects and is unaffected by eye opening or anti-epileptic medication. It may be precipitated by hyperventilation or blocked by attention. The discharge starts and ends abruptly, often lasting for tens of seconds. This phenomenon was formerly called "psychomotor variant" because of a supposed association with temporal lobe epilepsy but is of no known clinical significance.

Subclinical Rhythmic Epileptiform Discharge of Adults   Subclinical rhythmic epileptiform discharge of adults (SREDA) resembles RMTD but often develops from a run of sharp waves, increasing in frequency from 0.5 to 6 per second and is located further posteriorly in the temporoparieto-occipital region. It occurs in normal adults older than 50 and is not associated with epilepsy.

Midline Spikes   Midline spikes occurring at the vertex in the alert state must be distinguished from the vertex sharp transients of drowsiness. They are rare and weakly associated with epilepsy and occur mainly in normal subjects. Where epilepsy is present, seizures may arise from the supplementary motor area, but usually the phenomenon is of no clinical significance.

Frontal Slow Activity on Overbreathing   Young normal subjects up to age 30 commonly exhibit bifrontal slow activity after 3 minutes of vigorous hyperventilation. This normal finding is all too commonly reported by inexperienced interpreters as abnormal and supportive of epilepsy.

"Epileptic K-Complexes"   Arousal from deep sleep elicits sharp EEG transients near the vertex, notably so-called K-complexes, typically comprising a sharp wave, a slow wave, and a burst about 14 per second. Sometimes the initial sharp component is a spike or run of spikes. It is claimed that spiky K-complexes are associated with idiopathic generalized epilepsy;[40] certainly, such waveforms may be difficult to distinguish from SW discharges. There is, however, no convincing evidence that spiky K-complexes are associated with epilepsy.

Photosensitivity   Intermittent photic stimulation (IPS) elicits a range of EEG responses, from rhythmic posterior activity at the flash rate, through various normal variants, to generalized self-sustaining SW activity (see below). This last is strongly associated with epilepsy—more localized discharges, or spikes synchronous with the flashes, have little or no relationship to epilepsy.

These various spiky phenomena are normal or of little significance in relation to the diagnosis of epilepsy. The experienced observer should rarely have difficulty in identifying them by their characteristic morphology, topography, and circumstances of occurrence and in distinguishing them from those spiky phenomena that commonly occur in epilepsy and are conventionally described as "epileptiform."

Findings in Specific Epilepsies and Syndromes

Main Categories of Epilepsy

International seizure classification provides a means of communication about epileptic attacks, whereas that of epilepsies and syndromes provides a framework for describing the overall disease process. In addition to epileptiform activities related to seizure generation, the EEG may detect other abnormalities caused by more general interictal cerebral dysfunction or by underlying pathology and thus contribute to identification of the type of epilepsy or specific syndrome.

Idiopathic generalized epilepsy occurs in a structurally normal brain and does not generally give rise to any marked abnormalities of ongoing activity. The interictal and ictal EEG findings are those characteristic of the associated generalized seizure types, absences, tonic-clonic, and myoclonic seizures—i.e., generalized SW activity of various types.

Symptomatic and cryptogenic generalized epilepsies by definition reflect diffuse cerebral pathology or multiple lesions, which is likely to be reflected in abnormalities of the ongoing EEG, notably by slowing. Interictal discharges commonly occur at multiple foci together with generalized discharges, some of which may be secondarily generalized after a focal onset.

The idiopathic type of partial epilepsy is represented by the benign epilepsies of childhood, the most common form of which is characterized by high-amplitude, sharply focal spikes or SW complexes in the central or centrotemporal region of one or both hemispheres ("rolandic spikes," Figure 6.6). Typically there is a dipole field, the negative central spike being accompanied by a less conspicuous midfrontal positive component. Often the spikes occur many times per minute but their frequency increases during sleep and, early in the course of the disease, sleep recording may be necessary to demonstrate them. Indeed, activation by sleep may be regarded as a criterion for their identification. Another consideration in undertaking sleep recording is that some children with the clinical and electrographic features of benign epilepsy of childhood with rolandic spikes (BECRS) display almost continuous, generalized SW activity during slow-wave sleep. This implies the syndrome of electrical status epilepticus in slow sleep, a condition much less benign than BECRS. Interestingly, despite marked activation, rolandic spikes do not produce the disruption of sleep patterns usually seen in patients with frequent nocturnal epileptiform discharges.[41] The child usually has predominantly nocturnal seizures with focal features typically involving face and mouth at onset. The condition is easily controlled by antiepileptic drugs and resolves by age 16. Less com-

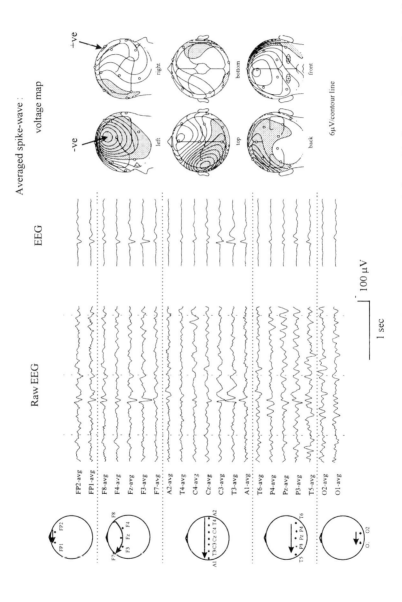

Figure 6.6 Rolandic spikes in benign childhood epilepsy. As in Figure 6.4, the raw electroencephalographic data are shown together with an average of the left centrotemporal spike and a corresponding voltage map. Note the typical dipolar distribution with a positive area in the frontal region corresponding to the negative centrotemporal spike.

mon variants are seen with temporal or frontal spikes or bioccipital SW or spike discharges with appropriate clinical concomitants. The occipital form is often associated with headache, nausea, and visual symptoms resembling those of migraine and probably accounts for most cases of so-called "basilar migraine" in children. The occipital discharges are usually suppressed by visual fixation and therefore activated by eye closure, darkness, or exposure to an unpatterned but illuminated visual field.

Finally, symptomatic partial epilepsy is caused by a localized structural abnormality of the brain producing partial seizures, the interictal and ictal EEG features of which have been described at some length above. In addition to abnormal discharges, there may be abnormalities of ongoing activity reflecting the underlying pathology, ipsilateral reduction of spontaneous and drug-induced beta activity, or focal slowing in the theta or delta ranges.

Epileptic Syndromes

Many epileptic syndromes produce characteristic EEG findings that often relate to the total cerebral disorder, of which epilepsy is not necessarily the most important feature. Most are age dependent, appearing in infancy or childhood, and are considered in Chapters 8 and 9. Only two will be selected for particular attention here, because they are among the most common and present characteristic EEG pictures.

In West syndrome the characteristic EEG picture of hypsarrhythmia is often seen. It is high voltage and chaotic, containing slow activity and focal and general epileptiform discharges of inconstant morphology and distribution, changing in sleep to bursts of high-amplitude activity alternating with low-amplitude activity. This pattern is not invariably found nor is it entirely specific to West syndrome (Figure 6.7). It generally improves during successful treatment. Seizures may be accompanied by generalized multiple spikes and slow waves or by a momentary reduction in amplitude of the EEG.

In Lennox-Gastaut syndrome, the general EEG findings are those of symptomatic generalized epilepsy with a severe disturbance of ongoing activity and multiple and generalized discharges but most characteristically a slow form of SW activity repeating approximately once per second (Figure 6.8). This may accompany the atypical absences, but may also persist when these are controlled by medication.

How to Use the Electroencephalogram Sensibly in Epilepsy

Diagnostic Sensitivity

Investigation of epilepsy with the electroencephalogram may provide evidence of cerebral pathology, anticonvulsant intoxication, and so forth, but the two main objectives are to support the diagnosis and to assist classification. Achieving these aims depends on finding epileptiform activity.

A single waking interictal EEG about 30 minutes in duration detects epileptiform activity in about 50% of people with epilepsy. This apparently poor sensitivity reflects a sampling problem resulting from the variability of the EEG in epilepsy. In repeated waking, interictal examinations, Ajmone Marsan and Zivin[42] found that 30% of subjects exhibited epileptiform activity in every record. By contrast, 11% consistently failed to do so despite multiple recordings. Fifty-nine percent exhibited discharges on some occasions only, with an overall yield of epileptiform activity in 43% for serial EEG recordings. Epileptiform activity was found in the first recordings from 55.5% of patients. These findings support the general proposition that a single waking EEG shows epileptiform activity in some 50% of patients, but also implies that by repeated EEG examination, inter-ictal discharges should be demonstrable in 89% of patients. It may be argued that the data of Ajmone Marsan and Zivin, from a tertiary center, were atypical, but a review of 100 consecutive EEG studies from a prospective study of newly diag-nosed, unmedicated patients showed a similar pattern.[43]

Sleep recording increases the prevalence of epileptiform activity, but it is uncertain what yield of additional information may be expected from its routine use. Most studies report sleep EEG recordings performed in patients whose wak-ing records proved inconclusive, confounding effects of sleep with those of repeating the EEG study However, an audit of 3,000 epileptic patients who had undergone at least three EEG examinations, including a sleep record,[43] gives some indication of sleep's role in a rational diagnostic strategy. In the interictal waking EEG recording, epileptiform activity was found consistently, intermit-tently, or never, in 33%, 53%, and 14% of subjects, respectively. In 51% of patients without discharges in the initial wake recording, a subsequent sleep EEG recording showed epileptiform activity in 63%, bringing the total yield to 81%. This increased with subsequent wake and sleep records to 92%. These results do not indicate the rate of activation by sleep as such, since some wake EEG recordings included spontaneous drowsiness, and the apparent yield from sleep may have been partly the result of repetition of the recording.

It follows that where an indication exists for diagnostic EEG examination, a sleep record is also indicated if the waking record is negative. There may, there-fore, be practical advantages in planning every diagnostic interictal EEG in epilepsy as a combined wake and sleep recording. An audit of this practice in 250 patients showed a yield at a single recording session of 80%.[43]

Specificity

Specificity is poor unless the sharp waveforms common in normal subjects are clearly distinguished from phenomena more strongly associated with epilep-sy. The best evidence of the prevalence of epileptiform activity in healthy adults is probably that from compulsory investigation of neurologically screened military personnel. Two such studies in a total of more than 21,000 airmen[44, 45] suggest a prevalence of only 2.4 per 1,000. A self-sustaining, gen-eralized photoparoxysmal response[46] was obtained in only 0.2 per 1,000 nonepileptic subjects.

The prevalence of epileptiform activity in nonepileptic patients is greater than in neurologically screened controls. Zivin and Ajmone Marsan[47] reported epilep-tiform activity in 2.2% of nonepileptic patients, but in 10% of those with cere-bral pathology. Similarly, in nonepileptic psychiatric patients the prevalence was

129

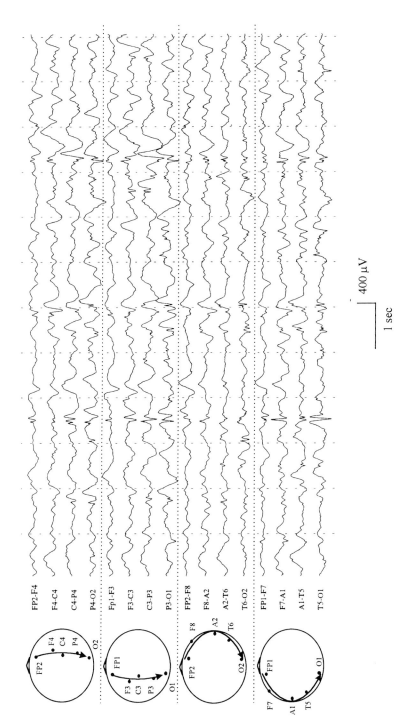

Figure 6.7 Hypsarrhythmia. Electroencephalographic recording of a 10-month-old girl with infantile spasms. It is severely disorganized with high-voltage slow activity and frequent spike-wave discharges of variable distribution. This recording uses a bipolar montage, so each channel displays the potential difference between the adjacent electrodes.

130

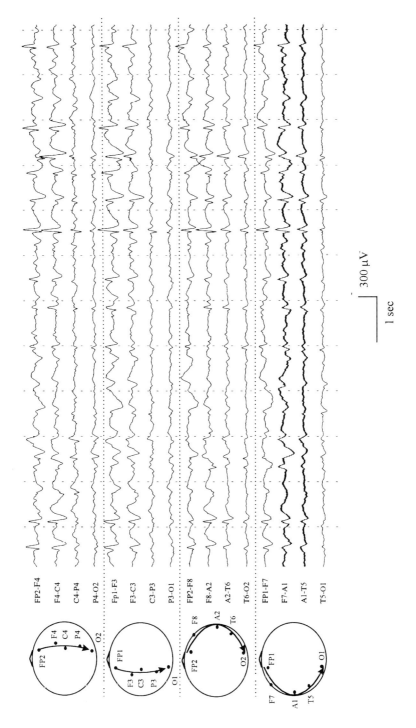

Figure 6.8 Lennox-Gastaut syndrome. This record, from a 13-year-old girl with a learning disability and a variety of seizure types, shows the characteristic generalized, slow spike-and-wave discharges at about 2 per second against a diffusely slowed background.

2.6%[48] but higher in particular categories, notably young adults with aggressive outbursts. The diagnostic significance of epileptiform activity thus depends on the clinical context. It is of little value for identifying epilepsy in the presence of cerebral pathologic entities but an important finding in a subject without other evidence of brain disease.

INTENSIVE MONITORING

Over many years, two competing technologies have been used for long-term monitoring of epilepsy: ambulatory recording by miniaturized portable recorders, and EEG telemetry by a cable or radio link, usually combined with video registration of behavior. These were often presented by their respective advocates as alternatives, misleadingly, as they had different advantages, drawbacks, and applications.

Applications

Differential Diagnosis

In most centers, the principal application of intensive monitoring in epilepsy is for the differential diagnosis of epileptic and nonepileptic seizures. If the clinical phenomenon in question is captured and is accompanied by appropriate ictal EEG changes, it can be confidently concluded that this event at least was epileptic. As noted above, in many seizures, and particularly those where the epileptic nature is most likely to be questioned, ictal EEG changes may be subtle or absent. When reviewing the EEG it is therefore important to know the precise timing of clinical events in order to identify subtle changes. Moreover, to interpret an absence of ictal EEG change, one needs to know whether the seizure was of such a type as to be compatible with an absence of changes in the scalp EEG. From these considerations, it follows that this application requires EEGs of high technical quality with synchronized video registration of clinical events.

Seizure Documentation and Classification

Simultaneous EEG and video monitoring has contributed importantly to understanding the phenomenology and semiology of epilepsy. In patients with intractable seizures, monitoring may be of clinical value for classifying seizures in order to select appropriate treatment.

Preoperative Assessment

Opinions differ concerning the role of ictal EEG in preoperative assessment of epilepsy. Where neuroimaging shows a potentially epileptogenic lesion at a site compatible with the nature of the seizures, and with interictal EEG and neuropsychological findings, further electrophysiologic investigation may be considered unnecessary. It may be argued, however, that scalp telemetry is obligatory in order to establish that therapy-resistant seizures are in fact epileptic, and some workers would insist that the epileptogenic zone can be defined only by intracranial ictal recording. Whatever use is made of electrophysiology in preoperative assessment, it is essential that ictal recordings employ appropriate technology. The number of channels required for reliable localization is at least 20 for scalp EEGs, and 32 to 128 or more for intracranial recordings. Simultaneous video registration is essential: If clinical ictal events precede the first electrographic changes, then the latter do not constitute reliable evidence of the site of onset of the seizure.

Detection of Subtle Seizures

Brief absences readily pass unrecognized, and monitoring may show their frequency to be 10 times greater than that reported by patients and caregivers. Partial seizures may also be difficult to detect, because the signs fall within the repertoire of normal behaviors, or because the clinical manifestations are confined to disturbances of psychological function that can be identified only if the subject is monitored while engaging in cognitive activity (see reference 49 for review). To monitor the occurrence of known ictal activity (for instance, to determine the frequency of absences), it may be sufficient to record a few channels of EEG. For identification of subtle ictal symptoms, video EEG, possibly with simultaneous psychological testing, may be required.

Seizure Precipitants

Besides those photosensitive subjects who clearly suffer from seizures precipitated by environmental stimuli, many patients report that attacks are triggered by more or less specific stimuli, cognitive activities, or situational factors. Unless these claims conform to established syndromes, such as primary reading epilepsy, they tend to be given little credence. Intensive monitoring with video recording as appropriate may be of value in investigating alleged seizure precipitants. Such studies may also be useful in detecting self-induction of attacks, which is particularly common but often overlooked in photosensitive patients.[50]

Ambulatory Recording

Ambulatory systems evolved from recorders originally developed for electrocardiographic applications. They used tape speeds so low that a 24-hour recording could be achieved on a single audiocassette. Their limited storage capacity restricted the number of channels to four and later to eight and dictated a dynamic range and frequency response barely adequate for reasonable EEG display. Moreover, these technical constraints presented problems in distinguishing abnormal EEG from artifacts, which readily occur in active subjects. This EEG registration technology could not conveniently be combined with video recording; documentation of clinical events depended on diaries kept by patients and caregivers, which did not allow precise, second-by-second comparison of clinical and EEG phenomena. Consequently, ambulatory monitoring with cassette recorders was rarely suitable for those applications considered above that demanded high-quality, multichannel EEG registration and accurate documentation of the nature and timing of clinical events. Their chief use was for recording known, easily recognized EEG phenomena in a particular environment; for instance, to determine the frequency of absence seizures at school.

Technical developments may expand the uses of ambulatory recording. Alternative mass storage devices, such as flash cards and miniature hard discs, offer greatly increased capacity, so that ambulatory recording of 32 channels is now feasible with bandwidth and dynamic range equal to those of a conventional EEG machine. Synchronized video monitoring is also possible.

Telemetry

There have been significant technologic advances in video-EEG telemetry, notably as a consequence of digital video compression, a dramatic fall in the cost of mass storage devices with capacities of tens of gigabytes, and development of optical disc recording. It is now feasible to store digitized video images with EEG data on random access devices, eliminating time consuming searching of video tapes to find salient events and allowing seizure records to be edited with a few keystrokes and archived on compact discs.

Manufacturers can now be expected to offer fully integrated systems for all forms of EEG using a common data storage format; archiving and review facilities for routine EEGs; and EEGs with video registration, telemetry, ambulatory monitoring, and polysomnography.

INTRACRANIAL RECORDING

Surgical treatment of epilepsy has been widely practiced for some four decades but has undergone a rapid expansion worldwide only in the past 10 years. The range of techniques available has also increased, but the procedures most commonly used involve resection or transection of an "epileptogenic zone" from which partial seizures arise. In practice, seizure relief is likely to be achieved only if the resected cortical tissue is structurally and functionally abnormal. The range and sensitivity of techniques for identifying epileptogenic structural abnormalities has been greatly increased by advances in neuroimaging, but these developments have not reduced the need for identification of the region of localized cerebral dysfunction. This is achieved by various methods of functional assessment, including clinical documentation of seizures (now enhanced by video monitoring), neuropsychological evaluation, positron emission tomography (PET), ictal single photon emission computed tomography (SPECT), and "functional" magnetic resonance imaging (fMRI). However, electrophysiology remains the cornerstone of functional assessment.

As indicated above, interictal and even ictal recording of the scalp EEG provides evidence of only limited reliability concerning the site of seizure onset. In typical temporal lobe epilepsy, the interictal EEG usually, but by no means invariably, identifies the affected lobe, whereas the ictal EEG is often nonlocalizing. In extratemporal epilepsies, the EEG is of less reliability. Interictal and ictal recording may show no abnormal activity in partial epilepsies of perirolandic origin, but usually give correct localization in those patients where focal discharges are found. In mesial and orbital frontal epilepsies, the EEG recording is rarely localizing and often nonlateralizing. In those patients where focal epileptiform EEG discharges are found and where these are concordant with the evidence of other functional and structural assessments, it may be reasonable to proceed to surgery without further investigation. Where EEG localization is not achieved or where it is not concordant with other data, more invasive methods may be required to establish the site of seizure onset.

Foramen ovale recording[51] provides a relatively noninvasive method of intracranial registration from mesial temporal structures. Multipolar electrodes are inserted bilaterally through the foramen ovale, coming to lie along the medial aspect of the parahippocampal gyrus. The procedure requires a general anesthetic and causes significant subsequent discomfort. Numbness or paresthesias in the trigeminal territory may persist for some weeks after removal of the electrodes. More significant morbidity is rare; fatalities caused by misplacement of electrodes have been reported, but we have encountered only one lasting hemiparesis and no deaths in more than 400 bilateral insertions. The electrodes do not record from the hippocampus itself, but because discharges usually spread rapidly to parahippocampal structures, high-frequency ictal activity can usually be seen very soon after onset of mesial temporal seizures (see Figure 6.5) and before involvement of neocortex is detectable in the scalp EEG recording. Conversely, in lateral temporal lobe seizures, discharges are detected first in the EEG recording, followed by slower, propagated spikes or SW activity at the foramen ovale electrodes.

Foramen ovale recording is of little value in extratemporal epilepsies except to establish that seizure onset is not temporal, which may itself be of considerable importance in planning further investigation of patients with symptoms caused by secondary temporal lobe involvement.

In extratemporal epilepsies known or presumed to arise from the convexity, subdural electrodes may be used to locate seizure onset and for functional mapping. This typically involves observing the clinical effects of electrical stimulation of neocortex through the subdural electrodes to locate functionally important areas of "eloquent" cortex that must be avoided in any resection. Sensory areas may also be mapped by evoked potentials recorded with subdural electrodes.

The electrodes themselves consist of small contacts mounted on plastic strips, which may be inserted through burr holes, or larger mats, which are placed through a craniotomy. There is a small but significant morbidity, particularly because of intracranial infection.

To record seizure onset from regions other than the convexity, it is necessary to use depth electrodes. This is necessary most often in epilepsies of suspected mesiobasal frontal origin and in complex partial seizures where foramen ovale recording has failed to establish whether onset is temporal or frontal. The electrodes are inserted by stereotaxy, most often using a lateral approach. However, the number of intracerebral electrodes required to achieve reliable localization may be reduced by using subdural contacts to record from the convexity.

Simultaneous insertion of subdural and depth electrodes is facilitated by inserting the latter from a central trephine hole[52] or by an occipital approach.

If seizure onset is sharply localized to the site of an electrode, as is often the case in mesial temporal epilepsies, high-frequency ictal activity is typically seen at seizure onset (Figure 6.9). If the onset is regional, as is often found in lateral temporal and mediobasal frontal epilepsies, or if the nearest contact is at some distance from the focus, the initial events may be sharp waves or SW complexes. In both cases, as the seizure evolves, the discharges become more widespread and less tightly synchronized, typically producing rhythmic sharp waves followed by SW activity.

Intracranial recording must not be used as an exploratory procedure and should be undertaken only to test a plausible hypothesis concerning the site of seizure onset. Partly as a consequence of advances in neuroimaging, depth recording is used in a steadily diminishing proportion of patients (currently some 8% in our practice). However, the increasing awareness of cortical dysgenesis as a cause of epilepsy treatable by surgery may create an increased demand for subdural recording, which is often essential to determine the extent of resection required and for functional mapping of areas that must not be resected.

TOPOGRAPHIC DISPLAYS: USES AND ABUSES

Displaying the scalp EEG presents a technical challenge, as it is a phenomenon existing in five dimensions (of potential, time, and three of space). Conventional EEG recordings use only the two dimensions of potential and time, and the observer is required to deduce the spatial characteristics by comparison of multiple channels recording from different electrodes. Alternative display methods highlight particular characteristics by eliminating other elements of the data. These have been known for several decades but have gained popularity with the advent of inexpensive computer graphics under the name of "brain mapping."

Isopotential Maps

By representing the surface of the scalp in only two dimensions and eliminating temporal information, the electrical field at any instant can be represented by a contour map (see Figure 6.4). Such a display provides no information that an expert observer cannot derive from a conventional EEG record using a common reference montage, but it presents this information in a permanent form independent of the skills of the interpreter.

In epileptologic practice, such displays have drawn attention to the characteristic bipolar topography of the rolandic spike (see Figure 6.6), the centrotemporal negative component of which is associated with a positivity in the midfrontal region.[53] It appears that children with presumed benign childhood epilepsy whose spikes do not show this topography are likely to have an atypical, and adverse, clinical course. Ebersole[24] has shown that temporal spikes in patients with seizures of mesial temporal origin also typically produce a bipolar field with pos-

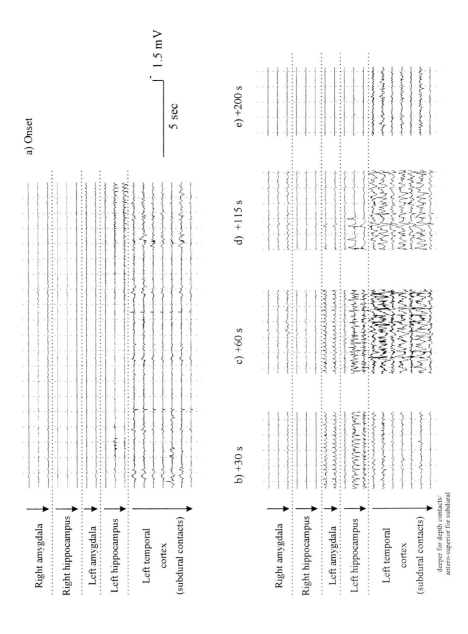

itivity in the contralateral central region. This is not usually seen in patients with neocortical temporal seizures (see Figure 6.4).

Spectral Mapping

An alternative method of data reduction discards information about instantaneous amplitude, polarity, and variation of the EEG record by presenting power in specified frequency bands as a contour map. The display supposedly presents the power recorded from each electrode, but depends on the overall topography of the electrical field between each electrode and a common reference point. The findings are dependent on the choice of reference and can be grossly misleading if this is inappropriate.[54] Spectral mapping has contributed little to the study of epilepsy.

Current Density Displays

The generators of the EEG record may be regarded as sources of potential difference; these give rise to currents in the brain, skull, and scalp, which in turn create a field of electrical potential that is recorded as the EEG pattern. The spread of the currents blurs the original potential sources but by application of an algorithm based on Laplace's theorem, the topography of these sources can be calculated. This principle is used to provide enhanced spatial resolution in conventional EEG recordings (so-called "source reference derivation") or in topographic displays as considered above. The clinical benefits and particular applications in epilepsy have yet to be established.

Equivalent Dipole Modeling

A region of cortex involved in synchronous discharge as described in the opening paragraph of this chapter may be regarded as a dipole, a source of potential

◀ *Figure 6.9*   Depth and subdural recording of complex partial seizure. Within each bundle of electrodes the sequence of channels (in direction of the arrows) is from superficial to deep for the intracerebral electrodes and from inferior to anterosuperior for the subdural (left temporal) contacts. All electrodes are referred to a right central common reference. Sixty-four channels were recorded from 92 electrodes available but for the sake of clarity only a selection of these are shown. (a) Seizure onset is heralded by a short burst of low-voltage fast activity at the middle contact of the left hippocampal bundle 2 seconds after the start of the excerpt. All activity is then attenuated at this site for 9 seconds (an electrodecremental event), and there follows a gradual buildup of activity at this and the adjacent hippocampal electrode. This activity is initially fast and of low amplitude but increases in voltage and declines in frequency over the remaining 8 seconds of the excerpt. (b) Left hippocampal activity has now evolved to rhythmic spiking at about 4 per second and has invaded the amygdaloid leads. (c) Sixty seconds into the seizure irregular spikes and slow waves are present at the left temporal subdural electrodes. (d) After 115 seconds, the deep spikes slow down and cease, but neocortical discharges continue. (e) Two hundred seconds after seizure onset, neocortical discharges have also subsided. In this seizure, no right-sided discharges were seen.

difference between two adjacent points. If the characteristics of such a dipole were known then, taking into account the electrical properties of the brain, skull, and scalp, it should be possible to determine what activity this would generate in the EEG recording. Conversely, given a known EEG phenomenon, it may be possible to determine the features and location of a cerebral dipole by which it *could* be generated. Computer programs are available that, usually by trial and error, identify single or multiple dipoles that could generate observed EEG phenomena. In view of the importance of epileptogenic sources at sites remote from the scalp electrodes, dipole modeling is of great potential significance in the management of epilepsy. Despite enthusiastic preliminary reports, two key issues need to be addressed before the clinical use of dipole modeling can be justified.

Firstly, the dipole modeling algorithms themselves are imperfectly validated. Under ideal conditions far simpler than those obtained in the human head—i.e., that of locating artificial dipoles in a spherical tank containing a homogeneous conducting medium—existing programs produce disappointing results. Single or superficial dipoles can be reliably located, but multiple or deep sources (critical for clinical use) cannot.[55] A more intractable problem, however, concerns the pathophysiology of EEG discharges. In patients with deep sources of epileptogenesis, spikes are not transmitted to the EEG electrodes by electrical conduction through the brain, skull, and scalp, but arise mostly from secondary activation of neocortex.[18] If computer modeling attributes these to a deep dipole generator, the result, even if correct, is fortuitous. Thus, for instance, the bipolar fields in mesial temporal epilepsies can be modeled by hippocampal dipoles, but it does not follow that such generators exist.

REFERENCES

1. Aarts JHP, Binnie CD, Smith AM, Wilkins AJ. Selective cognitive impairment during focal and generalized epileptiform EEG activity. Brain 1984;107:293.
2. Gloor P. Generalized corticoreticular epilepsies: some considerations on the pathophysiology of generalized bilaterally synchronous spike and wave discharge. Epilepsia 1968;9:249.
3. Stefan H. Pseudospontanbewegungen bei patienten mit petit-mal-anfaellen. Arch Psychiatr Nervenkr 1981;229:277.
4. Wilkins AJ, Binnie CD, Darby CE. Interhemispheric differences in photosensitive epilepsy: I. Pattern sensitivity thresholds. Electroencephalogr Clin Neurophysiol 1981;52:461.
5. Berkovic SF, Andermann F, Andermann E, Gloor P. Concepts of absence epilepsies: discrete syndromes or biological continuum? Neurology 1987;37:993.
6. Aird RB, Masland RL, Woodbury, DM. Hypothesis: the classification of seizures according to systems of the CNS. Epilepsy Res 1989;3:77.
7. Rodin E, Ancheta O. Cerebral electrical fields during petit mal absences. Electroencephalogr Clin Neurophysiol 1987;66:457.
8. Dondey M. Transverse topographical analysis of petit mal discharges: diagnostical and pathogenic implications. Electroencephalogr Clin Neurophysiol 1983;55:361.
9. Delgado-Escueta AV. Epileptogenic paroxysms: modern approaches and clinical correlations. Neurology 1979;29:1014.
10. Babb TL, Wilson CL, Isokawa-Akesson M. Firing patterns of human limbic neurons during stereoencephalography (SEEG) and clinical temporal lobe seizures. Electroencephalogr Clin Neurophysiol 1987;66:467.
11. Geiger LR, Harner RN. EEG patterns at the time of focal seizure onset. Arch Neurol 1978;35:276.
12. Alarcon G, Binnie CD, Elwes RDC, Polkey CE. Power spectrum and intracranial EEG patterns at seizure onset in partial epilepsy. Electroencephalogr Clin Neurophysiol 1994;95:326.

13. Falconer M, Kennedy WA. Epilepsy due to small focal temporal lesions with bilateral spike discharging foci: a study of seven cases relieved by operation. J Neurol Neurosurg Psychiatry 1961;24:205.
14. Morrell F, Whisler WW. Secondary Epileptogenic Lesions in Man: Prediction of Results of Excision of the Primary Focus. In R Canger, F Angelieri, JK Penry (eds), Advances in Epileptology: XIth Epilepsy International Symposium. New York: Raven, 1980;123.
15. Hughes JR. Long-term clinical and EEG changes in patients with epilepsy. Arch Neurol 1985;42:213.
16. Goldensohn ES. The relevance of secondary epileptogenesis to the treatment of epilepsy: kindling and the mirror focus. Epilepsia 1984;25:156.
17. Blume WT. Do epileptic foci in children migrate? The cons. Electroencephalogr Clin Neurophysiol 1990;76:100.
18. Alarcon G, Guy CN, Binnie CD, et al. Intracerebral propagation of interictal epileptiform activity in partial epilepsy: implications for source localization. J Neurol Neurosurg Psychiatry 1994;57;435.
19. Delgado-Escueta AV, Bascal FE, Treiman DM. Complex partial seizures on closed-circuit television and EEG. A study of 691 attacks in 79 patients. Ann Neurol 1982;11:292.
20. King DW, Ajmone Marsan C. Clinical features and ictal patterns in epileptic patients with EEG temporal lobe foci. Ann Neurol 1977;2:138.
21. So N, Gloor P, Quesney LF, et al. Depth electrode investigations in patients with bitemporal epileptiform abnormalities. Ann Neurol 1989;25:423.
22. Polkey CE. Prognostic Factors in Selecting Patients with Drug-Resistant Epilepsy for Temporal Lobectomy. In FC Rose (ed), Research Progress in Epilepsy. London: Pitman, 1983;500.
23. Binnie CD, Marston D, Polkey CE, Amin D. Distribution of temporal spikes in relation to the sphenoidal electrode. Electroencephalogr Clin Neurophysiol 1989;73:403.
24. Ebersole JS. Equivalent Dipole Modelling—A New EEG Method for Localisation of Epileptogenic Foci. In TA Pedley, BS Meldrum (eds), Current Problems in Epilepsy. London: Churchill Livingstone, 1992;51.
25. Lieb JP, Walsh GO, Babb TL, et al. A comparison of EEG seizure patterns recorded with surface and depth electrodes in patients with temporal lobe epilepsy. Epilepsia 1976;17:137.
26. Spencer SS, Williamson PD, Bridgers SL, et al. Reliability and accuracy of localization by scalp ictal EEG. Neurology 1985;35:1567.
27. Williamson PD, Spencer DD. Clinical and EEG features of complex partial seizures of extratemporal origin. Epilepsia 1986;27(Suppl 2):546.
28. Quesney LF, Constain M, Rasmussen T, et al. Presurgical EEG investigation in frontal lobe epilepsy. Epilepsy Res 1992;(Suppl 5):55.
29. Fegersten L, Roger A. Frontal epileptogenic foci and their clinical correlations. Electroencephalogr Clin Neurophysiol 1961;13:905.
30. Quesney LF. Seizures of frontal lobe origin. Electroencephalogr Clin Neurophysiol 1986;37 (Suppl):81.
31. Tükel K, Jasper H. The electroencephalogram in parasagittal lesions. Electroencephalogr Clin Neurophysiol 1952;4:481.
32. Ralston BL. Cingulate epilepsy and secondary bilateral synchrony. Electroencephalogr Clin Neurophysiol 1961;13:591.
33. Tharp BR. Orbital frontal seizures: an unique electroencephalographic and clinical syndrome. Epilepsia 1972;13:627.
34. Blume WT, Whiting SE, Girvin JP. Epilepsy surgery in the posterior cortex. Ann Neurol 1991;29:638.
35. Williamson D, Thadani VM, Darcey TM, et al. Occipital lobe epilepsy: clinical characteristics, seizure spread patterns, and results of surgery. Ann Neurol 1992;31:3.
36. Williamson D, Boon PA, Thadani VM, et al. Parietal lobe epilepsy: diagnostic considerations and results of surgery. Ann Neurol 1992;31:193.
37. Naquet R. The Clinical Significance of EEG in Epilepsy. In G Nistico, R De Perri, H Meinardi (eds), Epilepsy: An Update on Research and Therapy. New York: Liss, 1983;147.
38. Riley TL. Normal Variants in EEG that are Mistaken as Epileptic Patterns. In MG Ross (ed), Pseudoepilepsy. Lexington, MA: Heath, 1983;25.
39. Westmoreland BF, Reiher J, Klass DW. Recording small sharp spikes with depth electroencephalography. Epilepsia 1979;20:599.
40. Niedermeyer E. Sleep electroencephalogram in petit mal. Arch Neurol 1965;12:625.
41. Clemens B, Oláh R. Sleep studies in benign epilepsy of childhood with rolandic spikes: I. Sleep pathology. Epilepsia 1987;28:20.
42. Ajmone Marsan C, Zivin LS. Factors related to the occurrence of typical paroxysmal abnormalities in the EEG records of epileptic patients. Epilepsia 1970;11:361.
43. Binnie CD. Epilepsy in Adults: Diagnostic EEG Investigation. In J Kimura, H Shibasak (eds), Recent Advances in Clinical Neurophysiology. Amsterdam: Elsevier, 1996 (in press).

44. Robin JJ, Tolan GD, Arnold JW. Ten-year experience with abnormal EEGs in asymptomatic adult males. Aviat Space Environ Med 1978;49:732.
45. Gregory RP, Oates T, Merry RTG. Electroencephalogram epileptiform abnormalities in candidates for aircrew training. Electroencephalogr Clin Neurophysiol 1993;86:75.
46. Reilly EL, Peters JF. Relationship of some varieties of electroencephalographic photosensitivity to clinical convulsive disorders. Neurology 1973;23:1050.
47. Zivin L, Ajmone Marsan C. Incidence and prognostic significance of "epileptiform" activity in the EEG of non-epileptic subjects. Brain 1968;91:751.
48. Bridgers SL. Epileptiform abnormalities discovered on electroencephalographic screening of psychiatric inpatients. Arch Neurol 1987;44:312.
49. Binnie CD, Kasteleijn-Nolst Trenite DGA, Smit AM, Wilkins AJ. Interactions of epileptiform EEG discharges and cognition. Epilepsy Res 1987;1:239.
50. Binnie CD, Darby CE, De Korte RA, Wilkins AJ. Self-induction of epileptic seizures by eyeclosure: incidence and recognition. J Neurol Neurosurg Psychiatry 1980;43:386.
51. Wieser HG, Elger CE, Stodieck SRG. The "foramen ovale electrode": a new recording method for the preoperative evaluation of patients suffering from mesiobasal temporal lobe epilepsy. Electroencephalogr Clin Neurophysiol 1985;61:314.
52. Van Veelen CWM, Debets RM, Van Huffelen AC, et al. Combined use of subdural and intracerebral electrodes in preoperative evaluation of epilepsy. Neurosurgery 1990;26:93.
53. Wong PKH. Comparison of spike topography in typical and atypical benign rolandic epilepsy of childhood. Electroencephalogr Clin Neurophysiol 1985;61:S47.
54. Binnie CD, MacGillivray BB. Brain mapping   a useful tool or a dangerous toy? J Neurol Neurosurg Psychiatry 1992;55:527.
55. Holder D, Mansouri M, Binnie CD. Experimental validation of the localisation accuracy of inverse dipole modelling of the EEG in a saline filled spherical tank. Electroencephalogr Clin Neurophysiol 1996;98:2.

7
Partial Epilepsy Syndromes in Adults

Matthew Walker and Simon Shorvon

The impulse to classify epilepsy is not a modern phenomenon, but has developed over the ages to fulfill the needs, theories, and capacity of the time. Thus, the magicians of ancient Greece attributed different seizure types to individual gods so that it was clear to whom any sacrifice need be made.[1] "Mother of the Gods" was responsible if the patient imitated a goat, Poseidon if the cries were more violent so that the patient resembled a horse, Enodia for the passing of feces, and Hecate for twisting of the mind and falling. Hippocrates cast scorn on these ideas and considered epilepsy as one disease, "the so-called sacred disease."[1]

In 375 AD, Galen recognized that all epilepsy came from the brain but divided epilepsy into idiopathic (the brain was primarily affected) and sympathetic (the brain was healthy but had been affected by a disease originating in another part of the body). These terms persisted into the nineteenth century with the addition of "symptomatic epilepsy," which referred to epilepsy originating in the brain caused by an underlying cerebral lesion.[1] "Symptomatic" and "idiopathic" are terms still used in present classifications, but it is important to realize that their origins have a different physiologic viewpoint. Indeed, with the advances in modern imaging and genetics, the distinctions made by these terms are becoming less meaningful.

To understand the classifications that we have and the ways they have evolved, it is necessary to understand why we classify. Jackson, more than a century ago, realized that the requirement for a classification dictates its form. As he succinctly wrote, "Whilst it is convenient to consider a whale as a fish for legal purposes, it would never do to consider it so in zoology!"[2] We classify for four main purposes—communication, research, treatment, and prognosis—and we can classify in two broad fashions: empirically and scientifically. An empirical classification is one in which we group things purely according to our observations, and it is usually a classification of convenience. A scientific classification is one in which we group things according to an underlying hypothesis. In 1969, Gastaut proposed that epilepsy should be divided in an empirical and scientific fashion by classify-

Table 7.1　Summary of International League Against Epilepsy classification of seizures

I. Partial seizures
   A. Simple partial seizures
   B. Complex partial seizures
   C. Secondary generalized seizures
II. Generalized seizures
   A.1. Absence seizures (petit mal)
   A.2. Atypical absence seizures
   B. Myoclonic seizures
   C. Clonic seizures
   D. Tonic seizures
   E. Tonic-clonic seizures (grand mal)
   F. Atonic seizures
III. Unclassified epileptic seizures

Source: Adapted from Commission on the Classification and Terminology of the International League Against Epilepsy. Proposal for revised clinical and electroencephalographic classification of epileptic seizures. Epilepsia 1981;22:289.

ing it according to clinical and electroencephalographic (EEG) manifestations, anatomic substrate, age, etiology, interictal neuropsychiatric changes, response to treatment, and pathophysiology.[3] In 1981, as its first step toward classifying epilepsies, the International League Against Epilepsy (ILAE) proposed a classification of seizure types to rationalize and simplify the various classifications that were in common use (Table 7.1).[4] This classification was based on clinical form and interictal and ictal EEG findings. The classification had one underlying hypothesis—the differentiation of seizures into generalized and partial seizures—but in the main it was an empirical classification. Thus, it enables distinctions to be drawn between different seizures and for seizure type to be communicated in a universal fashion. It is pragmatic, although problems do exist (for example, how far does consciousness have to be impaired for a simple partial seizure to become a complex partial seizure), and it is not always certain under which category a particular seizure should be included (for example, many atonic seizures could be classified as complex partial seizures). It suffers from many limitations—it does not describe etiology, prognosis, or pathophysiology. These problems were realized, and in 1985 the ILAE proposed a classification of epilepsies and epilepsy syndromes (revised in 1989).[5, 6] This was a bold attempt to classify epilepsy in terms of anatomy, etiology, EEG findings, seizure type, precipitation, and syndromic features (Table 7.2). It had as its basis the same hypothesis that underlay the seizure classification—that is, the differentiation of partial from generalized seizures, which became the differentiation of partial from generalized epilepsies. The sharing of this hypothesis has created a certain amount of confusion, because many physicians confuse seizure type with epilepsy type and refer to such entities as complex partial epilepsy.[7] It is important to differentiate the nomenclative aims of the seizure classification from the nosologic aims of the epilepsies and epilepsy syndromes classification. Again, it is common for physicians' descriptions of epilepsies to proceed no further than the seizure type, and thus, unknowingly, they abandon the information that is possibly of greater use to the patient.

Table 7.2 Summary of the International League Against Epilepsy classification of epilepsies, epileptic syndromes, and related seizure disorders

1. **Localization related**
    1.1. Idiopathic
        Benign childhood epilepsy with centrotemporal spike
        Childhood epilepsy with occipital paroxysms
        Primary reading epilepsy
    1.2. Symptomatic
        Chronic progressive epilepsia partialis continua of childhood
        Syndromes characterized by seizures with specific modes of precipitation
        Temporal lobe epilepsies
        Frontal lobe epilepsies
        Parietal lobe epilepsies
        Occipital lobe epilepsies
    1.3. Cryptogenic
        As 1.2, but etiology is unidentified
2. **Generalized**
    2.1. Idiopathic
        Benign neonatal familial convulsions
        Benign neonatal convulsions
        Benign myoclonic epilepsy in infancy
        Childhood absence epilepsy (pyknolepsy)
        Juvenile absence epilepsy
        Juvenile myoclonic epilepsy (impulsive petit mal)
        Epilepsies with grand mal seizures on awakening
        Other generalized idiopathic epilepsies
        Epilepsies with seizures precipitated by specific modes of activation (reflex
            epilepsies)
    2.2. Cryptogenic or symptomatic
        West syndrome (infantile spasms, Blitz-Nick-Salaam-Krämpfe)
        Lennox-Gastaut syndrome
        Epilepsy with myoclonic-astatic seizures
        Epilepsy with myoclonic absences
    2.3. Symptomatic
        2.3.1. Nonspecific etiology
            Early myoclonic encephalopathy
            Early infantile epileptic encephalopathy with suppression bursts
            Other symptomatic generalized epilepsies
        2.3.2. Specific syndromes
            Epileptic seizures may complicate many disease states
3. **Undetermined epilepsies**
    3.1. With generalized and focal features
        Neonatal seizures
        Severe myoclonic epilepsy in infancy
        Epilepsy with continuous spike-waves during slow wave sleep
        Acquired epileptic aphasia (Landau-Kleffner syndrome)
        Other undetermined epilepsies
    3.2. Without unequivocal generalized or focal features
4. **Special syndromes**
    4.1. Situation-related seizures (Gelegenheitsanfälle)
        Febrile convulsions
        Isolated seizures or isolated status epilepticus
        Seizures occurring only when there is an acute or toxic event due to factors such
            as alcohol, drugs, eclampsia, or nonketotic hyperglycemia

Source: Adapted from Commission on Classification and Terminology of the International League Against Epilepsy. Proposal for revised classification of epilepsies and epileptic syndromes. Epilepsia 1989;30:389.

INTERNATIONAL LEAGUE AGAINST EPILEPSY CLASSIFICATION OF EPILEPSIES AND EPILEPSY SYNDROMES

Differentiation of partial epilepsies—in which the seizure activity commences in one part of the cerebrum—from generalized epilepsies—in which the epileptic activity involves wide areas of cerebral hemispheres simultaneously from the onset of the attack with no evidence of an anatomic or functional focus—seems clear and simple. A third category, however, had to be introduced for epilepsies and syndromes in which the seizure activity is undetermined—that is, whether it is focal or generalized (usually because both types of seizure are present). This uncertainty, however, is not confined to the epilepsies described in the classification (see Table 7.2), as cases of absence epilepsy have been associated with frontal and temporal lobe lesions and these cases are thus probably partial epilepsies.[8] Indeed, the distinction between partial and generalized epilepsy, which is mainly an electroclinical one, will possibly have to be redefined in light of modern imaging techniques and physiologic theories (e.g., the view that a seizure depends on a neural network and not a focus). There is also a fourth category of special syndromes, which, although epileptic in nature, do not usually carry the diagnosis of epilepsy. This is because there is an acute precipitating factor (e.g., metabolic or toxic events) or the seizure is an isolated event. Within each category, the epilepsies are divided into idiopathic, symptomatic, and cryptogenic (an underlying lesion is presumed but not discovered). As alluded to earlier, these divisions are becoming less helpful. Underlying structural and genetic causes are being revealed for syndromes that were previously classified as idiopathic.

Idiopathic epilepsies are defined according to clinical and EEG characteristics and, importantly, age-related onset. There is often a family history. There has been constant debate about how far to take the subdivision of idiopathic epilepsies and whether to include separate subgroups as separate syndromes.[9] Again, such divisions need to be justified by the difference they make to prognosis, treatment, and the elucidation of underlying genetic cause. It has been found in other neurologic conditions that often a detailed clinical subdivision needs to be made before accurate and worthwhile genetic analysis can take place, and this is a justification in itself.

The idiopathic epilepsies usually have a favorable response to antiepileptic drug therapy, a relatively benign prognosis (spontaneous remission with time is common), and are rarely associated with psychiatric or other mental disorders. These epilepsies are well and easily defined, and their prognosis and treatment are well established. This is not the case with symptomatic epilepsies, which, because of their diverse etiologic and physiologic substrates, have poorly defined prognoses and treatments. The situation is further complicated by the failure of antiepileptic drug trials to differentiate partial epilepsies (the majority of the symptomatic epilepsies) according to the ILAE classification or according to etiology.[10] Thus, useful information on treatment and prognosis is lost. Furthermore, the ease with which idiopathic syndromic analysis is applied as indicated by syndromic classifications of childhood epilepsies (usually idiopathic epilepsies) in which more than 90% of patients' epilepsies can be classified, does not hold for adult epilepsies (usually cryptogenic or symptomatic) in which only a third fall into a "diagnostic" ILAE category as opposed to nonspecific categories.[11]

Table 7.3 Summary of anatomic subdivisions of partial epilepsy syndromes in the International League Against Epilepsy classification

---

Seizures arising from temporal lobe
    Mesiobasal limbic
    Lateral temporal
Seizures arising from frontal lobe
    Supplementary motor
    Cingulate
    Anterior frontopolar
    Orbitofrontal
    Dorsolateral
    Opercular (includes regions in temporal and frontal lobes)
    Perirolandic (may include symptoms from pre- and postcentral regions)
Seizures arising from parietal lobe
Seizures arising from occipital lobe

Source: Adapted from Commission on Classification and Terminology of the International League Against Epilepsy. Proposal for revised classification of epilepsies and epileptic syndromes. Epilepsia 1989;30:389.

It is in this light that we review the partial epilepsy syndromes of adults and conclude with a review of the possible role of this syndromic classification.

PARTIAL EPILEPSIES ARISING IN DIFFERENT ANATOMIC REGIONS

Defining the region of origin of a seizure is not a clear-cut or simple matter. There are at least three defining methods: clinical history and scalp EEG findings, neuroimaging, and electrocorticography. Each of these may point to a different anatomic region for seizure onset. There are a number of reasons for this: The fact that seizures arising in one particular area spread quickly to other regions; the fact that seizures can be caused by an abnormality in a distant location; the fact that seizures may have a basis in a neural network and not in a focus; and the fact that some underlying abnormalities are widespread with microscopic abnormalities not evident on macroscopic imaging. Furthermore, the features of seizures originating from different regions overlap. Although each method of distinguishing the partial epilepsies has its own value, neuroimaging is growing in importance in identifying the region for resection in epilepsy surgery.[12] The electroclinical method of anatomic differentiation has a less well-defined role, although it is easier to apply. The extent to which it helps in localization, prognosis, response to drug treatment, and neuropsychological and psychiatric outcomes are subjects to which we will return. Descriptions and modifications of the electroclinical localization of seizures used by the ILAE classification (Table 7.3)[6] are contained in a number of extensive reviews and patient series. Rather than repeat exactly what is included in those, we will describe the salient features, happy in the knowledge that, as the adage goes, "to take from one source is plagiarism, but to take from two is research." For greater detail, we refer the reader back to one of

Table 7.4   Summary of clinical features of seizures by lobe

Temporal lobe	Longer than frontal lobe seizures; auras are common; autonomic changes occur; slow evolution of seizure; prominent motor arrest; automatisms are rarely violent; postictal confusion
Central region	No loss of consciousness; contralateral jerking; contralateral dystonia; posturing; speech arrest; contralateral sensory symptoms
Other frontal regions	Frequent attacks; clustering; brief; sudden onset; rapid evolution; posturing; violent and bizarre automatisms; absent postictal confusion; history of status epilepticus
Parietal lobe	Somatosensory symptoms; sensation of immobility; illusions of change in body shape; vertigo; gustatory aura
Occipital lobe	Elementary visual hallucinations; visual distortions; amaurosis; blinking/eyelid fluttering; nystagmus; head turning

these comprehensive reviews. The anatomic lobar subclassification is one that is generally used and one that we will use here. However, certain anatomic regions lie in more than one lobe (e.g., the opercular region), and the spread of seizures may result in neighboring regions having identical symptoms despite their location in different lobes (e.g., central epilepsies can result from pre- or postcentral lesions). A summary of the clinical features by lobe is contained in Table 7.4.

Temporal Lobe Epilepsy

Approximately 60% of complex partial seizures have their origin in the temporal lobe, the rest being extratemporal.[6, 13–19] Attempts have been made to subclassify the temporal lobe epilepsies in terms of more specific anatomic structures. Jackson was one of the first to describe the "uncinate group of epileptic fits," which comprised crude sensations of smell and taste, oroalimentary automatisms, and, in some cases, a dreamlike state.[2] This led to the concept of limbic epilepsy, of seizures involving the limbic lobe, and this was later differentiated from seizures arising in the lateral temporal lobe. Indeed, the classification of Wieser divided temporal lobe seizures into opercular, temporal polar, and basal or limbic.[13] To what extent this subclassification has any actual anatomic validity or any usefulness are matters of debate. This complex subclassification is also onerous to apply; a subclassification into mesiobasal limbic and lateral neocortical types is more pragmatic. Although the distinction between lateral and mesial temporal seizures may at times be blurred (spread of seizure activity within the temporal lobe is common), this discrimination remains useful at a pragmatic level and can be justified by the extensive neuroanatomic, neurophysiologic, and neurochemical distinctions between these areas.

Mesiobasal Limbic

Mesiobasal limbic seizures involve the hippocampus and are occasionally referred to as hippocampal seizures. Various pathologic entities of the hippocampus can underlie these seizures, such as tumors, arteriovenous malformations, neuronal migration defects, and hippocampal sclerosis, which is the most common underlying pathologic state. Hippocampal sclerosis is associated with a history of complex febrile convulsions, but whether it is the result or cause is unknown. Prolonged seizures cause similar damage in animal models, lending weight to the supposition that it is the result of the febrile convulsion. Conversely, in some patients, features of the hippocampus suggest the existence of a congenital dysplasia, in which case the hippocampal abnormality is the substrate of the febrile convulsion. These two possibilities are not mutually exclusive, and it is possible that a pre-existing hippocampal abnormality results in the prolonged febrile convulsion, which then results in hippocampal cell death.[20] Indeed, there are animal data to suggest that hippocampal sclerosis may be a progressive condition.[21, 22]

Seizures take the form of complex partial seizures and, less commonly, simple partial seizures. The seizure usually has a gradual evolution over 1–2 minutes (substantially longer than extratemporal seizures) and lasts longer (2–10 minutes) than complex partial seizures originating in extratemporal sites. The most common aura is that of a rising epigastric sensation. Other gastrointestinal auras can occur, especially nausea, borborygmus, and belching. Auras can also consist of olfactory-gustatory hallucinations, autonomic symptoms, affective symptoms, or dysmnesic symptoms. Cephalic symptoms of vague dizziness, headache, strange "heady" feelings, etc., can occur but are more typical of a frontal lobe focus. The olfactory aura is usually intense and unpleasant and is especially characteristic of seizures originating in the sylvian region. Autonomic symptoms include changes in heart rate and blood pressure, pallor or flushing of the face, pupillary dilatation, and piloerection. Speech arrest can occur, but, conversely, repetitive vocalizations can be present (especially if the seizure originates in the nondominant temporal lobe). Affective symptoms typically take the form of fear (the most common and often very intense), depression, anger, and irritability. Euphoria and erotic thoughts have also been described. Dreamy states, such as described by Jackson, and feelings of depersonalization commonly occur. Déjà vu, déjà entendu, and other dysmnesic symptoms, such as recollections of childhood or even former lives, can also be present in this form of epilepsy.

In the early stages of the seizure, motor arrest and absence are prominent and certainly more so than in extratemporal lobe epilepsy. The automatisms of mesiobasal temporal lobe epilepsy can be prolonged, are usually less violent than those of frontal lobe epilepsy, and are typically oroalimentary (e.g., lipsmacking, chewing) or gestural (e.g., fidgeting, undressing, walking). Dystonic posturing is usually contralateral to the focus, and unilateral automatisms are usually ipsilateral. Vocalizations are common, and recognizable words suggest a focus in the nondominant temporal lobe. Secondary generalization is less common than in extratemporal lobe epilepsy. Postictal confusion is typically longer than in frontal lobe epilepsy, and postictal headache also occurs. There is complete amnesia for the absence and automatism. Postictal dysphasia may follow seizures originating in the dominant temporal lobe. Postictal psychosis may also occur,[23] during which auditory and visual hallucinations are prominent and are characteristically paranoiac. Severe depression has also been described, as well as hypomania in association with right-sided foci. These episodes develop within 24 hours of a seizure and last from 24 hours to 3 months. They tend to occur in an older population, usually those between 30 and 40 years old.

Interictal EEG findings may be normal, may demonstrate intermittent or persistent slow activity over the temporal lobe, or interictal spikes may be present. The spikes are usually anterior or midtemporal, and superficial sphenoidal or zygomatic electrodes may be necessary for their detection. Bilateral independent interictal spikes are common, even when well-lateralized pathologic features are present. Ictal scalp EEG findings correlate well with the findings of depth EEG recordings, with lateralization being determined by the onset of unilateral temporal/sphenoidal rhythmic discharge of 5 hertz (Hz) or above within 30 seconds of the ictus.[24]

Lateral Temporal Neocortex

There is considerable overlap between the characteristics of the seizures from mesiobasal temporal lobe foci and from lateral temporal foci because of the rapid spread of seizure activity to neighboring areas. It is usual to find a structural lesion underlying seizures originating in the lateral temporal neocortex. The most common are glioma, angioma, neuronal migration defects, posttraumatic change, hamartoma, and dysembryoplastic neuroepithelial tumor. Consciousness is usually preserved longer than in mesiobasal temporal lobe seizures. The aura is more likely to comprise structured visual, auditory, gustatory, and olfactory hallucinations, and illusions especially of size (micropsia and macropsia) are typical. The affective and psychic auras that are typical of mesiobasal temporal lobe foci are less common. Although the automatisms have more prominent motor manifestations, the subsequent course and postictal phenomena are indistinguishable from mesiobasal temporal lobe epilepsy. The interictal EEG often shows spikes over the lateral convexity of the temporal lobe rather than from inferomesial electrodes, and spikes are of a shorter duration than those from mesiobasal foci. Occasionally, large temporal lobe lesions may be associated with ictal and interictal EEG changes that are predominant over the contralateral temporal lobe.[24]

Psychological Aspects

There are certain neuropsychological aspects that are characteristic of temporal lobe epilepsy; for example, problems with verbal memory with left-sided temporal lobe lesions and problems with nonverbal memory with right-sided temporal lobe lesions.[25] However, the existence of temporal lobe epilepsy leading to a specific temporal lobe personality syndrome is a matter of debate. Particular traits of humorlessness, dependence, circumstantiality, obsessionality, preoccupation with religious and philosophical concerns, and hyperemotionality were found in patients with temporal lobe epilepsy when compared with healthy controls and patients with different neurologic diagnoses.[26] It was suggested by Geschwind that some patients with temporal lobe epilepsy showed hyposexuality, hyperreligiosity, and hypergraphia and that these may be characteristic of a temporal lobe personality syndrome.[27] Whether these are related to epilepsy itself is contentious; a number of groups have pointed out that these personality changes are more likely related to psychosis and psychiatric illness. Indeed, the same pathologic state that underlies epilepsy may be the substrate of the psychopathologic features rather than there being a direct link.[28] Furthermore, social and demographic factors are likely to play a part. This could also be true for interictal psychosis and interictal aggression, which are said to be related to temporal lobe epilepsy. In the case of the latter, there is good evidence to suggest that it is related to the degree of brain damage rather than the severity of the epilepsy.[28]

Frontal Lobe Epilepsy

Frontal lobe epilepsy accounts for approximately 30% of partial epilepsy syndromes in adults.[6, 29–32] Attempts have been made to subclassify frontal lobe epilepsy on the basis of distinct anatomic regions. These subclassifications are in many ways more difficult to justify than the subclassifications of temporal lobe epilepsy. Indeed, many of the manifestations of frontal lobe epilepsies are not the result of the origin, but are the result of the pattern and rate of seizure spread. Electroclinical features of these seizures overlap considerably with temporal lobe seizures because of the extensive interconnections between frontal and temporal lobes. Nevertheless, a division of frontal lobe epilepsies into those arising from the central region (precentral gyrus or supplementary motor area [SMA]) and those arising from other areas of the frontal lobe is justified.

Epilepsy Arising from the Central Region

Epilepsy arising from the central region can be divided into seizures from the precentral gyrus and seizures from the SMA. The precentral gyrus, or motor cortex, carries a topographic representation of muscle groups as a homunculus, and stimulation of this part of the cortex results in the relaxation and contraction of muscles necessary to perform a single movement of a part of the body relating to the homunculus.[33] The homunculus emphasizes the relatively large representation of hands, feet, and mouth. Thus, seizures often begin with brief unilateral tetanic contractions involving one of these areas. The seizure activity then spreads, producing clonic movements according to the sequence of cortical representation. The spread is typically slow, leading to a "jacksonian" march of seizure activity from one part of the body to another. If a seizure begins in the hand, it typically spreads up the arm and down the leg, while seizures starting in the foot typically spread up the leg and down the arm. Consciousness is usually well preserved. There may be a postictal localized paralysis in the affected limbs (Todd's paralysis), which is typically short-lived but may persist for days.[34] Seizure spread from central regions may result in sensory manifestations of tingling, numbness, formication, and frequently pain. Seizures arising from the precentral gyrus can have sensory symptoms that progress in a similar fashion to the motor component (i.e., as a jacksonian march).

Seizures originating in the SMA are brief, frequently occurring in clusters, and predominantly nocturnal. They are sometimes precipitated by startle. The seizures may begin with an aura of often an ill-defined jolt or shock sensation, followed by sudden asymmetric posturing. Typically, this posturing consists of abduction, external rotation, and flexion at the elbow of the contralateral arm with the head and eyes deviated toward the upraised hand. The ipsilateral arm is often held down in rigid extension, the contralateral leg is typically extended, and the foot plantar flexed. Other postures occur frequently, however. Stereotypical vocalizations and speech arrest can occur, although speech can be preserved during the seizures (this is probably of little localizing value). Strikingly, consciousness is preserved during thes<e seizures, although this is sometimes not appreciated in patients with speech arrest. Secondary generalization may occur, following which there is often rapid return of alpha activity in the EEG recording in contrast to the prolonged postictal suppression and slow activity seen after other secondary generalized seizures. Although the features of seizures arising from the SMA are said to serve localization and lateralization, seizures arising from areas adjacent to and distant from the SMA may mimic the typical SMA seizure, and spread to the SMA from other areas is common. The ictal and interictal EEG recordings of patients with seizures arising from central regions are usually disappointing, and often appear normal, as the focus may be well buried within the central gyri.

Other Frontal Lobe Epilepsies

Frontal lobe seizures have a number of common distinguishing features. The seizures are frequent and brief (usually <30 seconds) and have a marked tendency to cluster. The gradual evolution so typical of temporal lobe seizures is rare with frontal lobe seizures, which tend to have an abrupt onset. In some cases, the seizures predominantly occur at night with brief, dystonic seizures occurring during sleep.

The aura is typically of a cephalic type with nonspecific dizziness or a strange feeling in the head. The typical psychic auras of temporal lobe epilepsy are absent unless there is early seizure spread to temporal lobe structures. Forced thinking and ideational and emotional manifestations can also occur. There is then rapid evolution with early loss of awareness. Motor arrest and absence are not a major feature and if present are usually very brief.

Automatisms of frontal lobe epilepsy typically differ from those of temporal lobe epilepsy. Temporal lobe automatisms are typically oroalimentary or gestural, with coordinated and well-structured movements of the upper limbs. Mimicry and ambulation can also be present. In contrast, automatisms of frontal lobe epilepsy often consist of bilateral motor automatisms affecting the lower limbs, such as cycling, stepping, dancing, and kicking. Also in contrast to temporal lobe automatisms, frontal lobe automatisms tend to be violent and often bizarre, so that confusion with nonepileptic attacks with a psychological basis is commonplace. This misdiagnosis is abetted by the frequent absence of EEG changes during complex partial seizures originating in the frontal lobe (see below). Ictal posturing and tonic spasms are a prominent feature of frontal lobe epilepsy. Vocalization is usual, typically consisting of a shrill, loud cry, although fragments of speech do also occur. Version of the head and eyes, although typical of frontal lobe epilepsy, can also be seen in temporal lobe epilepsy and is common in occipital lobe epilepsy. When version occurs at the onset of the seizure while the patient is conscious, the seizure focus is usually in the contralateral frontal dorsolateral convexity; in all other circumstances the direction of version is of no help in determining the laterality of the seizure onset.[35] Adversion of the body can also occur, resulting in circling. Autonomic symptoms can occur in frontal lobe seizures—indeed, seizures with an orbitofrontal focus may have autonomic symptoms as their only manifestation. Sexual automatisms with pelvic thrusting, obscene gestures, and genital manipulations have also been reported in seizures supposedly originating in the orbitofrontal region. Dysphasia can also occur, often accompanied by adversive or clonic movement. With seizures originating in the sylvian areas, the aphasia can be preceded by numbness in the mouth and a choking sensation in the throat. Evolution to secondary generalized seizures is common in frontal lobe epilepsy, and certainly this tendency is much more marked than in the case of temporal lobe epilepsy. Convulsive and nonconvulsive status epilepticus are well-recognized complications of frontal lobe epilepsy. Postictal confusion is brief. Rapid recovery can confound the diagnosis, resulting in confusion with nonepileptic attacks with a psychological basis.

The misdiagnosis of frontal lobe epilepsy is typical and often results from the indistinct phases that occur. As opposed to temporal lobe epilepsy, the differentiation of simple from complex partial seizure in frontal lobe epilepsy is rarely well defined. Seizures can occur with clonic jerking or bilateral motor activity (jerking or posturing) with retained or only mildly impaired consciousness. Furthermore, rapid spread, especially of seizures originating in the cingulate or dorsolateral cortex, can lead to tonic-clonic seizures with no warning or lateralizing features; this can lead to confusion with primary generalized epilepsies. Secondarily generalized tonic and atonic seizures can occur that are clinically indistinguishable from their primary generalized counterparts. Mesial frontal lobe epilepsy can result in blank spells with associated spike-wave discharges that can be difficult to discern from typical absences.

Two factors confound the EEG localization in frontal lobe epilepsy. First, the frontal lobe is poorly served by scalp electrodes (medial and inferior surfaces are inaccessible and few electrodes cover the other surfaces). Second, seizures spread rapidly within the frontal lobe from one frontal lobe to the other or from the frontal lobes to other parts of the brain. Thus, the EEG results are often disappointing with even ictal EEG recordings failing to demonstrate or poorly defining the focus. Generalized EEG disturbances (polyspikes, synchronous spike-and-wave, etc.) are not uncommon EEG findings that, although often with an anterior predominance, can be confused with EEG features from generalized epilepsies. Ictal and interictal slow activity, which may be generalized or focal, can be the only EEG finding.

Psychological Findings

As can be seen, the frontal lobes are far from being an homogeneous entity, and seizures from these lobes spread rapidly from one side to the other and to temporal lobe and other cortical structures. It is thus not surprising that difficulties can be encountered in delineating the neuropsychological characteristics of frontal lobe epilepsy. In looking at a well-defined population of frontal lobe epilepsy compared with temporal lobe epilepsy, a number of distinguishing characteristics can be found.[36] The performance of patients with frontal lobe epilepsy in neuropsychological tests to an extent mirrors that of patients with frontal lobe dysfunction; a deficit in executive skills is frequently present. In certain tasks, however, the lateralization of the focus rather than its lobar localization seemed to be of greater importance in determining the degree of dysfunction. Conversely, in other tasks, it was the lobar localization rather than the lateralization that was of greater importance. These results emphasize the difficulties that can be encountered.

Parietal Lobe Epilepsy

Parietal lobe epilepsy probably makes up less than 5% of all partial epilepsy syndromes in adults.[32, 37] Seizures originating from parietal lobes are associated with subjective sensations, but seizure spread can result in complex partial and generalized seizures that are indistinguishable from seizures originating in other areas. Furthermore, as described above, spread of seizures arising especially in the central region and from the temporal lobes can result in seizure semiology more typical of parietal lobe epilepsy. Consciousness is usually lost late in the seizure, but this may partly be because rapidly evolving parietal lobe seizures are easily confused with seizures originating in other areas. Somatosensory symptoms commonly consist of elementary paraesthesia of tingling or numbness, which may begin and progress similar to the jacksonian march of seizures originating in the precentral region. Motor activity similar to a precentral gyrus seizure can be associated with this somatosensory march. Pain may also be an associated or an isolated feature. Abdominal pain and headache have also been described. Seizures with a sexual content can occur, but this usually consists of an unpleasant genital sensation rather than the pleasurable sexual auras of temporal lobe epilepsy or the masturbatory automatisms of frontal lobe epilepsy. Other somatosensory auras consist of ideomotor apraxia and illusions of distortion, including swelling, shrinking, lengthening, or shortening of a part of the body. Ictal apraxia, acalculia, alexia, and aphemia have been reported. Seizures originating in the suprasylvian region are associated with gustatory aura and with ictal vertigo. Automatisms are indistinguishable from other partial epilepsy syndromes. Postictal persistence of numbness or an inability to move a body part can occur.

EEG features may again be unhelpful or misleading. Ictal and interictal EEG recordings can appear normal, especially in the context of simple partial seizures. In other cases, interictal and ictal spikes have been observed in frontal and temporal regions.

Occipital Lobe Epilepsy

Occipital lobe epilepsy probably makes up about 8% of partial epilepsies in adults.[37] Its major manifestations are elementary visual hallucination, including colors, shapes, flashes, and patterns. Hallucinations can be intermittent, stationary, or moving. They can occur in the entire visual field or in one hemifield and may commonly occur in a blind or damaged field. They can be differentiated from the visual hallucinations of migraine by their brevity and character; migrainous auras are typically black and white zigzag patterns, while multicolored circular patterns are typical of occipital lobe epilepsy.[38] However, prolonged atypical elementary hallucinations and headache that were initially misdiagnosed as migraine have been described in occipital lobe epilepsy.[39]

More complex visual hallucinations can also occur and are usually stereotyped. Visual illusions of spatial orientation, size, shape, color, continuity, and movement have been reported. Palinopsia (persistence or recurrence of visual images after the stimulus has been removed) is also observed in a defective field or more typically in seizures in a normal visual field. Ictal amaurosis is also well recognized in occipital lobe seizures and may be restricted to a hemifield, may spread to the entire field, or may affect the entire field from onset. In association with these visual symptoms, forced head and eye movements can occur in which the patients feel that they are voluntarily tracking the visual hallucination. Rapid blinking and eyelid flutter have been reported to be reliable indicators of occipital lobe onset if they occur at the start of the seizure. Contraversive nystagmus has also been described.[40] Progression to complex partial and secondary generalized seizures is common. Postictal amaurosis can occur and can be prolonged.

Interictal and ictal EEG recordings can be normal or misleading. Poorly localized discharges, usually over the posterior temporal lobe, are not uncommon. Photosensitivity can occur in up to one-third of patients, but a true photoconvulsive response is much rarer.

LOCALIZATION BY SEMIOLOGY OR BY IMAGING

Jackson originally pointed out that foreign tissue could not itself be the origin of seizure discharges,[2] and thus the question remains whether a lesion is the cause of the seizures even if seizure expression would suggest an origin from a distant site. The current and gradually more accepted belief is well summarized by Williamson[29]—"The older teaching that the relationship between the lesion and seizures needs to be electrographically verified is obsolete. Unless there is strong reason to believe otherwise, such a lesion should be considered the cause of the epilepsy." This is supported by the growing number of studies showing that complete removal of a well-circumscribed lesion is associated with seizure elimination in the majority of patients.[29] Electroclinical diagnoses have thus taken on more of a supporting role in epilepsy surgery and tend to provide evidence of a lesion's epileptogenicity. It is, however, becoming increasingly important to determine how well semiologic classifications localize seizures—through the subsequent success of epilepsy surgery or through correlation with modern neuroimaging—in order to define more properly the role of such classifications. This question has been addressed in a prospective analysis of ictal clinical manifestations correlated with neuroimaging abnormalities that was carried out in 352 seizures.[41] The conclusions reached were interesting and pertinent. Using cluster analysis, 14 clinical groups could be identified. Of these, four were predominantly related to temporal lobe abnormalities: fear/olfactory/gustatory, absence with no focal features, experiential, and visual. The fear/olfactory/gustatory group had in association with these symptoms epigastric sensations, pallor, and pupillary dilatation. The group with absences with no focal features was clinically indistinguishable from the group with petit mal, but was not associated with generalized spike and wave discharges. The experiential group had experiential phenomena typical of temporal lobe epilepsy, such as déjà vu and jamais vu. The visual group had formed and unformed hallucinations as well as micropsia/macropsia as symptoms. Two groups were related to frontal lobe seizures, version/posturing and motor agitation, and were typical of frontal phenomena described above. Interestingly, all these groups, whether showing a frontal or temporal predominance, would still include some patients with lesions of the other lobe. Somatosensory and jacksonian motor seizures, however, were very specific for lesions in the central regions. Further analysis was also carried out in order to see which clinical features (signs or symptoms) were associated with pure frontal and temporal lobe lesions. This analysis supported to some extent the cluster analysis and also demonstrated a strong association of oroalimentary automatisms with temporal lobe abnormalities. Very frequent (>50 per day) or very short (<10 seconds) seizures were associated with pure frontal lobe lesions, and sensitivity to startle was rarely but solely a frontal lobe phenomenon. Interictal EEG spikes and ictal EEG onset tended to be consistent with or more diffuse than lesion localization rather than frankly discordant. It thus seems that few symptom groups can have their lesions localized accurately by seizure semiology, and even in those cases in which there is a correlation, there is still a minority of patients for whom it falsely localizes the lesion.[41] Seizure semiology is thus deficient in this respect and cannot replace localization by neuroimaging. The question arises, "What purpose can an electroclinical diagnosis serve?" and we return to the possible criteria laid down in the introduction: localization, prognosis, response to drug treatment, and neuropsychological and psychiatric outcomes. Although neuroimaging is more accurate for localization, the epileptogenic zone may be larger than the visible lesion. This is because abnormalities may exist at a synaptic or microscopic level well beyond the visible lesion. Indeed, cases of secondary epileptogenesis occurring far from the site of a lesion have been reported.[42] There are also instances in which neuroimaging in patients with partial epilepsy may be reported as normal despite the existence of surgically resectable lesions.[12] This has been noted in some patients with histologically proven end-folium sclerosis and amygdala sclerosis in which a magnetic resonance imaging (MRI) scan can appear normal.[43] In these instances, reliance has to be placed on electroclinical data. Advances in neuroimaging techniques will, however, result in greater sensitivity in detecting such lesions, and thus electroclinical data could take on an almost exclusively confirmatory role.

What of the use of electroclinical diagnosis in determining prognosis, response to drug treatment, and neuropsychological and neuropsychiatric outcomes? There is a dearth of data on each of these, and especially on the response to drug treatment and on the prognosis. This has arisen partly because of the reticence of physicians to apply the ILAE classification and the difficulties in distinguishing partial epilepsy types because of seizure spread and the blurring of anatomic distinctions. Useful information may be missed. Although anatomicopathologic distinctions appear most useful for epilepsy surgery and possibly eventual prognosis, they may not be the determinant of response to antiepileptic drugs. Antiepileptic drugs are known to concentrate in specific brain regions, and it is unknown whether their main action is on brain in the vicinity of the lesion or on the part of the brain that determines the seizure semiology (as has been discussed, these regions may be distinct). Reason would dictate that drugs act where the seizure activity is greatest, i.e., on the area that is most affected—possibly the area determined by electroclinical diagnosis. Similar arguments could be used for neuropsychological and neuropsychiatric outcomes. Thus, although the semiologic classification of epilepsies is taking on a secondary role in determining the localization of resection in epilepsy surgery, it may find a new position in determining response to drug treatment and, to some extent, prognosis. Trials are needed in these areas, and, more important, prospective trials involving cluster analysis such as was performed by Manford et al.[41] are needed to determine a useful, easily applicable, and accurate semiologic classification. In the end, it is not what we believe or hold to be true, but what we find to be true that will best determine clinical practice. It is likely that electroclinical data, neuroimaging, and determination of etiology will all have roles to play in understanding and treating epilepsy.

Acknowledgments

We thank the Wellcome Trust for supporting the work of Dr. Walker.

REFERENCES

1. Temkin O. The Falling Sickness: A History of Epilepsy from the Greeks to the Beginnings of Modern Neurology (2nd ed). Baltimore: John Hopkins, 1971.
2. Jackson JH. In J Taylor (ed), Selected Writings of John Hughlings Jackson. London: Staples, 1958.
3. Gastaut H. Clinical and electroencephalographic classification of epileptic seizures. Epilepsia 1969;10:S2.
4. Commission on Classification and Terminology of the International League Against Epilepsy. Proposal for revised clinical and electroencephalographic classification of epileptic seizures. Epilepsia 1981;22:289.
5. Commission on Classification and Terminology of the International League Against Epilepsy. Proposal for classification of epilepsies and epileptic syndromes. Epilepsia 1985;26:268.
6. Commission on Classification and Terminology of the International League Against Epilepsy. Proposal for revised classification of epilepsies and epileptic syndromes. Epilepsia 1989;30:389.
7. Benbadis SR, Luders HO. Generalized epilepsies. Neurology 1996;46:1194.
8. Fish DR. Blank Spells That are not Typical Absences. In JS Duncan, CP Panayiotopoulos (eds), Typical Absence and Related Epileptic Syndromes. Edinburgh: Churchill Livingstone, 1995;253.
9. Reynolds EH, Andermann F, Panayiotopoulos CP, et al. Debate on the Classification of Epileptic Syndromes with Typical Absences. In JS Duncan, CP Panayiotopoulos (eds), Typical Absence and Related Epileptic Syndromes. Edinburgh: Churchill Livingstone, 1995;300.
10. Walker MC, Sander JW. The impact of new antiepileptic drugs on the prognosis of epilepsy: seizure freedom should be the ultimate goal. Neurology 1996;46:912.
11. Manford M, Hart YM, Sander JW, Shorvon SD. The national general practice study of epilepsy: partial seizure patterns in a general population. Neurology 1992;42:1911.
12. Cook M, Sisodiya SM. Magnetic Resonance Imaging Evaluation for Epilepsy Surgery. In S Shorvon, F Dreifuss, D Fish, D Thomas (eds), The Treatment of Epilepsy. Oxford: Blackwell Science, 1996;589.
13. Wieser HG. Electroclinical Features of the Psychomotor Seizures. Stuttgart: Fisher/Butterworths, 1983.
14. Wieser HG, Kauser W. Limbic Seizures. In HG Wieser, CE Elgar (eds), Presurgical Evaluation of Epileptics: Basis, Techniques, Implications. Berlin: Springer-Verlag, 1987.
15. Wieser HG, Muller RU. Neocortical Temporal Seizures. In HG Wieser, CE Elgar (eds), Presurgical Evaluation of Epileptics: Basis, Techniques, Implications. Berlin: Springer-Verlag, 1987.

16. Delgado-Escueta AV, Bascal FE, Treiman DM. Complex partial seizures on closed circuit television and EEG: a study of 691 attacks in 79 patients. Ann Neurol 1982;11:292.
17. Duncan JS, Sagar HJ. Seizure characteristics, pathology and outcome after temporal lobectomy. Neurology 1987;37:405.
18. Maldonado HM, Delgado-Escueta AV, Walsh GO, et al. Complex partial seizures of hippocampal and amygdala origin. Epilepsia 1987;29:420.
19. Kotagal P, Luders H, Williams G, et al. Temporal lobe complex partial seizures: analysis of symptom clusters and sequences. Epilepsia 1988;29:661.
20. Raymond AA, Fish DR, Sisodiya SM, Shorvon SD. The Developmental Basis of Epilepsy. In S Shorvon, F Dreifuss, D Fish, D Thomas (eds), The Treatment of Epilepsy. Oxford: Blackwell Science, 1996;20.
21. Cavazos J, Sutula TP. Progressive neuronal loss induced by kindling: a possible mechanism for mossy fiber synaptic reorganization and hippocampal sclerosis. Brain Res 1990;527:1.
22. Mathern GW, Babb TL, Vickrey BG, et al. The clinical-pathogenic mechanisms of hippocampal neuron loss and surgical outcomes in temporal lobe epilepsy. Brain 1995;118:105.
23. Trimble MR. The Psychoses of Epilepsy. New York: Raven, 1991.
24. Fish DR. The Role of Scalp Electroencephalography in Presurgical Evaluation. In S Shorvon, F Dreifuss, D Fish, D Thomas (eds), The Treatment of Epilepsy. Oxford: Blackwell Science, 1996;542.
25. Jones-Gotman M. Psychological Evaluation for Epilepsy Surgery. In S Shorvon, F Dreifuss, D Fish, D Thomas (eds), The Treatment of Epilepsy. Oxford: Blackwell Science, 1996;621.
26. Bear D, Fedio P. Quantitative analysis of inter-ictal behavior in temporal lobe epilepsy. Arch Neurol 1977;34:451.
27. Geschwind N. Behavioral changes in temporal lobe epilepsy. Psychol Med 1979;9:217.
28. Fenwick P. Psychiatric Disorder and Epilepsy. In A Hopkins, S Shorvon, G Cascino (eds), Epilepsy. London: Chapman & Hall, 1995;453.
29. Williamson PD. Frontal lobe epilepsy: some clinical characteristics. Adv Neurol 1995;6:127.
30. Chauvel P, Trottier S, Vignal JP, Bancaud J. Somatosensory seizures of frontal lobe origin. Adv Neurol 1992;57:185.
31. Bancaud J, Talairach J. Clinical semiology of frontal lobe seizures. Adv Neurol 1992;57:3.
32. Mauguiere F, Courjon J. Somatosensory epilepsy. Brain 1978;101:307.
33. Penfield W, Jasper HH. Functional Anatomy of the Human Brain. Boston: Little, Brown, 1954.
34. Todd RB. Clinical Lectures on Paralysis, Disease of the Brain and Other Afflictions of the Nervous System. London: Churchill, 1854.
35. Ochs R, Gloor P, Quesney F, et al. Does headturning during a seizure have lateralizing or localizing significance? Neurology 1984;34:884.
36. Upton D, Thompson PJ. General neuropsychological aspects of frontal lobe epilepsy. Epilepsy Res 1996;23:169.
37. Sveinbjornsdottir S, Duncan JS. Parietal and occipital lobe epilepsy: a review. Epilepsia 1993;34:493.
38. Panayiotopoulos CP. Elementary visual hallucinations in migraine and epilepsy. J Neurol Neurosurg Psychiatry 1994;57:1371.
39. Walker MC, Smith SJM, Sisodiya SM, Shorvon SD. A case of simple partial status epilepticus in occipital lobe epilepsy misdiagnosed as migraine: clinical, electrophysiological and magnetic resonance imaging characteristics. Epilepsia 1995;36:1233.
40. Furman JRM, Crumrine PK, Reinmuth OM. Epileptic nystagmus. Ann Neurol 1990;27:686.
41. Manford M, Fish DR, Shorvon SD. An analysis of clinical seizure patterns and their localizing value in frontal and temporal lobe epilepsies. Brain 1996;119:17.
42. Morrell F. Secondary epileptogenic lesions. Epilepsia 1960;1:538.
43. Van Paesschen W, Sisodiya SM, Connelly A, et al. Quantitative hippocampal MRI and intractable temporal lobe epilepsy. Neurology 1995;45:2233.

8
Malignant Syndromes of Childhood Epilepsy

Fritz E. Dreifuss

One of our early forebears in neurology, Samuel Auguste Tissot, in his "Traité de L'Épilepsie,"[1] recognized that symptomatic epilepsies frequently had a grave prognosis. He stated, "If the seizures persist after the first year, if they recur frequently and are triggered by minor incidents, if they seem to overwhelm the child, if there is a site of the body that in all seizures is afflicted first, if there remain features of astonishment in the physiognomy, if the faculties do not develop as one might hope, then one has to fear that the epilepsy will continue forever."[2] Tissot described a patient suffering from what we now call the Lennox-Gastaut syndrome. West[3] first described "a peculiar form of infantile convulsions" in his own son, and in this heart-wrenching manner kindled awareness of the West syndrome. William Lennox in 1945,[4] and subsequently Henri Gastaut and colleagues in 1966,[5] recognized the syndromic nature of the Lennox-Gastaut syndrome. Ohtahara in 1978[6] described early myoclonic encephalopathy with tonic seizures and suppression burst on electroencephalography. Jean Aicardi et al.[7] described the syndrome that bears his name. Rasmussen et al.[8] in 1958 described a chronic progressive continuous focal epilepsy. Patry et al.[9] in 1971 described epileptic status in slow wave sleep in children.

The classification of childhood epilepsies by syndromes became common practice in the 1980s,[10, 11] and the concept of many epilepsies as syndromes was dignified by International League Against Epilepsy acceptance in 1989.[12]

It soon became evident that the prognosis of epileptic seizures, which are the symptoms with which the patient presents, is not so much a function of the nature of the seizures nor of their treatment but rather is predicated on the etiology, and very frequently on the nature, of the syndrome that the seizures represent. It rapidly became evident that many childhood epileptic syndromes—for example, benign epilepsy in childhood with rolandic spikes, benign occipital epilepsy, simple febrile convulsions, and pyknoleptic petit mal with childhood absence seizures—generally have a benign outcome. On the other hand, the syndromes mentioned in the introductory section present the opposite outcome, namely, severe and intractable disorders with striking morbidity and mortality.

157

These were well described by Renier[13] as "the malignant epilepsies of childhood and adolescence."

INDIVIDUAL SYNDROMES

Traditionally, childhood syndromes are considered age-related phenomena.

Seizures in the Neonate

In the neonatal period, the only well-described syndromes are benign, familial, and sporadic, or they are malignant by virtue of the severity of the underlying disorder—be it the result of intrauterine disease or malformation, birth-related injury, or a metabolic disorder that manifests during neonatal age.

Intrauterine disorders appearing in the neonatal period and responsible for a malignant course include infections, such as cytomegalic inclusion disease, toxoplasmosis, or congenital rubella. Perinatal problems include ischemic hypoxic encephalopathy and the results of immaturity, such as germinal matrix hemorrhages. Severely hypoxic children frequently suffer from hypoglycemia or hypocalcemia, which can further lead to severe repercussions. Metabolic disorders in the neonatal period include galactosemia or nonketotic hyperglycinemia. Results of cerebral ischemia may include cerebral infarction, and this may be the end result of maternal drug abuse.

Results of migration disorders of gray matter, various cerebral dysgenesis syndromes, and other malformations caused by genetic or gross chromosomal abnormalities usually manifest themselves later in infancy.

Early Infantile Epileptic Encephalopathies

It is not clear how many distinct entities exist under the rubric of early infantile epileptic encephalopathy (EIEE). The condition described by Ohtahara as EIEE is characterized by onset between the ages of 4 weeks and around 2 years. The seizures consist of tonic extensor spasms, which may look like infantile spasms of particularly early onset. The disease is extremely serious, and many children die within the first year of life. The electroencephalographic (EEG) pattern is characterized by suppression bursts and later may appear as hypsarrhythmia. The cause of this condition is frequently severe cerebral malformation with dysgenesis, but it may also be the result of glycine encephalopathy or other metabolic defects. The finding of hyperglycinemia may dictate treatment with benzodiazepine drugs, which tend to bind to glycine receptors.

Early myoclonic encephalopathy (EME) is characterized by frequent myoclonic and partial seizures. Here the onset is usually between 2 weeks and 3 months of age. The EEG recording again shows suppression bursts, and the pathologic entity is frequently a subcortical cystic brain atrophy. Hypoxic-ischemic encephalopathy or nonketotic hyperglycinemia have been etiologically implicated.

If there is indeed a difference in these two conditions, Ohtahara's disease is more likely to be associated with malformations and EME with metabolic causation.[14]

Pyridoxine Dependency Seizures

Pyridoxine dependency seizures enter into the differential diagnosis of the intractable epilepsies, although it yields to the administration of appropriate amounts of pyridoxine, which rapidly reverses the intractable seizures even in the form of status epilepticus. Prolonged therapy is indicated.[15] Seizures associated with this condition have rarely occurred in utero as the earliest manifestations of an epileptic proclivity.

West Syndrome

Over the years, West syndrome has been recognized for its presenting symptom—infantile spasms—a condition that has to a large degree continued to defy etiologic speculation and therapeutic intervention. The signal symptom is the occurrence of infantile spasms, which are usually flexion spasms of a lightning-like nature that then become tonic, lasting for a few seconds. The flexion seizures are often known as salaam seizures, spasmes salutatoires, or Blitz-Nick-Salaam-Krämpfe. Some patients have extensor spasms rather than the massive jackknife movements, and the tonic extensor spasms are sometimes known as "cheerleader seizures." Characteristically, the condition begins at approximately 3–5 months of age, and about that time there is a halt or reversion of developmental progress. The EEG recording usually shows hypsarrhythmia, and the individual spasms are frequently characterized by a period of voltage depression. It has been said that after attacks, the hypsarrhythmia immediately recommences, but if it does not, the prognosis is much worse.[16] Many causes may be represented by this syndrome, including idiopathic epilepsy (probably on a genetic basis), cryptogenic epilepsy (in which the cause remains obscure, although behaving as a symptomatic epilepsy with evidence of cerebral deficits over and above those associated with seizures), and a clearly symptomatic group, often exemplified by seizures that have a focal signature, a focally abnormal EEG pattern, and stigmata of such conditions as cerebral dysgenesis or tuberous sclerosis. Aicardi's syndrome, which comprises agenesis of the corpus callosum, lacunar retinal degeneration, and a predilection for girls, and syndromes associated with lissencephaly are other conditions of which infantile spasms may be symptomatic.

The EEG pattern in Aicardi's syndrome is not usually truly hypsarrhythmic. There is usually a so-called split-brain abnormality of asymmetry between the two hemispheres. The lissencephalies vary in genetic expression as well as in cortical appearance between simple pachygyria and a smooth cortical surface with underlying band heterotopias, double cortex, nodular subependymal heterotopias, and a variety of other expressions. Hemimegalencephaly is characterized by predominantly unilateral cortical neuronal dysplasia, which may be amenable to hemispherectomy. Tuberous sclerosis is a common etiologic cerebral abnormality associated with the symptomatic form of infantile spasms. The severity of the neurologic syndrome is not necessarily paralleled by the number, location, or size of cortical tubers. In fact, there may only be cutaneous areas of depigmentation. This is similar to other neurocutaneous syndromes, such as hypomelanosis of Ito. On the other hand, in tuberous sclerosis, the tip-off to a severely localized dysmorphic appearance is the presence of asymmetry in the clinical seizure presentation. The finding of a focal brain malformation by magnetic resonance imaging (MRI) or positron emission tomography (PET) scanning in the form of interictal hypometabolism has led to effective surgical intervention.[17]

There is occasionally a relationship between infantile spasms and Down syndrome. The prognosis of spasms in Down syndrome is for especially severe retardation. There has been a suspicion that treatment of hypotonia with serotonin may precipitate the onset of spasms, but this has not been confirmed.[18] There may be an overlap between West syndrome and early infantile encephalopathies, previously described, in terms of age of onset and progression.

The infantile spasms frequently occur in series of 20–40, are usually worse at the time of awakening and sometimes during or after feeding, and the individual seizure may cause the child discomfort sufficient enough to cause crying with each episode. Spasms gradually abate over the course of 10–30 minutes and remain in abeyance for several hours. Treatment of the condition is still quite unsatisfactory. Treatment of choice consists of corticotropin or prednisone, failing which valproic acid, with or without benzodiazepines, may be instituted. This condition affects the age group that is at highest risk for hepatic toxicity with valproic acid, so that the risk/benefit equation of its use has to be carefully considered. Cytomegalic inclusion disease should be excluded before corticotropin is used because of the danger of exacerbating the underlying disease.[19] If the infantile spasms are associated with tuberous sclerosis, vigabatrin may be the drug of choice, as recommended by Chiron et al.[20] Partial seizures, myoclonic seizures, tonic-clonic seizures, or hemiconvulsive seizures have been reported at times to be associated with infantile spasms, and the semiology of the condition is that it frequently evolves into Lennox-Gastaut syndrome with atypical absence, sudden drop attacks, tonic axial seizures, and even generalized tonic-clonic convulsions, which may occur in prolonged attacks.

Type I neurofibromatosis may be associated with infantile spasms, and in this concatenation, the infantile spasms are frequently relatively benign. Before subjecting an infant to a corticotropin regimen with the potential side effects of Cushing's syndrome and hypertension, growth changes, and diminished resistance to infection, a trial of high-dose pyridoxine is frequently recommended. Definitive therapy should not be long withheld, however, as there is some evidence that intellectual prognosis is better with early intervention.

Severe Myoclonic Epilepsy of Infancy

Severe myoclonic epilepsy of infancy was described in detail by Dravet et al.[21] It begins during the first year of life, usually with febrile seizures during the first few months, and there is often a family history of febrile seizures. Seizures may be partial motor seizures or myoclonic attacks. Developmental progress is frequently slowed. The EEG recording shows generalized spike-and-wave (SW) and polyspike and wave activity, early photosensitivity, and some focal abnormalities, usually in the form of excessively slow activity. The seizures are quite resistant to medication, and the patients often become significantly developmentally delayed.

Lennox-Gastaut Syndrome

Lennox-Gastaut syndrome is an epileptic encephalopathy, most commonly observed in childhood, but occasionally appearing in adult life, and consisting of seizures that are axial tonic seizures, atypical absence attacks, atonic drop attacks, or occasionally myoclonic falling spells. The EEG pattern consists of fast (10 counts per second) bursts in sleep and frequently a slow spike wave (1.5–2.5 counts per second) in the waking state, a slowed interictal background, and occasionally prolonged episodes of atypical absence status. The condition may evolve from preceding West syndrome or from an ongoing encephalopathic illness, or it may develop de novo without any antecedent mental or personality impairment.

A slow spike wave was described by Gibbs et al. in 1939[22] but was linked with an epileptic encephalopathy by Lennox and Davis in 1950.[23] Gastaut et al.[5] characterized the disorder in detail in 1966.

Etiology is variable, and it is likely that it is the end result of a variety of encephalopathic disturbances, including static encephalopathies, developmental disorders, encephalitis, porencephaly of vascular origin, and various metabolic disorders. On the other hand, it does suddenly appear in previously normal, healthy children.

The evolution of the syndrome is usually unfavorable, and the individual seizures are extremely resistant to pharmacologic therapy. Although defects in development and neural migration disorders may play an etiologic role in some instances, ablative surgery is usually not indicated by virtue of multifocal encephalopathic involvement as evidenced in MRI and PET scans.

The worst clinical feature is the tendency to drop attacks, which frequently result in cranial and facial trauma and occasionally in broken bones. Occasionally, there are myoclonic manifestations, but these are more common in Lennox-Gastaut syndrome variants rather than the characteristic disease. The condition usually becomes chronic, and although the seizures may lessen over time, the retardation and encephalopathic behavior usually continue. Speech is usually extremely delayed and imperfect. The children are frequently impervious to meaningful contact, have difficulty maintaining their nutrition, and tend to salivate excessively.

Pharmacologic polytherapy is the rule in an attempt at treatment. Valproate occasionally helps in controlling atypical absence attacks, and felbamate has been found to be useful in assuaging all forms of seizures as well as the atypical absence episodes and the drop attacks. This medication is fraught with the hazards of aplastic anemia or hepatic toxicity. Resection of the corpus callosum, in its anterior half or totally, may be helpful in lessening or even obviating the atonic episodes.[24] Lamotrigine, which has not been approved for this purpose in the United States, has been recommended as potentially helpful in European reports. Where a focus can be determined, surgical resection of the affected area may be considered. Clobazam and nitrazepam, among the benzodiazepine drugs, have resulted in transient palliation, but the development of tolerance has usually put a time limit on any beneficial effects with these agents. The ketogenic diet has occasionally been successfully used in alleviating many of the seizures[25] but appears to impart little long-term benefit. Only about 4% of patients with Lennox-Gastaut syndrome achieve remission of seizures and intellectual recovery.

Landau-Kleffner Syndrome

Landau-Kleffner syndrome was first described in 1957[26] and is characterized by a childhood-onset epilepsy associated with receptive aphasia. While the aphasia is usually acquired, it may on occasion present as a developmental aphasia with paroxysmal EEG abnormalities.[27] Seizures characteristically appear but are inconstantly related to the aphasia and appear to bear little immediate relation to it. Usually, there is loss of acquired language, mainly receptive. At the same time, there is a change in developmental progress, and this may progress to an autism-like state. The EEG abnormalities vary from multifocal spikes, which usually become more marked during sleep and involve REM sleep, to a picture that merges into one suggestive of epilepsy with continuous SW during slow wave sleep (ESES), in which there is electrographic status replacing slow wave sleep.

Characteristically, the prognosis for speech development is uncertain, whereas seizures usually respond well to antiepileptic drug therapy. Rarely, seizures and the speech abnormality recover pari passu.[28] Usually, the speech recovery may await the administration of steroids,[29] and there have been reports of successful surgical intervention in the form of multiple subpial transections, usually performed unilaterally on the side of the more pronounced electrographic abnormalities.[30]

Epilepsy With Continuous Spike-and-Wave During Slow Wave Sleep

First described by Patry et al.,[9] epilepsy with ESES is characterized by continuous SW activity occurring during slow wave sleep and occupying no less than 85% of slow wave sleep time. The seizures accompanying this condition may be unilateral or generalized and frequently occur during sleep. EEG abnormalities are frequently present in the waking state in the form of short bursts of generalized SW activity with or without eyelid twitching but become quite marked during slow wave sleep, and they continue in this fashion for months or years, relatively impervious to the administration of antiepileptic drugs. Overt seizure frequency varies from rare to very frequent.

With the passage of time, patients undergo regression in psychomotor development characterized by a decline in IQ scores and the emergence of behavioral disturbances.

Although Landau-Kleffner syndrome enters the differential diagnosis, there may be a specific relationship between the two conditions.

OTHER DISEASES ASSOCIATED WITH A MALIGNANT EPILEPTIC COURSE

Rasmussen's Syndrome

Rasmussen's syndrome[31] is characterized by a progressive, predominantly unilateral encephalopathy with epilepsia partialis continua leading to a hemiplegia. The age of onset is between 14 months and 14 years and in about one-half of cases there is a preceding inflammatory illness. Beginning as simple or complex partial seizures, these gradually lengthen or generalize. The next phase includes increasing hemiparesis and enlargement of the ventricular system on the affected side, and a progressive dementia ensues. The EEG recording begins with unilateral abnormality but ultimately the abnormalities may spread to the contralateral side. The pathologic features are reminiscent of a viral encephalitis involving predominantly cortex with lymphocytic infiltration and perivascular cuffing. Only hemispherectomy offers any tangible benefit, although the use of plasmapheresis and intravenous immune globulin has also been attempted. The finding of abnormalities in glutamate receptor antibody formation promises an awakened interest in this area.[32]

Progressive Myoclonic Epilepsies

Neuronal Storage Diseases

Myoclonic seizures may occur as part of generalized gray-matter disorders. The lipid storage disorders include recessively inherited disorders with ganglioside deposition. GM2 gangliosidosis is Tay-Sachs disease, which is caused by a hexosaminidase-A deficiency. It begins in the first year of life with seizures and decreasing vision. The macular cherry-red spot and the rapid downhill progression are characteristic. Hypotonia and an excessive response to startle occur. In GM1 gangliosidosis, visceromegaly also occurs, the onset is later, and hexosaminidase A and B are involved. Between the ages of 2 and 4 years are seen early ceroid lipofuchsinosis (Batten disease) with macular pigmentary changes, myoclonic seizures, and a progressive dementia. Histologically, curvilinear bodies are seen. Several varieties are described characterized by age of onset and rapidity of progression from early infantile to late juvenile. The sialidoses range from cherry-red spot myoclonus syndrome type 1 with neuraminidase deficiency to galactosialidosis with betagalactosidase defect and an intention tremor in addition to the above. In Gaucher's disease, the storage is beta-cerebroside, and in Niemann-Pick disease, sphingomyelin.

Other generalized gray-matter disorders include Alpers' disease or progressive poliodystrophy, which is characterized by progressive decline with myoclonic and generalized tonic-clonic seizures. One of the important considerations in this condition is the frequency of hepatic cirrhosis, which is often made symptomatic by sodium valproate and may account for a considerable proportion of valproate-associated hepatic failure.

Subacute sclerosing panencephalitis is a measles-related disease with clinical characteristics almost identical to those of progressive poliodystrophy, but the clinical course varies in its duration and may plateau for considerable periods.

Mitochondrial encephalomyopathy, lactic acidosis, and strokelike episodes (MELAS) and myoclonic epilepsy with ragged red fibers (MERRF) are disorders of mitochondrial inheritance that affect respiratory chain enzymes. In addition to ataxia and myoclonus, the clinical findings vary from family to family and include changes in muscle tone and reflexes, the presence or absence of deafness, optic atrophy, neuropathy, lactic acidosis, and alternating hemiplegias and headache.

Lafora's disease is a progressive myoclonic epilepsy with developing dementia and ataxia that usually commences early in childhood and progresses to death early in the third decade. The pathologic marker is the intracytoplasmic poly-glycan inclusion that is found in biopsy specimens of brain, liver, muscle, or the sweat-gland duct epithelium from an axillary full-thickness skin biopsy speci-men. As in most progressive myoclonic epilepsies, the electroencephalographic findings are the occurrence of SW or polyspike-wave generalized bursts of dis-charges on a pathologically slow background.

Unverricht-Lundborg disease is a progressive myoclonic epilepsy with, ulti-mately, an ataxic and a dementing component that is considerably slower in pro-gression than is Lafora's disease. The principal genetic finding is a gene alteration on chromosome 21, and this is common to the Baltic and Mediterranean varieties, suggesting that they are indeed identical in etiology if not in the ethnic groups predominantly involved.

In all of these conditions, an intractable malignant type of epileptic disturbance may be the presenting feature and it certainly supervenes during the evolution of the illness, but ultimately the prognosis is determined by the etiology rather than the epileptic disturbance.

Although therapeutic intervention is frequently futile in assuaging the epilep-tic process in cases of malignant childhood epilepsies, there is much that can be achieved in palliative pursuits as well as in education of the family, genetic coun-seling, and producing some relief with a relatively limited set of expectations. It is quite touching to see a child with Lennox-Gastaut syndrome hugging his or her mother and kissing her goodnight, perhaps the only therapeutic success, and to see how this modest act elicits visible delight in the recipient of the embrace.

REFERENCES

1. Tissot SA. Traité de l'épilepsie faisant le tome troisiemedu traite des nerfs et de leurs maladies. Paris: PF Didot, 1772.
2. Karbowski K. Developments in Epileptology in the 18th and 19th Century Prior to the Delineation of the Lennox-Gastaut Syndrome. In E Niedermeyer, R Degen (eds), The Lennox-Gastaut Syndrome. New York: Liss, 1988.
3. West WJ. On a peculiar form of infantile convulsions. Lancet 1841;1:724.
4. Lennox WG. The petit mal epilepsies; their treatment with Tridione. JAMA 1945;129:1069.
5. Gastaut H, Roger J, Soulayrol R, et al. Childhood epileptic encephalopathy with diffuse slow-spike waves (otherwise known as "petit mal variant") or Lennox syndrome. Epilepsia 1966;7:139.
6. Ohtahara S. Clinico-electrical delineation of epileptic encephalopathies in childhood. Asian Med J 1978;21:499.
7. Aicardi J, Chevrie J-J, Rousselie F. Le syndrome spasmes en flexion, agenesie calleuse, anomalies chorioretiniennes. Arch Fr Pediatr 1969;26:1103.
8. Rasmussen T, Olszewski J, Lloyd-Smith D. Focal seizures due to chronic localized encephalitis. Neurology 1958;8:435.
9. Patry G, Lyagoubi S, Tassinari CA. Subclinical "electrical status epilepticus" induced by sleep in children. Arch Neurol 1971;4:242.
10. Dreifuss FE. Pediatric Epileptology. Boston: John Wright/PSG, 1983.
11. Roger J, Dravet C, Bureau M, et al. Epileptic Syndromes in Infancy, Childhood and Adolescence. London: John Libbey, 1985.
12. Commission on Classification and Terminology of the International League Against Epilepsy. Proposal for revised classification of epilepsy and epileptic syndromes. Epilepsia 1989;30:389.
13. Renier WO. The Malignant Epilepsies of Childhood and Adolescence. In AP Aldenkamp, FE Dreifuss, WO Renier, TPBM Suurmeijer (eds), Epilepsy in Children and Adolescents. Boca Raton, FL: CRC Press, 1995;43.

14. Aicardi J. Early Myoclonic Encephalopathy (Neonatal Myoclonic Encephalopathy). In J Roger, M Bureau, C Dravet, et al. (eds), Epileptic Syndromes in Infancy, Childhood and Adolescence (2nd ed). London: John Libbey, 1992;13.

15. Goutières F, Aicardi J. Atypical presentations of pyridoxine-dependency seizures: a treatable cause of intractable epilepsy in infants. Ann Neurol 1985;17:117.

16. Dulac O, Plouin P, Jambaque I. Predicting favorable outcome in idiopathic West syndrome. Epilepsia 1993;34:747.

17. Chugani HT, Pinard J-M. Surgical Treatment. In O Dulac, HT Chugani, B Dalla Bernadina (eds), Infantile Spasms and West Syndrome. London: Saunders, 1994.

18. Coleman M. Infantile spasms associated with 5-hydroxy-tryptophan-administration in patients with Down's syndrome. Neurology 1971;21:911.

19. Riikonen R. A long-term follow-up study of 214 children with the syndrome of infantile spasms. Neuropediatrics 1987;17:117.

20. Chiron C, Dulac O, Luna D. Vigabatrin in infantile spasms. Lancet 1990;1:363.

21. Dravet C, Bureau M, Roger J. Severe Myoclonic Epilepsy in Infants. In J Roger, C Dravet, M Bureau, et al. (eds), Epileptic Syndromes in Infancy, Childhood and Adolescence. London: John Libbey, 1985.

22. Gibbs FA, Gibbs EL, Lennox WG. The influence of the blood sugar level on the wave and spike formation in petit mal epilepsy. Arch Neurol Psychiatry 1939;41:1111.

23. Lennox WG, Davis JP. Clinical correlates of the fast and the slow spike-wave electroencephalogram. Pediatrics 1950;5/4:626.

24. Andermann F, Olivier O, Gotman J, Sergent J. Callosotomy for the Treatment of Patients with Intractable Epilepsy and the Lennox-Gastaut Syndrome. In E Niedermeyer, R Degen (eds), The Lennox-Gastaut Syndrome. New York: Liss, 1988.

25. Wilder RM. Effects of ketonuria on the course of epilepsy. Mayo Clin Proc 1921;2:307.

26. Landau WM, Kleffner FR. Syndrome of acquired aphasia and convulsive disorder in children. Neurology 1957;7:523.

27. Sato S, Dreifuss FE. Electroencephalographic findings in a patient with developmental expressive aphasia. Neurology 1973;23:181.

28. Deuel RK, Lenn NJ. Treatment of acquired epileptic aphasia. J Pediatr 1977;90:959.

29. Lerman P, Lerman-Sagie T, Kivity S. Effect of early corticosteroid therapy for Landau-Kleffner syndrome. Dev Med Child Neurol 1991;33:257.

30. Morrell F, Whistler W, Bleck T. Multiple sub-pial transections: a new approach to the surgical treatment of focal epilepsies. J Neurosurg 1989;70:231.

31. Andermann F (ed). Chronic Encephalitis and Epilepsy: Rasmussen's Syndrome. Boston: Butterworth–Heinemann, 1991.

32. Andrews PI, Lewis DV, McNamara JO. Clinical and electroencephalographic evidence for epileptogenic autoantibodies in Rasmussen's encephalitis. Epilepsia 1995;36(Suppl 4):107.

9
Benign Syndromes in Childhood Epilepsy

Olivier Dulac

Epileptic disorders in childhood offer a wide diversity of clinical expression and prognosis, ranging from the most benign, with recovery in a few days, to the most severe, with major cognitive and motor deterioration. Epilepsy syndromes have been widely studied over the years, classified by the International League Against Epilepsy,[1] and reviewed in detail.[2] Yet new syndromes are being described, and some patients remain unclassifiable within the presently recognized classification of epileptic syndromes, particularly those syndromes beginning in infancy. Some syndromes are malignant because of the intractability of seizures and deterioration of cognitive function. Other syndromes leave severe cognitive sequelae, although the seizure disorder dies out after a few months or years of evolution. Others exhibit a favorable outcome for seizures and cognitive function throughout their course or although the course of the seizure disorder seems very alarming at some point. Only the latter conditions deserve being qualified as "benign."

Benign epilepsy syndromes comprise neonatal and infantile convulsions, idiopathic generalized epilepsies (IGEs), idiopathic partial epilepsies, and rare cases of epileptogenic encephalopathies.

BENIGN NEONATAL AND INFANTILE EPILEPTIC SYNDROMES

Benign Neonatal Convulsions

Benign neonatal convulsions (NCs) are defined as NCs showing a favorable outcome—i.e., a normal psychomotor development without secondary epilepsy.[3] Following a workshop in Marseille, France, in 1983, two benign epileptic syndromes with convulsions occurring in the first week of life were recognized: benign idiopathic neonatal convulsions (BINNCs), and benign familial neonatal convulsions (BFNNCs). Both are difficult to confirm without prolonged follow-up. To overcome these difficulties, several clinical and electroencephalographic (EEG) cohort studies were conducted that aimed at determining early prognostic features in neonatal seizures with unknown etiology.

Benign Idiopathic Neonatal Convulsions

The incidence of BINNCs ranges from 2% to 7% of all NCs. In a review of series of NCs published before 1979, Plouin[3] found that the outcome was favorable in 120 of the 195 cases with unknown etiology in which the outcome was mentioned. Cases with unknown etiology and favorable outcome accounted for 6.6% of all NCs (range, 0–28%). Sixty-two percent of patients are boys. In 1977, Dehan et al.[4] reported a series of term newborns with NCs of unknown etiology and with favorable outcome. They found that there were two major characteristics: age of onset mainly around the fifth day of life and a particular interictal EEG pattern that they called "théta pointu alternant."

The epidemiologic study performed between 1980 and 1985 in the Oise area of France included 217 epileptic patients having a first seizure within the first 10 years of life. Patients were followed for more than 6 years, disclosing 16 patients with BINNCs.[5, 6] North et al.[7] insisted that no case was observed in their department between 1982 and 1989, raising the question of an epidemic having occurred in the 1970s.

First seizures appear between 1 and 7 days of life; 97% appear between days 3 and 7. A few patients with similar characteristics may begin seizures by the end of the first month of life.[8] The seizures are clonic, mostly partial, affecting one side and then the other, or apneic, but not tonic. Apneic seizures involved 31% of patients of one series.[7] Seizures last 1–3 minutes and are repeated frequently during 2 hours to 3 days (mean, 20 hours). Patients are interictally normal at onset but become progressively drowsy and hypotonic, partly because of drug administration, and they remain so for several days after the last seizures before recovering.

Interictal EEG recordings show in 60% of cases a dominant theta activity, alternating or discontinuous, unreactive, with sharp waves and frequent interhemispheric asynergy. This nonspecific aspect may be seen in cases of convulsions related to hypocalcemia, meningitis, and subarachnoid hemorrhage, and it correlates with good prognosis. The ictal pattern consists of rhythmic spikes and rhythmic slow waves, localized in any area, but mostly unilateral rolandic and most often involving alternately both hemispheres, unilateral before becoming generalized, or immediately generalized. There is no alpha-like ictal pattern. Seizures are electroclinical at onset but may become subclinical in the course of the cluster.

The etiology remains unknown, since infectious, toxic, and metabolic causes and malformations have been excluded. Acute zinc deficiency was suggested but not confirmed.[9] Treatment is usually poorly effective. Long-term outcome data are poor since follow-up rarely exceeds a few years (6 months to 6 years). Psychomotor retardation, simple febrile convulsions, afebrile seizures, and microcephaly are on record, which raises a question about the term "benign."

Benign Familial Neonatal Convulsions

More than 25 families with BFNNCs have been reported with autosomal dominant transmission over one to five generations.[3] Birth is at full term without any sign of distress and with a free interval before the first seizures. In 80% of cases, convulsions occur on the second or third day of life, although in occasional cases onset at up to 3 months of age has been reported. Seizures are motor clonic, unilateral or bilateral, apneic, or eventually tonic as shown by video-EEG recording.[10] They last 1–3 minutes, frequently are repeated for a few days, and then become occasional for a few weeks. The interictal EEG recording rarely shows "théta pointu alternant" tracing. No pattern suggesting poor prognosis, such as a paroxysmal or inactive EEG pattern, has been reported. Although the outcome is favorable, 10–15% of the patients exhibit rare nonfebrile seizures later in life and fewer have febrile convulsions (FCs), with a rate similar to that of the general population. In several families, the disorder is linked to chromosome 20q.[11, 12] In 15–20% of families, the disorder is not linked to chromosome 20q: In one family, it was linked to chromosome 8.[13]

Thus, BFNNCs differ from BINNCs in many respects: genetic background, age of onset and cessation of convulsions, and occurrence of epilepsy.

Benign Infantile Convulsions (Idiopathic Partial Epilepsy of Infancy)

Japanese authors have reported benign infantile convulsions (idiopathic partial epilepsy of infancy). Patients exhibit clusters of seizures over a few days, between the ages of 3 and 20 months, and have favorable outcomes.[14, 15] Seizures are focal or secondarily generalized, are repeated three to five times a day for 1–3 days, the cluster itself being eventually repeated 1–3 months later. The interictal EEG pattern is normal. Ictal discharges show rhythmic activity localized to the parietal or occipital areas in patients with secondarily generalized seizures and to the temporal area in those with complex partial seizures. One-half of the cases have first-degree relatives with afebrile seizures in the same age range. The latter probably belong to the syndrome described as "benign familial infantile convulsions" (BFICs).

Benign Familial Infantile Convulsions

BFICs were first reported in Italy[16] and later in Japan[15] and France[17] as clusters of focal seizures eventually shifting from one side of the body to the other beginning between 3 and 8 months of age and transmitted as an autosomal dominant trait. Between seizures, the EEG pattern is normal. The outcome is excellent. Thirty-one cases could be collected in France, with the patients beginning nonsymptomatic convulsions between 1 and 12 months of age (mean, 6 months).[18] Seizures were brief (less than 5 minutes in most cases), occurring in clusters of up to 12 a day during 1–4 days. Seizures were of a single type, most often secondarily generalized. Partial onset seizures were confirmed on ictal EEG discharges recorded in six cases. Between seizures during a cluster, the EEG pattern showed focal spikes in 19 of 27 recordings, involving various areas depending on ictal manifestations. Following the cluster, the EEG pattern was normal. Recurrence of seizures was exceptional, with or without treatment. Familial recurrence involved one-third of the cases, suggesting an autosomal dominant mode of inheritance. Malafosse et al.[19] showed in Italian families that this condition was not genetically linked to BFNNCs but to chromosome 19.[20]

Benign infantile convulsions (BICs) do not seem to differ from BFICs, and, indeed, the first Japanese cases of BFICs were reported within a series of non-familial cases.[14, 15] Molecular biology studies are necessary to determine whether sporadic and familial cases have similar etiologies. BFNNCs and BFICs are heterogenous, but further data are needed to determine whether the clinical expression—i.e., partial versus generalized seizures—is linked to the gene involved within a single age range.

IDIOPATHIC GENERALIZED EPILEPSIES

IGEs were the first to be identified as epileptic syndromes. IGEs share generalized seizures and spike waves (SWs) and usually a favorable outcome.[21] They comprise cases with absence, myoclonic, and tonic-clonic seizures. Cases with absences are distinguished in childhood and juvenile absences, based on age of onset, seizure semiology and frequency, and outcome differences. Cases with myoclonic seizures were first identified in adolescence, then in infancy, but cases in childhood are being identified. Cases with tonic-clonic seizures were first recognized in adolescence as awakening epilepsy (generalized grand mal [GMA]), but cases are now being identified in childhood. In addition to cases with a single or predominant seizure type, in many patients several seizure types are combined—i.e., juvenile absence and myoclonic epilepsy or juvenile myoclonic (JME) and GMA. The most striking condition is myoclonic astatic syndrome, which often combines the three seizure types and in which only one-half of the patients experience a favorable outcome, thus sharing clinical and EEG features of IGE.

Benign Myoclonic Epilepsy of Infancy

Benign myoclonic epilepsy of infancy is rare. The incidence seems to be less than 1% of all epilepsies in childhood. However, these data are based on studies performed in tertiary reference centers, which mainly deal with intractable cases, and therefore may underestimate the number of benign cases. Boys are affected twice as often as girls. The rate of familial antecedents in a combined series of 37 cases was 31% for febrile convulsions and 25% for epilepsy.[22] Febrile convulsions occur in 28% of patients, most often before the first myoclonic fits.

First seizures occur between 4 months and 3 years of age. They consist of brief, generalized myoclonic attacks (MAs) of varying intensity. They appear as head nodding or loss of tone, exceptionally causing the patient to fall. On video-polygraphy they appear as massive myoclonic jerks, with upward outward movements of the upper limbs, flexion of the head and lower limbs, and, eventually, rolling of the eyes. Mild jerks only produce forward movements of the head. Severe ones produce falls or projections of objects held by the child. The attacks are brief (1–3 seconds), rarely longer (5–10 seconds), especially in older children and consist of rhythmically repeated jerks with mild or no reduction of alertness. On EEG recordings, MAs consist of bursts of generalized SWs or polyspike waves (PSWs), isolated or in brief clusters of two or three. Jerks are correlated to the spike or polyspike and may be followed by a brief atonia correlated to the slow wave. Bursts are occasionally triggered by intermittent light stimulation, more often by drowsiness. The background activity is normal, and there seldom are SWs without concomitant clinical manifestations.

There are no other types of seizures. Psychomotor development and neurologic examination findings are normal in most instances. Valproate (VPA) and ethosuximide (ESM) monotherapy are effective treatments. The outcome is usually favorable. However, a small proportion of patients exhibit mental retardation with behavioral problems during the course of the disease, particularly in those with early onset or when the diagnosis is overlooked, in whom it is difficult to assess development before the first seizures. Similar cases with onset in childhood have been reported.[23]

Reflex Myoclonic Epilepsy in Infancy

In one series, six infants started experiencing massive myoclonic jerks between 6 and 20 months of age.[24] They consisted of 5 to 20 generalized jerks each day as the only seizure type, isolated or as brief bursts lasting a fraction of a second to a few seconds, and correlated with generalized SWs on EEG recordings. Auditory and tactile stimuli were precipitating factors, not light stimulation. Spontaneous jerks were rare. There were few interictal paroxysmal abnormalities. Three patients ceased having seizures spontaneously after 4–7 months: the others had them controlled with VPA.

Eyelid Myoclonia with Absences

Eyelid myoclonia with absences is an often overlooked condition mainly involving girls; prevalence is unknown.[25, 26] Onset is between 2 and 4 years of age. The condition consists of jerks of the eyelids and eventually the head, lasting 1–3 seconds. It is difficult to determine whether there is loss of consciousness. The seizures recur several times a day with clear photosensitivity. Occasional generalized tonic-clonic seizures (GTCSs) occur between 6 and 20 years of age.

Ictal EEG recordings show generalized bursts of PSWs and SWs, often triggered by photic stimulation. Interictal EEG recordings appear normal. Carbamazepine (CBZ) may worsen the condition, whereas VPA and ESM alone or in combination may control seizures. There is no tendency to spontaneous recovery. The term "benign" is therefore disputable.

Myoclonic Astatic Epilepsy

Myoclonic astatic epilepsy (MAE) was first identified by Doose[27] as a group with mixed seizure types and psychomotor deterioration that could be distinguished from Lennox-Gastaut syndrome, since there were EEG characteristics of IGE—i.e., 3-hertz (Hz) generalized SWs. However, in contrast to other types of IGEs, MAE shows a wide range of outcomes, including severe mental deterioration with persistence of intractable seizures in a sizable number of patients. Nevertheless, one-half of the patients recover completely after a few months or years, suggesting that in some cases the course is indeed that of a benign epilepsy of idiopathic origin.

In a retrospective review of 62 children with epilepsy and myoclonus 1–10 years old, Dulac et al.[28] identified 16 patients with mixed seizure types who had stopped having seizures for more than 2 years at the end of followup. Onset ranged from 18 months to 4 years of age with generalized tonic-clonic or clonic seizures. A mean 3 months later, massive epileptic myoclonus occurred together with absences. This period with mixed seizures lasted a mean 10 months during which seizure frequency fluctuated and the patients were ataxic and hyperkinetic. Eleven patients had an episode of absence status lasting a few hours to a few days. The EEG recordings showed rhythmic slow activity notched with spikes, which is different from the slow SW pattern of Lennox-Gastaut syndrome. There was no photosensitivity. The overall duration of seizures was 16 months, with a few nocturnal convulsive seizures at the end.

In a complementary study, it was shown that this group with a favorable outcome could be distinguished from other patients whose seizure disorder began the same way but evolved unfavorably. Indeed, the latter suffered, a few months after onset, from long-lasting episodes of myoclonic status during which the patient had erratic myoclonus of the face and extremities, generalized vibratory tonic seizures, and obtundation.[29] During these episodes, which lasted several months, the patient suffered considerable deterioration of cognitive functions. Factors triggering these episodes of status remain to be identified. However, various antiepileptic compounds, mainly CBZ[30] and vigabatrin (VGB),[31] seem to be major contributors. Outcome is unfavorable, with persistence of intractable tonic seizures occurring in clusters at the end of each night's sleep.

The use of CBZ, phenytoin (PHT), and phenobarbital (PB), which are shown to eventually worsen myoclonic or absence seizures, should undoubtedly be avoided in treatment.[30, 32] VPA contributes to reduce tonic-clonic and absence seizures, and ESM reduces myoclonic and absence seizures. Therefore, this combination is the base of treatment. It must take into account metabolic interactions for the choice of the dose of ESM. Benzodiazepines may also contribute during episodes of daily seizures.

Epilepsy with Generalized Tonic-Clonic Seizures in Childhood

Epilepsy with GTCSs is less frequent in childhood than in adolescence, is evenly distributed in patients between 3 and 11 years old, often begins with FCs, has a low-seizure frequency, and has an excellent prognosis for seizures. One-half of the patients exhibit generalized SWs. GTCSs can be associated with absences, from the onset, in which case the group is no different from GTCSs occurring alone, or the absences can precede the occurrence of the GTCSs, in which case the absences are frequent, rarely preceded by FCs, and have a higher recurrence rate on withdrawal of medication.[33]

Childhood Absence Epilepsy

Childhood absence epilepsy (CAE) consists of frequent typical absences as a single seizure type, beginning in early childhood, mainly in girls with previously normal development and no evidence of brain damage. Onset is between 3 and 12 years of age, with a peak at 6–7 years. Seizures last 5–10 seconds, rarely more than 30 seconds. The onset and end are abrupt and the patient carries on her activity as if nothing had happened. Cessation of activity and of awareness are characteristic of simple absences.[34] A mild clonic component involves the upper eyelids or the chin, lips, and face. Rarely, jerks of the upper limbs raise the possibility of myoclonic absences in the differential diagnosis. Atonic, tonic, or version components are most unusual. Some patients exhibit autonomic features, such as urination or automatisms, that may be perseveration of ongoing activity or occurring de novo. Seizures are frequent, ranging from 10 to 200 a day. Precipitating factors include release of attention, drowsiness, emotion, and especially hyperventilation, which is practically constant.

Ictal EEG recordings show rhythmic bilateral synchronous 3-Hz SWs with abrupt onset and mild slowing down at the end, around 2.5–2.0 Hz.[35] Moderate variations in amplitude and rhythm and the presence of PSWs do not modify the prognosis.

The interictal EEG pattern comprises normal background activity and brief bursts of bilateral SWs, particularly during nonrapid eye movement (NREM) sleep. Some children exhibit bursts of posterior rhythmic, usually asymmetric, 3-Hz slow waves that are blocked by opening the eyes and enhanced by hyperventilation.

Outcome is favorable in a majority of patients, the proportion of which is difficult to determine with presently available medications. Indeed, prognosis depends on drug choice.[36] In addition, subsequent occurrence of GTCSs involves about 40% of patients. The latter begin at 10–15 years of age, eventually later in adulthood, are infrequent, and are easily controlled. Factors predisposing to GTCSs are late-onset absences (after the age of 8 years), male sex, type of drug prescribed, poor response to treatment, and the presence of photosensitivity on EEG recordings, whereas bursts of posterior rhythmic slow waves are seldom followed by GTCSs. Early-onset GTCSs, before 15 years of age, would tend to be more frequent than later-onset GTCSs.[37, 38] Social prognosis once was considered unfavorable in these children with previously normal development, but polymedication may have played a role in these old studies.[39]

Treatment involves VPA, ESM, and lamotrigine (LTG). VPA may be preferred because of the later risk of GTCSs. However, most often GTCSs occur several years after absences have ceased and treatment has been withdrawn. ESM is equally effective and should be given as monotherapy, since the risk of GTCSs is low at this age. Both drugs carry a risk of idiosyncratic side effects, and there is no evidence that one drug is safer than the other. Thus, whereas VPA is preferred in Europe, ESM in more often prescribed in the United States. In case of inefficacy, the alternate monotherapy or eventually a combination is usually effective. In the latter case, it is important to lower the dose of ESM because of metabolic interaction. Benzodiazepines—i.e., clobazam and clonazepam—are rarely helpful because of side effects and potential intolerance. LTG seems very effective, including in patients with seizures intractable to VPA and ESM[40] alone and even more so combined with VPA.[41] The main restriction is high cost, making it a third choice in the armamentarium.

Juvenile Absence Epilepsy

Juvenile absence epilepsy (JAE) was first differentiated from CAE by Janz and Christian[42] and by Doose et al.[43] based on the lower frequency of absences, their occurrence in clusters, the combination with tonic-clonic seizures, and the peak of onset between 10 and 12 years of age. Whether JAE is neurobiologically different from CAE or part of a single spectrum remains open to question.[44, 45] The incidence of JAE is unknown but is supposed to be considerably lower than that of CAE. There is a slight preponderance of males with CAE, in contrast to JAE. Although there is clearly a moderately increased incidence of familial cases, the family picture is less homogenous than that of JME.

Age of onset is difficult to determine, depending on whether the cohorts studied were treated at pediatric or adult neurology centers. It peaks at the end of the first decade and the beginning of the second. Ictal manifestations consist of absences with less consciousness impairment and less retropulsive phenomena compared with CAE.[46, 47]

The proportion of patients with GTCSs is high but difficult to determine, since many JAE patients seek medical advice after the first GTCS, sometimes long after the first absences. Most GTCSs occur on awakening. In addition, 16% of patients exhibit myoclonic seizures of the type of JME. Other seizure types have not been reported.

The background EEG activity is usually normal. SW frequency is high (3.5–4.0 Hz) and precipitated by sleep deprivation and hyperventilation. The slow wave is often preceded by two or three spikes. Panayiotopoulos et al.[48] found JAE absences to be longer (16.3 ± 7.15) than those of CAE or JME and to show fragmentation unlike that in CAE. Photosensitivity is infrequent, occurring in 7.5–18% of patients.

Treatment with ESM and VPA is usually effective for absences and for GTCSs in more than 80% of cases.[49] Sometimes both need to be combined. LTG is also effective, but studies with this compound did not distinguish JAE from CAE.[40, 41]

Juvenile Myoclonic Epilepsy

JME was first described by Herpin[50] but studied with particular detail by Janz and Christian.[42] The prevalence is between 4% and 5% of epileptic patients, and around 15% of those with IGE.[51, 52] The sex ratio distribution is equal.

Mean age of onset is 15 years, three-fourths of patients being between 12 and 18 years old; the age at onset is slightly younger for those who are photosensitive than for those who are not. However, the precise age is often difficult to determine, since the disorder is often overlooked for months before medical attention is sought; a mean 13-year delay has been reported.[53] Jerks are bilateral, not always symmetric, single or in repetition, rapid, and of variable amplitude. They mostly involve the upper limbs and rarely cause the patient to fall. Sleep deprivation is a precipitating factor. Whereas only 10% of patients are clinically sensitive to light stimulation, 90% of patients also have GTCSs, two-thirds of which occur on awakening, often preceded by a series of myoclonic jerks; 20–30% of the patients also have absences, most of whom have had JAE, although 3–4% have had CAE.

Interictal EEG recordings show normal background activity. Generalized PSWs are combined with clinical jerks, the intensity of which is correlated with the number of spikes of the PSW complex. When PSWs are interictal, there are no more than two or three spikes. Only patients with previous CAE may also exhibit 3-Hz SWs.[54] Twenty-five to forty percent of patients are photosensitive, which is the highest rate in idiopathic epilepsy. Precipitation of PSWs and jerks by eye closure occurs in 20% of patients. Polygraphic studies have shown that the highest rate of PSWs is in nocturnal awakening, followed by morning awakenings.[55]

One-fourth of the patients have a family history of epilepsy, the relatives having GTCSs (85%), myoclonic epilepsy (14%), JAE (12%), and CAE (3–4%).[51] The rate seems higher for girls than boys. Polygenic[51] and autosomal recessive inheritance[56] have been suggested, the latter in a highly consanguineous population. A linkage to chromosome 6p has been suggested[57] but still remains to be confirmed. There may be genetic heterogeneity, and several loci may be involved. Another open question is whether the same genes are involved for all or several types of IGEs, since there is clear overlap between different syndromes, particularly in adolescence.

VPA seems at present to be the most effective drug, with more than 85% of patients controlled in monotherapy.[58] PB and acetazolamide may also be effective,[59] as may LTG.[60] Clonazepam is effective on myoclonic seizures but disappointing on concomitant GTCSs.[61] Although good control is often obtained, the disorder is not cured, since more than 90% of patients relapse, often when withdrawal is attempted. This is the highest relapse rate among epilepsy syndromes;[62] the term "benign" is therefore disputable.

Epilepsy with Grand Mal on Awakening

First identified by Gowers in 1885,[63] awakening epilepsy was described in detail by Janz.[64] Epilepsy with grand mal on awakening (GMA) consists of generalized tonic-clonic seizures occurring mostly on awakening, sometimes in late afternoon. The incidence varies between 22% and 37% of patients with GTCSs, with a slight male preponderance. There are significantly more familial antecedents for GMA (12%) than for other types of GMs.[54]

Onset is usually at the end of the first decade, 78% of patients having the first seizure between 6 and 12 years of age.[65] In other GMs, there is no clear peak of age of onset.

Seizures are generalized tonic-clonic and some patients also have absences or myoclonic seizures, sometimes preceding the GTCS.

Leder[66] has reported particular psychological characteristics, based on Rorschach and Szond tests—patients were extroverted, unable to renounce, and they followed simultaneously irreconcilable aims without being aware of difficulties. This could explain the poor compliance with treatment and irregular lifestyle that often characterize these patients and contribute to provoked seizures.[67] Sleep deficit, excessive alcohol intake, and sudden external arousal are the major precipitating factors.[63] Whether menstruation contributes remains controversial.[64, 68] Precipitating factors involve three-fourths of the patients.

EEG recordings show generalized SWs in one-half of the patients with pure GMA. Seventy percent of patients with additional myoclonus or absences have SWs. Wolf and Inoue[46] found that sleep organization was affected by antiepileptic drugs: There was more than an average amount of NREM sleep in the first cycle with PB, and a decrease of stage II and of cycle duration with PHT. This suggests that sleep is particularly unstable and affected by external stimuli. Patients with persisting seizures exhibit a secondary change in circadian seizure distribution, with seizures occurring in the evening instead of on awakening.[69] Published neuropathologic data concern eight patients, seven of whom showed various microdysgenesic features, with significant differences when compared with controls.[70] However, the pathogenetic significance of these findings remains disputed.[71]

PB and VPA[58] seem to be better than PHT and CBZ for the treatment of GMA.

Photosensitive Epilepsies

Among the various abnormal responses produced by intermittent photic stimulation (IPS), generalized SW activity is correlated with the occurrence of epileptic seizures, the highest risk being when photoconvulsive reaction (PCR; i.e., SW) is self-sustained and continues for more than 100 ms after cessation of stimulation.[72] More than 70% of patients with PCR exhibit seizures,[73] the figure reaching 95% for self-sustained PCR. Sensitivity to linear patterns involves 30% of IPS-sensitive patients.[74] The highest range of sensitivity is 15–18 Hz, and sensitivity is increased by linear pattern and reduced by monocular fixation. Five percent of epileptic patients and 25% of those with IGE are photosensitive;[75, 76] the age of highest incidence being between 12 and 14 years. Two-thirds of patients are girls. In 80% of cases, seizures are triggered by environmental stimuli, television, flickering sunlight, or video games.

Forty percent of patients have purely photosensitive epilepsy without spontaneous seizures; 84% consist of GTCSs, 62% of absences, 2.5% of partial seizures, and 1.5% of myoclonic seizures.[77] In addition to the other 60% of patients having spontaneous epilepsy and photosensitivity, a number of photosensitive patients never have seizures.

Attention has been called to video game epilepsy. It begins in the second decade, with an incidence of 1–5 per 100,000, involving 10% of new epilepsy cases in this age range. In the United Kingdom, one-third of photosensitive patients had their first seizure triggered by video games.[78] In addition, 5% of patients in this epidemiologic study were not conventionally photosensitive, although they had recurrent GTCSs triggered by video games.

There is a high genetic predisposition to photosensitivity, 40% of siblings also being photosensitive.[79] JME is the idiopathic epilepsy syndrome in which the prevalence of photosensitivity is the highest—more than 30%,[80] followed by CAE (18%) and GMA (13%), but the incidence of photosensitivity is higher for severe epilepsies, including severe myoclonic epilepsies of infancy, Lafora's body disease, Gaucher's disease, and, particularly, Baltic myoclonus. It also involves 5% of cryptogenic and symptomatic epilepsies.[77]

Self-induction may be seen in mentally retarded patients by waving a hand in front of the eyes, or, in patients with normal intelligence, by closing the eyes slowly. The latter condition may be difficult to distinguish from the eyelid myoclonia syndrome.

Photosensitivity is controlled acutely by various drugs, and this is used as a test to detect antiepileptic potentials of new compounds.[81] For chronic administration,

VPA is the most effective. In practice, it may be preferable to avoid the causative stimulus: Television should be viewed under bright ambient light at a distance of more than 2 meters, and one eye should be covered when approaching the set, or a set with a small screen should be used.[82] More sophisticated methods, such as use of Polaroid spectacles, are difficult in practice.

The prognosis for seizure control varies in the different IGE syndromes, the best being for CAE. The prognosis for psychosocial integration and schooling is also variable, even for patients who have complete seizure control. Desguerre et al.[6] in an epidemiologic study found that patients who had recovered from IGE with convulsive seizures experienced more schooling difficulties than patients with infantile absence or idiopathic partial epilepsies.

IDIOPATHIC PARTIAL EPILEPSIES IN CHILDHOOD

The group of idiopathic partial epilepsies in childhood shares age of onset, partial seizures, focal interictal spikes, and favorable outcome. The diagnosis is based on clinical and EEG grounds, and, in order to avoid misdiagnosis, it is important to be very strict when gathering the various diagnostic criteria given by Dalla Bernardina et al.[83]: lack of neurologic or cognitive defect, age of onset after 18 months, a single type of seizure in a given patient, no tonic or reflex seizures, and normal interictal clinical condition. The frequency of seizures may be high at onset, but it never increases. Status epilepticus may occur as the initial event. The EEG recordings show normal background activity and focal or multifocal spikes that are activated by sleep but remain with similar morphology. There are no PSWs or periods of suppression of activity following the spikes. Continuous SWs during slow sleep may develop, particularly with CBZ therapy, and this condition may be combined with atypical absences and cognitive deterioration. Evoked potentials, somatosensory or visual according to the type of epilepsy, are occasionally giant, but their latency and morphology are unchanged.[84, 85]

Benign Partial Epilepsy with Centrotemporal Spikes

Benign partial epilepsy with centrotemporal spikes (BECT) is the most frequently observed, accounting for 10–20% of all cases of childhood epilepsy.[5, 86] Centrotemporal spikes were first recognized by Gastaut as not being related to a focal lesion.[87] The clinical symptoms observed in patients with these spikes were reported by Nayrac and Beaussart,[88] Faure and Loiseau,[89] and Gibbs and Gibbs.[90] Gibbs et al.[91] were the first to notice that centrotemporal spikes could occur in children without seizures, and Cavazzuti et al.[92] found that this was the case in 2% of school-age children and that they tended to disappear by the end of the first decade.

Past history is usually uneventful. Febrile convulsions in 7–9%, neonatal difficulties in 6–10%, and mild head injuries in 4–5% do not seem to contribute to the epilepsy. The sex ratio is 3 boys to 2 girls.

The age of onset ranges from 3 to 13 years; in 76% of patients onset is between 5 and 10 years with two peaks at 4 and 10 years. Most seizures occur only during sleep, whereas only 12–20% occur in the waking state only. Typical seizures occur on awakening in a 5- to 10-year-old child who is conscious, starting with numbness in the tongue, gums, or cheek on one side and speech loss before a few hemifacial jerks occur. The seizure eventually spreads to the upper limb, rarely to the lower one. In younger children, 2–5 years old, generalization merely happens when seizures occur in sleep, and long seizures are rare. Ictal abdominal pain, vertigo, flashing lights, blindness, and absences have been reported.[93, 94] Seizures last a few seconds to 2 minutes. Nocturnal seizures tend to be longer.

Interictal EEG recordings disclose normal background activity and sleep organization and diphasic, high-voltage, blunt, centrotemporal spikes, at times followed by a slow wave and often occurring in clusters. In 60% of cases, the focus is unilateral, sometimes shifting from one side to the other. Spikes are activated by sleep and tend to become generalized, and occasionally activation may lead to continuous SWs during slow sleep.[95] Sometimes centrotemporal spikes can only be recorded during sleep. In addition to centrotemporal spikes, some patients have generalized SWs: 40% during drowsiness.[96] Occipital spikes are also occasionally recorded. In all patients, EEG activity normalizes within 6 months to 6 years.[97] There is no correlation between the intensity of spike discharges and the frequency of seizures.

The ictal EEG activity was recorded in a nocturnal stage II seizure.[98] It showed rhythmic spikes in the left central region, then involving the vertex and temporal regions, while the patient was showing tonic contraction and clonic jerks of the right facial area. A similar seizure was reported during daytime.[99]

A genetic predisposition is highlighted by up to 40% of close relatives having a history of convulsions or epilepsy. In a genetic study of 19 probands, Heijbel et al.[100] could show that centrotemporal spike loci were transmitted as an autosomal dominant trait. However, it is most likely that the epilepsy itself is transmitted in a multifactorial mode.

For diagnosis, the combination of clinical and EEG characteristics, when indisputable, is sufficient. Radiologic investigations, even computed tomographic (CT) scans, are superfluous. Rare cases of BECT in patients with brain lesions, including callosal agenesis or hemiparesis, have been reported as a coincidental occurrence.[101, 102] However, in all cases, clinical findings indicated additional neurologic abnormalities.

Drug treatment is only required in cases where the seizures are frequent or socially disabling—i.e., in less than one-fourth of the cases—and usually after the third seizure. Although the use of PHT[99] and CBZ[30] has been advised, these drugs produce more side effects than VPA[103] and clobazam,[104] which have been shown to be similarly effective. In addition, CBZ may produce a major increase of SW activity in sleep, with atypical absences and drop attacks during the day.[30]

Status epilepticus has been reported early in the disease.[105] After a first seizure, there is an 85% risk of recurrence, but more than two-thirds of patients have few seizures, recurring once every 2–12 months, and they do not require any treatment.[106, 107] Although in up to 20% of patients seizures persist despite treatment, the course is favorable in all cases[108] since seizures do not recur beyond adolescence.

A particular type of BECT has been reported by Dalla Bernardina et al.[109] and later called "atypical BECT" by Aicardi and Chevrie.[110] It begins between the ages of 2 and 6 years and comprises atypical absences and drop attacks in addition to earlier partial motor fits combined with continuous SWs in slow sleep after the initial pattern of centrotemporal spikes. In fact, most patients experienced worsening after the administration of CBZ.[30]

The psychosocial impact of the disease has been shown to depend on the quality of information the parents and teachers receive.[97] The overall social prognosis is good when a good prognosis has been given early in the course of the disorder.

Benign Partial Epilepsy of Childhood with Occipital Paroxysms

Diagnosis of benign partial epilepsy of childhood with occipital paroxysms (EOP) may be difficult because the nosologic limits are unclear. EOP is five times less frequent than BECT. It is characterized by the combination of visual or motor seizures with occipital SWs attenuated when opening the eyes.

The age of onset ranges from 2 to 5 years, with more than 30% of the patients having a family history of seizures and 15% of migraine. As in BECT, a history of febrile convulsions and perinatal distress, although slightly higher than in the general population, does not seem to have contributed to occurrence of the syndrome.

Seizures are visual or motor. Visual symptoms account for 30% of the cases.[111] They consist of amaurosis, usually preceded by partial loss of visual field, elementary hallucinations, or complex visual hallucinations or illusions. Motor seizures consist of hemiclonic fits or generalization: some patients exhibit dysphasia, dysesthesia, or adversive events. After the seizure, 33% of patients suffer headache. A small proportion have other symptoms of migraine, including nausea and vomiting.

The frequency and severity of the seizures vary. Several authors have called attention to the occasional presentation with status epilepticus,[112] and a number of patients end up in the intensive care unit although the outcome is most often benign: loss of consciousness for up to 12 hours is combined with tonic lateral deviation of the eyes followed by unilateral or generalized convulsion.

Panayiotopoulos[113] distinguished two groups of patients with idiopathic occipital epilepsy. In one group, the disease begins between the ages of 2 and 8 years, with a peak at 5 years and remission before age 12. A similar group was reported by Vigevano et al.,[114] with seizures beginning between 2 and 6 years of age. Seizures are prolonged and comprise nausea and vomiting, lateral deviation of the eyes, impaired consciousness, and hemiconvulsion. Lack of visual symptoms is striking, although occasional patients suffer from dizziness and visual illusions. The seizures are nocturnal, lasting 15–120 minutes, depending on the time lag to treatment administration. They are often sporadic, with one-third of the patients experiencing no recurrence after the first seizure and other patients exhibiting no seizure after the age of 12 years. Some patients also have rare oropharyngeal clonic seizures. In one case, ictal EEG recordings showed widespread 1- to 2-Hz temporo-occipital waves intermingled with spikes.[115] Interictal EEG recordings show high-amplitude occipital spikes sometimes followed by a slow wave contralateral to the clinical manifestation. They occur with the eyes open and closed. Photic stimulation is ineffective. Some patients also have rolandic spikes. In these patients, treatment may not be warranted.

The second group has a later onset with mainly diurnal seizures with visual symptoms followed by hemiconvulsion and headache. The prognosis is not always good. Seizures occur in clusters, sometimes whatever the treatment, but there is no tendency to progressive worsening. They may recur when treatment is stopped, even after a 2-year, seizure-free period.[116] The interictal clinical condition is normal. Interictal EEG recordings show SWs (80%) or sharp waves of high amplitude localized to the occipital region rhythmically repeated at 1–3 Hz in bursts or in trains. These SWs disappear with opening of the eyes in 94% of patients. There is no significant effect of photic stimulation, sleep, or hyperventilation. In 38% of patients, these SWs are associated with generalized SWs or centrotemporal spikes.[117]

A third group was defined by Dalla Bernardina et al.[118] The disease in this group consists of partial occipital seizures often spreading to motor areas with focal or hemiclonic features and with occipital SWs dramatically increased by sleep.

The differential diagnosis with symptomatic cases is based on clinical and radiologic grounds. Cryptogenic cases may be more difficult to distinguish; however, the presence of types of seizures other than visual or motor and of EEG manifestations other than occipital spikes, rolandic or generalized SWs, and a normal background are likely to exclude EOP. This pattern must be distinguished from that of symptomatic epilepsy, particularly caused by mitochondrial encephalomyopathy, lactic acidosis, and strokelike episodes (MELAS) syndrome, or by occipital calcifications linked to gluten intolerance.[119]

Idiopathic Partial Epilepsy with Affective Seizures

Idiopathic partial epilepsy with affective seizures (benign psychomotor epilepsy) is even less frequent than EOP and may be difficult to identify.[120] Seizures begin between the ages of 2 and 9 years with two peaks, one between 2 and 5 years, the other between 6 and 9 years. Their main characteristic is an expression of terror with screaming or hiding. This is eventually combined with chewing or swallowing movements, laughter, arrest of speech or salivation, pallor, sweating, or abdominal pain but no motor manifestation. There is usually loss of contact but not complete unconsciousness. There is no postictal deficit. Seizures are brief, lasting 1–2 minutes, and occur during daytime and at night with high frequency at onset. Apart from rare orofacial clonic seizures, there are no other types of seizures, particularly no tonic or tonic-clonic seizure. EEG recordings show normal background activity and sleep organization and focal temporal or rolandic spike and slow waves activated by sleep. Early in the course of the disease, one-half of the patients exhibit rhythmic sharp waves in the frontotemporal or parietotemporal area. Generalized SWs occasionally occur during drowsiness. Ictal EEG recordings showed frontotemporal, centrotemporal, or parietal discharges, but sometimes no focal onset could be recognized. The ictal pattern is similar whether the patient is awake or asleep. Treatment is usually effective, although infrequent attacks may persist for a few months. CBZ[120] and clobazam[104] seem to be the most efficient. This type of epilepsy should therefore be considered a variant of BECT.

Benign Partial Epilepsy with Extreme Somatosensory Evoked Potentials

One percent of school-age children with no evidence of brain damage were found to have giant evoked potentials when the sole of their foot was tapped.[121, 122] These potentials predominated in the parietal and parasagittal area. They were giant but with normal latency and morphology, as in other types of idiopathic partial epilepsy, and contrasted to the shorter latency giant potentials observed in progressive myoclonic epilepsy.[123] In a number of these patients, follow-up showed spontaneous spikes to occur a few years later during sleep and later when awake. Between the ages of 4 and 8 years, 10% of the 8-year-olds exhibited a few spontaneous seizures over a 1- or 2-year period. These seizures consisted of lateral rotation of the head and hypertonia of the upper limb with occasional jerks. In this series, a single seizure was recorded and surface EEG recordings failed to show any focal onset. The outcome was favorable, including motor and cognitive functions. Therefore, this type of epilepsy seems to differ from BECT by the seizure type, the duration of the period of seizures, and the EEG aspects, although other characteristics are shared by both conditions.

CONCLUSIONS

The concept of epileptic syndromes is a useful tool in everyday practice of childhood epileptology provided the user adheres to very strict diagnostic criteria. It contributes to the proper choice of antiepileptic drug therapy and is useful for research regarding nosology, etiology, mechanisms of cognitive impairment, and basic mechanisms.

Recognition of idiopathic epileptic syndromes is most useful in order to determine management, these benign syndromes being age-related in terms of onset and cessation of the seizure disorder. However, even a benign syndrome may become troublesome if it is misdiagnosed and mistreated (for example, childhood absences or myoclonic astatic epilepsy treated with CBZ). In addition, recognition of idiopathic epilepsies will contribute to the search for etiology, especially the genetic predisposition that seems central to these syndromes. The next decade should tell us how their molecular biology determines the spectrum of clinical phenotypes, their neurophysiology, and mechanisms.

REFERENCES

1. Commission on Classification and Terminology of the International League Against Epilepsy. Proposal for a revised classification of epilepsies and epileptic syndromes. Epilepsia 1989;30:389.
2. Roger J, Bureau M, Dravet C, et al. (eds). Epileptic Syndromes in Infancy, Childhood and Adolescence (2nd ed). London: John Libbey, 1992.
3. Plouin P. Benign Idiopathic Neonatal Convulsions (Familial and Non-Familial). In J Roger, M Bureau, C Dravet, et al. (eds), Epileptic Syndromes in Infancy, Childhood and Adolescence (2nd ed). London: John Libbey, 1992;3.

4. Dehan M, Quillerou D, Navelet Y, et al. Les convulsions du cinquième jour de vie: un nouveau syndrome? Arch Fr Pediatr 1977;34:730.
5. Luna D, Chiron C, Pajot N, et al. Epidemiologie des Épilepsies de L'Enfant dans le Département de L'Oise (France). In P Jallon (ed), Epidémiologie des Épilepsies. Paris: John Libbey, 1988;41.
6. Desguerre I, Chiron C, Loiseau J, et al. Epidemiology of Idiopathic Generalized Epilepsy. In A Malafosse, P Genton, E Hirsch, et al. (eds), Idiopathic Generalized Epilepsies: Clinical, Experimental and Genetic Aspects. London: John Libbey, 1994;19.
7. North KN, Storey GNB, Handerson-Smart DJ. Fifth day fits in the newborn. Aust Pediatr J 1989;25:284.
8. Dulac O, Cusmai R, De Oliveira K. Is there a partial benign epilepsy in infancy? Epilepsia 1989;30:798.
9. Goldberg HJ, Sheehy EM. Fifth day fits: an acute zinc deficiency syndrome? Arch Dis Child 1983;57:633.
10. Hirsch E, Velez A, Sellal F, et al. Electroclinical signs of benign neonatal familial convulsions. Ann Neurol 1993;34:835.
11. Leppert M, Anderson VE, Quattlebaum T, et al. Benign familial neonatal convulsions linked to genetic markers on chromosome 20. Nature 1989;337:647.
12. Malafosse A, Leboyer M, Dulac O, et al. Confirmation of linkage of benign neonatal convulsions to D20S19 and D20S20. Hum Genet 1992;89:54.
13. Ryan SG, Wisnitger M, Hollman C, et al. Benign familial neonatal convulsions: evidence for clinical and genetic heterogeneity. Ann Neurol 1991;29:469.
14. Watanabe K, Yamamoto N, Negoro T, et al. Benign complex partial epilepsics in infancy. Pediatr Neurol 1987;3:208.
15. Watanabe K, Negoro T, Aso K. Benign partial epilepsy with secondarily generalized seizures in infancy. Epilepsia 1993;34:635.
16. Vigevano F, Fusco L, Di Capua M, et al. Benign infantile familial convulsions. Eur J Pediatr 1992;151:608.
17. Echenne B, Humbertclaude V, Rivier F, et al. Benign infantile epilepsy with autosomal dominant inheritance. Brain Dev 1994;16:108.
18. Gautier A, Pouplard F, Bednarek N, et al. Benign infantile convulsions [abstract]. Epilepsia 1995;36(Suppl 3):S200.
19. Malafosse A, Beck C, Bellet H, et al. Benign infantile familial convulsions are not an allelic form of the benign familial neonatal convulsions gene. Ann Neurol 1994;35:479.
20. Guipponi M, Rivier F, Vigevano F, et al. Linkage mapping of benign familial infantile convulsions (BFIC) to chromosome 19q. Hum Mol Genet (in press).
21. Malafosse A, Genton P, Hirsch E, et al. (eds). Idiopathic Generalized Epilepsies: Clinical, Experimental and Genetic Aspects. London: John Libbey, 1994.
22. Dravet C, Bureau M, Roger J. Benign Myoclonic Epilepsy in Infants. In J Roger, M Bureau, C Dravet, et al. (eds), Epileptic Syndromes in Infancy, Childhood and Adolescence (2nd ed). London: John Libbey, 1992;67.
23. Guerrini R, Dravet C, Gobbi G, et al. Idiopathic Generalized Epilepsies with Myoclonus in Infancy and Childhood. In A Malafosse, P Genton, E Hirsch, et al. (eds). Idiopathic Generalized Epilepsies: Clinical, Experimental and Genetic Aspects. London: John Libbey, 1994.
24. Ricci S, Cusmai R, Fusco L, Vigevano F. Reflex myoclonic epilepsy in infancy: a new age-dependent idiopathic epileptic syndrome related to startle reaction. Epilepsia 1995,36.342.
25. Jeavons PM. Nosological problems of myoclonic epilepsies in childhood and adolescence. Dev Med Child Neurol 1977;19:3.
26. Appleton RE, Panayiotopoulos CP, Acomb BA, Beirne M. Eyelid myoclonia with typical absences: an epilepsy syndrome. J Neurol Neurosurg Psychiatry 1993;56:1312.
27. Doose H. Das akinetische petit mal. II. Verlaufsformen und beziehungen zu den Blitz-Nick-Salaam-Krämpfen und den absencen. Arch Psychiat Nervenkr 1964;205:637.
28. Dulac O, Plouin P, Chiron C. Forme "benigne" d'épilepsie myoclonique chez l'enfant. Neurophysiol Clin 1990;2:77.
29. Dulac O, Plouin P, Chiron C. Nonprogressive myoclonic epilepsy in childhood [abstract]. Epilepsia 1994;35(Suppl 8):119.
30. Lerman P. Seizures induced or aggravated by anticonvulsants. Epilepsia 1986;27:706.
31. Lortie A, Chiron C, Mumford J, Dulac O. The potential for increasing seizure frequency, relapse, and appearance of new seizure types with vigabatrin. Neurology 1993;43(Suppl 5):S24.
32. Snead OC, Hosey LC. Exacerbation of seizures in children by carbamazepine. N Engl J Med 1985;313:916.

33. Oller-Daurella L, Oller LF-V. Epilepsy with Generalized Tonic-Clonic Seizures in Childhood. Does a Childhood "Grand Mal" Syndrome Exist ? In J Roger, M Bureau, C Dravet, et al. (eds), Epileptic Syndromes in Infancy, Childhood and Adolescence (2nd ed). London: John Libbey, 1992;161.
34. Penry JK, Porter RJ, Dreifuss FE. Simultaneous recording of absence seizures with video tape and electroencephalography. A study of 374 seizures in 48 patients. Brain 1975;98:427.
35. Lennox WG, Lennox MA. Epilepsy and Related Disorders. Boston: Little, Brown, 1960.
36. Bergamini L, Bram S, Broglia S, Alessandro R. L'insorgenza tardive di crisi grande male nal piccolo male puro. Studio catammestico di 78 casi. Arch Suisses Neurol Neurochirug Psichiat 1965;96:306.
37. Dietrich E, Baier WK, Doose H, Tuxhorn J. Longterm follow-up of childhood epilepsy with absences. I: Epilepsy with absences at onset. Neuropediatrics 1985;16:149.
38. Dietrich E, Doose H, Baier WK, Fichsel H. Longterm follow-up of childhood epilepsy with absences. II: Absence-epilepsy with initial grand mal. Neuropediatrics 1985;16:155.
39. Beaumanoir A. Les épilepsies infantiles. Problèmes de diagnostic et de traitement. Bâle: Éditions Roche, 1976.
40. Schlumberger E, Chavez F, Palacios L, et al. Lamotrigine in the treatment of 120 children with epilepsy. Epilepsia 1994;35:359.
41. Panayiotopoulos CP, Ferrie CD, Knott C, Robinson RO. Interaction of lamotrigine with sodium valproate. Lancet 1993;341:445.
42. Janz D, Christian W. Impulsiv-petit mal. J Neurol 1957;176:346.
43. Doose H, Volzke E, Scheffner D. Verlaufsformen kindelicher epilepsien mit spike-wave-absencen. Arch Psychiat Nervenkr 1965;207:394.
44. Berkovic SF, Howell RA, Hopper JI, et al. A twin study of the epilepsies. Epilepsia 1990;31:813.
45. Janz D, Beck-Mannagetta G, Spröder B, et al. Childhood Absence Epilepsy (Pyknolepsy) and Juvenile Absence Epilepsy: One or Two Syndromes? In P Wolf (ed), Epileptic Seizures and Syndromes. London: John Libbey, 1994;115.
46. Wolf P, Inoue Y. Therapeutic response of absence seizures in patients of an epilepsy clinic for adolescents and adults. J Neurol 1984;231:225.
47. Panayiotopoulos CP, Obeid T, Waheed G. Differentiation of typical absence seizures in epileptic syndromes. Brain 1989;112:1039.
48. Panayiotopoulos CP, Obeid T, Waheed G. Absences in juvenile myoclonic epilepsy: a clinical and video-electroencephalographic study. Ann Neurol 1989;25:391.
49. Wolf P. Juvenile Absence Epilepsy. In J Roger, M Bureau, C Dravet, et al. (eds), Epileptic Syndromes in Infancy, Childhood and Adolescence (2nd ed). London: John Libbey, 1992.
50. Herpin TH. Des accès incomplets d'épilepsie. Paris: Baillière, 1867.
51. Tsuboi T. Primary Generalized Epilepsy with Sporadic Myoclonias of Myoclonic Petit Mal Type. Stuttgart: Thieme, 1977.
52. Mai R, Canevini MP, Pontrelli V, et al. L'épilepsia mioclonica giovanile di Janz: analisi prospettiva di un campione di 57 pazienti. Boll Lega Ital Epil 1990;70/71:307.
53. Salas-Puig J, Gonzalez C, Tunon A, et al. Epilepsia mioclonica juvenile: aspectos electroclinicos. Boll Lega Ital Epil 1988;62/63:199.
54. Janz D. Die Epilepsien. Stuttgart: Thieme, 1969.
55. Touchon J. Effect of Awakening on Epileptic Activity in Primary Generalized Myoclonic Epilepsy. In MB Sterman, MN Shouse, P Passouant (eds), Sleep and Epilepsy. New York: Academic, 1982;239.
56. Panayiotopoulos CP, Obeid T. Juvenile myoclonic epilepsy. An autosomal recessive disease. Ann Neurol 1989;25:440.
57. Delgado-Escueta AV, Greenberg DA, Weissbecker K, et al. Gene mapping in the idiopathic generalized epilepsies: juvenile myoclonic epilepsy, childhood absence epilepsy, epilepsy with grand mal seizures, and early childhood myoclonic epilepsy. Epilepsia 1990;31(Suppl 3):S19.
58. Feuerstein J, Revol M, Roger J, et al. La monotherapie par le valproate de sodium dans les épilepsies généralisées primaires. Sem Hôp Paris 1983;59:1263.
59. Resor SR, Resor LD. Chronic acetazolamide monotherapy in the treatment of juvenile myoclonic epilepsy. Neurology 1990;40:1677.
60. Richens A, Yuen AW. Overview of the clinical efficacy of lamotrigine. Epilepsia 1991;32(Suppl 2):S13.
61. Obeid T, Panayiotopoulos CP. Clonazepam in juvenile myoclonic epilepsy. Epilepsia 1989;30:603.
62. Janz D, Kern A, Mössinger HJ, Puhlmann HU. Rückfallprognose während und nach Reduktion der Medikamente bel Epilepsiebehandlung. In H Rehmschmidt, R Rentz, J Jungmann (eds), Epilepsie. Stuttgart: Thieme, 1981;53.

63. Gowers WR. Epilepsy and Other Chronic Convulsive Diseases: Their Causes, Symptoms and Treatment (reprint 1966). New York: Dover, 1885.
64. Janz D. "Aufwach"-Epilepsien (als Ausdruck einer den "Nacht"-oder "Schlaf"-Epilepsien gegenuberzustellenden verlausform epileptischer Erkrankungen). Arch Psychiat Nervenkr 1953;191:73.
65. Tsuboi T, Christian W. Epilepsy: a clinical, electroencephalographic and statistical study of 466 patients. Berlin: Springer, 1976.
66. Leder A. Zur Psychopathologie der Schlaf- und Aufwachepilepsie (eine psychodiagnostische Untersuchung). Nervenarzt 1967;38:434.
67. Wolf P. Epilepsy with Grand Mal on Awakening. In J Roger, M Bureau, C Dravet, et al. (eds), Epileptic Syndromes in Infancy, Childhood and Adolescence (2nd ed). London: John Libbey, 1992;329.
68. Loiseau P. Crises epileptiques survenant au réveil et épilepsie du réveil. Sud Médical et Chirurgical 1964;99:11492.
69. Janz D. The grand mal epilepsies and the sleeping-waking cycle. Epilepsia 1962;191:73.
70. Meencke HJ, Janz D. Neuropathological findings in primary generalized epilepsy: a study of eight cases. Epilepsia 1984;25:8.
71. Lyon G, Gastaut H. Considerations on the significance attributed to unusual cerebral histological findings recently described in eight patients with primary generalized epilepsy. Epilepsia 1985;26:365.
72. Reilly EL, Peters JF. Relationship of some varieties of electroencephalographic photosensitivity to clinical convulsive disorders. Neurology 1973;13.1050.
73. Kasteleijn-Nolst Trénité DGA, Binnie CD, Neinardi H. Photosensitive patients: symptoms and signs during intermittent photic stimulation and their relation to seizures in daily life. J Neurol Neurosurg Psychiatry 1987;50:1546.
74. Wilkins AJ, Binnie CD, Darby CE. Visually-induced seizures. Prog Neurobiol 1980;15:85.
75. Jeavons PM, Harding GFA. Photosensitive Epilepsy. London: Heinemann, 1975.
76. Kasteleijn-Nolst Trenité DGA. Photosensitivity in epilepsy, electrophysiological and clinical correlates. Master's thesis, University of Utrecht, 1989.
77. Binnie CD, Jeavons PM. Photosensitive Epilepsies. In J Roger, M Bureau, C Dravet, et al. (eds), Epileptic Syndromes in Infancy, Childhood and Adolescence (2nd ed). London: John Libbey, 1992;299.
78. Quirk JA, Fish DR, Smith SJM, et al. First seizures associated with playing electronic screen games: a community-based study in Great Britain. Ann Neurol 1995;37:733.
79. Doose H, Gerken H. On the genetics of EEG-anomalies in childhood. IV. Photoconvulsive reaction. Neuropediatrie 1973;4:162.
80. Binnie CD, Jeavons PM. Photosensitive Epilepsies. In J Roger, M Bureau, C Dravet, et al. (eds), Epileptic Syndromes in Infancy, Childhood and Adolescence (2nd ed). London: John Libbey, 1992.;299.
81. Binnie CD, Kasteleijn-Nolst Trenité DGA, de Korte R. Photosensitivity as a model for acute antiepileptic drug studies. Electroencephalogr Clin Neurophysiol 1986;63:35.
82. Binnie CD, Darby CE, de Korte RA, et al. EEG sensitivity to television: effects of ambient lighting. Electroencephalogr Clin Neurophysiol 1980;50:329.
83. Dalla Bernardina B, Sgrò V, Fontana E, et al. Idiopathic Partial Epilepsies in Children. In J Roger, M Bureau, C Dravet, et al. (eds), Epileptic Syndromes in Infancy, Childhood and Adolescence (2nd ed). London: John Libbey, 1992;173.
84. Farnarier G, Bureau M, Mancini J, Regis H. Etude des potentiels évoqués multimodalitaires dans les épilepsies partielles de l'enfant. Neurophysiol Clin 1988;18:243.
85. Plasmati R, Michelucci R, Salvi F, et al. Potenziali evocati somestesici giganti nelle epilessie idiopathiche dell'infanzia. Boll Lega Ital Epil 1990;70/71:199.
86. Cavazzuti GB. Epidemiology of different types of epilepsy in school age children of Modena, Italy. Epilepsia 1980;21:57.
87. Gastaut Y. Un élément déroutant de la symptomatologie électroencéphalographique: les pointes prérolandiques sans signification focale. Rev Neurol 1952;87:488.
88. Nayrac P, Beaussart M. Les pointes-ondes prérolandiques: expression EEG très particulière. Rev Neurol 1958;99:201.
89. Faure J, Loiseau P. Une corrélation particulière des pointes-ondes sans signification focale. Rev Neurol 1960;102:399.
90. Gibbs EL, Gibbs FA. Good prognosis of mid-temporal epilepsy. Epilepsia 1959–60;1:448.

91. Gibbs EL, Gillen HW, Gibbs FA. Disappearance and migration of epileptic foci in children. Am J Dis Child 1954;88:596.
92. Cavazzuti GB, Capella L, Nalin A. Longitudinal study of epileptiform EEG patterns in normal children. Epilepsia 1980;21:43.
93. Loiseau P, Beaussart M. The seizures of benign childhood epilepsy with rolandic paroxysmal discharges. Epilepsia 1973;14:381.
94. Beaumanoir A, Ballis T, Varfis G, Ansari K. Benign epilepsy of childhood with rolandic spikes. Epilepsia 1974;15:301.
95. Dalla Bernardina B, Bondavalli S, Colamaria V. Benign Epilepsy of Childhood with Rolandic Spikes (BERS) During Sleep. In MB Sterman, MN Shouse, P Passount (eds), Sleep and Epilepsy. New York: Academic, 1982;495.
96. Dalla Bernardina B, Beghini G. Rolandic spikes in children with and without epilepsy (20 subjects polygraphically studied during sleep). Epilepsia 1976;17:161.
97. Lerman P, Kivity S. Benign focal epilepsy of childhood. A follow-up study of 100 recovered patients. Arch Neurol 1975;23:261.
98. Dalla Bernardina B, Tassinari CA. EEG of a nocturnal seizure in a patient with "benign epilepsy of childhood with rolandic spikes." Epilepsia 1975;16:497.
99. Lerman P. Benign Partial Epilepsy with Centro-Temporal Spikes. In J Roger, M Bureau, C Dravet, et al. (eds), Epileptic Syndromes in Infancy, Childhood and Adolescence (2nd ed). London: John Libbey, 1992;189.
100. Heijbel J, Blom S, Rasmuson M. Benign epilepsy of childhood with centro-temporal EEG foci: a genetic study. Epilepsia 1975;16:285.
101. Ambrosetto G. Unilateral opercular macrogyria and benign childhood epilepsy with centrotemporal (rolandic) spikes: report of a case. Epilepsia 1992;33:499.
102. Santanelli P, Bureau M, Magaudda A, et al. Benign partial epilepsy with centrotemporal (or rolandic) spikes and brain lesion. Epilepsia 1989;30:182.
103. Chaigne D, Dulac O. Carbamazepine versus valproate in partial epilepsies of childhood. Adv Epileptol 1980;17:198.
104. Dulac O, Figueroa D, Rey E, Arthuis M. Monotherapie par le clobazam dans les épilepsies de l'enfant. Presse Med 1983;12:1067.
105. Fejerman N, Di Blasi AM. Status epilepticus of benign partial epilepsies in children: report of 2 cases. Epilepsia 1987;28:351.
106. Ambrosetto G, Giovannardi-Rossi P, Tassinari CA. Predictive factors of seizure frequency and duration of antiepileptic treatment in rolandic epilepsy: a retrospective study. Brain Dev 1987;9:300.
107. Hamada Y, Okuno T, Hattori H, Mikawa H. Indication for antiepileptic drug treatment of benign childhood epilepsy with centro-temporal spikes. Brain Dev 1994;16:159.
108. Loiseau P, Duché P, Cordova S, et al. Prognosis of benign childhood epilepsy with centro-temporal spikes: a follow-up study of 168 patients. Epilepsia 1988;29:229.
109. Dalla Bernardina B, Tassinari CA, Dravet C, et al. Épilepsie partielle bénign et état de mal électroencéphalographique pendant le sommeil. Rev EEG Neurophysiol 1978;8:350.
110. Aicardi J, Chevrie JJ. Atypical benign partial epilepsy of childhood. Dev Med Child Neurol 1982;24:281.
111. Kivity S, Lerman P. Benign Partial Epilepsy of Childhood with Occipital Discharges. In J Manelis, E Bental, JN Loeber, FE Dreifuss (eds), Advances in Epileptology (Vol XVII). New York: Raven, 1989;371.
112. Kivity S, Lerman P. Stormy onset with prolonged loss of consciousness in benign childhood epilepsy with occipital paroxysms. J Neurol Neurosurg Psychiatry 1992;55:45.
113. Panayiotopoulos CP. Benign nocturnal childhood occipital epilepsy: a new syndrome with nocturnal seizures, tonic deviation of the eyes and vomiting. J Child Neurol 1989;4:43.
114. Vigevano F, Ricci S, di Capua M, et al. Vomito, deviazione oculare, emiconvulsione: una particolare forma di stato epilettico nel bambino. Boll Lega Ital Epil 1989;66/67:315.
115. Vigevano F, Ricci S. Benign Occipital Epilepsy of Childhood with Prolonged Seizures and Autonomic Symptoms. In F Andermann, A Beaumanoir, L Mira, et al. (eds), Benign Occipital Epilepsy of Childhood with Prolonged Seizures and Autonomic Symptoms. London: John Libbey, 1993;133.
116. Guerrini R, Battaglia A, Dravet C, et al. Outcome of Idiopathic Childhood Epilepsy with Occipital Paroxysms. In F Andermann, A Beaumanoir, L Mira, et al. (eds), Benign Occipital Epilepsy of Childhood with Prolonged Seizures and Autonomic Symptoms. London: John Libbey, 1993;165.
117. Gastaut H. Benign Epilepsy of Childhood with Occipital Paroxysms. In J Roger, M Bureau, C Dravet, et al. (eds), Epileptic Syndromes in Infancy, Childhood and Adolescence (2nd ed). London: John Libbey, 1992;201.

118. Dalla Bernardina B, Fontana E, Cappellaro O, et al. The Partial Occipital Epilepsies in Childhood. In F Andermann, A Beaumanoir, L Mira, et al. (eds), Benign Occipital Epilepsy of Childhood with Prolonged Seizures and Autonomic Symptoms. London: John Libbey, 1993;173.
119. Andermann F, Beaumanoir A, Mira L, et al. Benign Occipital Epilepsy of Childhood with Prolonged Seizures and Autonomic Symptoms. London: John Libbey, 1993;133.
120. Dalla Bernardina B, Colamaria V, Chiamenti C, et al. Benign Partial Epilepsy with Affective Symptoms ("Benign Psychomotor Epilepsy"). In J Roger, M Bureau, C Dravet, et al. (eds), Epileptic Syndromes in Infancy, Childhood and Adolescence (2nd ed). London: John Libbey, 1992;219.
121. De Marco P, Negrin P. Parietal spikes evoked by contralateral tactile somatotopic stimulations in four non-epileptic subjects. Electroencephalogr Clin Neurophysiol 1973;34:308.
122. Tassinari CA, De Marco P. Benign Partial Epilepsy with Extreme Somato-sensory Evoked Potentials. In J Roger, M Bureau, C Dravet, et al. (eds), Epileptic Syndromes in Infancy, Childhood and Adolescence (2nd ed). London: John Libbey, 1992;225.
123. Karigi R, Shibasaki H. Generator mechanisms of giant somatosensory evoked potentials in cortical reflex myoclonus. Brain 1987;110:1359.

10
Nonepileptic Seizures

A. James Rowan

Nonepileptic seizures (NESs) have been well described since the time of Charcot and Gowers in the latter half of the nineteenth century.[1] In Charcot's clinic and during his well-publicized demonstrations, the classic manifestations of opisthotonos (*arc de circle*) were the object of great interest and said to be characteristic in young women. Since that time, the subject surfaced in sporadic case reports, and NESs were recognized as manifestations of psychiatric illness. Various treatments were prescribed, usually individual psychotherapy, with varying degrees of success. Little attention, however, was paid NESs by the neurologic and psychiatric communities until the last 25 years when, with the growth of multidisciplinary epilepsy centers abroad and in the United States, the extent of the problem became well known. The use of intensive electroencephalographic (EEG)-video monitoring allowed the diagnosis to be made with relative certainty and made it possible to study the phenomenology of these events. We now recognize that NESs are quite common, occurring in epileptic and nonepileptic populations. Moreover, it became clear that the manifestations of NESs constitute a rich fabric of clinical signs—far beyond those originally described. Of greater importance has been the growing understanding of the range of psychiatric problems that underlie the seizures themselves.

DEFINITIONS

The term *hysterical seizures*, by which these events were known for many years, derived from the Greek *hustere* or womb. Hysteria itself was a psychiatric condition thought to affect women and to derive from a disorder of the uterus. These false notions have been relegated to the dust bin of history, yet some physicians still refer to hysteria or a hysterical personality. These terms should not be used.

The term *pseudoseizures* gained popularity earlier in this century, mainly because the observed events were not epileptic but indeed simulated epilepsy.[2]

187

Because the seizures were not "real," by definition they were false or "pseudo." The *American Heritage Dictionary* defines *pseudo* as false, deceptive, sham. Like the term *hysteria*, the term pseudoseizure deserves to be discarded, for patients suffering from these events are ill, and deception does not underlie the often alarming and always disabling symptoms.

The term that best describes the clinical problem is *nonepileptic seizures*. This has the clear connotation of episodic events that resemble epileptic seizures but are not manifestations of epilepsy. The patient comes to neurologic attention because of this resemblance; thus, the term recognizes the serious nature of the illness without containing an intrinsic pejorative.

NESs are not always an overt manifestation of psychiatric illness. Indeed, many physiologic conditions result in clinical events that resemble epileptic seizures. To distinguish between the two, NESs are classified into two main categories: psychogenic NESs and physiologic NESs. In this chapter the abbreviation NES refers to a psychogenic NES. Each will be discussed in subsequent sections.

EPIDEMIOLOGY

NESs are more common than generally appreciated. In the absence of specialized diagnostic procedures such as EEG-video monitoring, patients often receive a diagnosis of epilepsy based on descriptions provided by relatives or others or based on historical data provided by the patient. Details of the events are often obscured by their often frightening manifestations, and it is understandable that many patients with NESs receive a diagnosis of epilepsy and therefore are treated with antiepileptic drugs (AEDs). In a recent series of 79 patients diagnosed as having psychogenic NESs in our EEG-video monitoring unit, 51 (65%) were taking AEDs at the time of study and an additional five had been treated with AEDs in the past.[3]

There are relatively few data on the prevalence or incidence of NESs. Scott[4] estimated that 5% of his patients in an epilepsy clinic suffered from NESs, although he did not have the benefit of EEG-video monitoring. Gates et al.[5] reported that 20% of patients entered into a comprehensive epilepsy center had NESs. The coexistence of epilepsy and NESs has been estimated by other authors at 10–58%.[6, 7] The wide range of these figures may be explained by varying referral patterns, the availability of monitoring, and perhaps the specialized interest of the investigators. In any case, it is clear that NESs are quite common, and it is reasonable to assume that increased sensitivity to the possibility of NESs by all neurologists will lead to more accurate diagnosis.

CLASSIFICATION

A widely accepted classification system of psychogenic NESs has yet to be devised. The most commonly used classification follows the International Classification of Epileptic Seizures, based on the idea that NESs may resemble generalized tonic-clonic convulsions, complex partial seizures, or absence attacks.[8] While true in a general sense, there are so many exceptions to this categorization that it has little practical utility. Moreover, this system contains no recognition of the associated psychiatric conditions that are variable in their type and extent, nor does it take into account any underlying brain disease that may contribute to the overall syndrome.

A more suitable system would combine clinical manifestations and psychiatric diagnoses. Gates and Erdahl have suggested using *Diagnostic and Statistical Manual* (DSM)-III-R (now DSM-IV) psychiatric diagnoses to categorize patients with NESs.[9] NES is essentially a somatoform disorder[10]—that is, a disorder with primarily somatic manifestations. In addition, patients with NESs often meet criteria for additional disorders (for example, depression or panic disorder).[11] Such a classification has implications for treatment and prognosis and better portrays the clinical status of the patient. When used in conjunction with descriptive phenomenology, this schema represents an advance in our understanding of NESs. It does not, however, meet the problem of attempting to match types of NESs with types of epileptic seizures as defined by the International Classification.

In our review of 79 consecutive patients with NESs documented by EEG-video monitoring, several general types of seizure phenomenology were observed, ranging from vigorous, chaotic motor activity to unresponsive staring.[3] It was further noted that some events truly resembled epileptic seizures (for example, generalized tonic-clonic convulsions), whereas many did not. It was possible to classify patients into two broad categories: active events and passive events, with subdivisions of each. Conceptually, it would appear that the particular phenomenology of NESs may be related to the underlying psychiatric disorder. Furthermore, the presence or absence of organic brain dysfunction may play a role in seizure manifestations and resultant disability.[12] Thus, a multiaxial classification for NESs based on symptoms, psychiatric diagnosis, and neurologic and neuropsychological findings may allow a broader understanding of an individual's illness and improve communication among clinicians and investigators (Table 10.1).

CHARACTERISTICS OF PSYCHOGENIC NONEPILEPTIC SEIZURES

As outlined above, psychogenic NESs may or may not closely resemble true epileptic seizures. Although the diagnosis may be difficult without the availability of monitoring, there are historical and phenomenologic features that can suggest the diagnosis. None, however, are pathognomonic.

Historical Features Suggestive of Psychogenic Nonepileptic Seizures

The history of patients with psychogenic NESs usually contains important clues regarding the true nature of the events. If the seizures are of relatively recent onset, inquiry into any surrounding social or emotional factors may suggest a correlation with onset of the illness. Seizures may occur only when the patient is alone, or, conversely, only when the patient is in the company of others (for exam-

Table 10.1   Proposed multiaxial classification of psychogenic nonepileptic seizures

Axis I.   Event phenomenology
   I.   Active events
      A. Chaotic motor activity
         1. Bilateral
         2. Unilateral or clearly asymmetrical
      B. Minor motor activity
         1. Bilateral
         2. Unilateral
         3. Wandering
      C. Ocular/facial motor activity
      D. Events strikingly similar to epileptic seizures
         1. Generalized tonic-clonic; tonic; clonic
         2. Complex partial
         3. Myoclonic
      E. Unclassifiable
Each of the above categories modified with:
      a.   Apparent altered consciousness i. Emotional
      b.   Without altered consciousness ii. Nonemotional
   II. Passive events
      A. Staring/unresponsive
      B. Sleeplike, motionless
      C. Subjective
Axis II.   Underlying psychiatric disorder (partial listing)
   I.   Somatization disorder
   II.   Undifferentiated somatoform disorder
   III.   Conversion disorder
   IV.   Mood disorder
   V.   Panic disorder without agoraphobia
   VI.   Panic disorder with agoraphobia
   VII.   Schizophrenia
   VIII. Malingering
Axis III.   Associated organic brain dysfunction
   I.   Epilepsy
      A. Current
      B. Remote
   II. Brain dysfunction as manifested by
      A. Clinical examination findings
      B. Electroencephalographic findings
         1. Focal slowing (specify location)
         2. Diffuse slowing
         3. Epileptiform activity (specify)
      C. Neuroimaging results
         1. Focal abnormality
         2. Diffuse abnormality
      D. Neuropsychological testing results
         1. Localized abnormality (specify)
         2. Global abnormality

Note: Using Axis I of the proposed classification, we were able to classify 75 of 77 consecutive patients. With respect to active events, some form of chaotic motor activity was found in 26, minor motor activity in 30, pure ocular manifestations in two, and events strikingly similar to epileptic seizures in only eight. Thirteen patients had passive events, and two were unclassifiable. Insufficient data were available to classify patients according to axes II and III. A prospective study will be required to determine the utility of this system for the purposes of professional communication, planning therapy, and determining prognosis.
Source: M Muxfeldt, H Price, SH Dane, et al., unpublished observations, 1995.

ple, family members). Such selectivity might be regarded with suspicion. Precipitating emotional factors for each event may or may not be present. If the patient is receiving AEDs, a careful assessment of response is required. A history of lack of response to AEDs, regardless of type or dose, may arouse suspicion, as may an increase in seizures as the AED dose is increased. Another clue is intolerance to any AED in spite of slow and careful dose escalation.

Patients with NESs may suffer a relatively high seizure frequency; sometimes many in the course of a day. High seizure frequency is also seen in patients with epilepsy, especially those with seizures originating in the supplementary motor area of the frontal lobe. Incontinence and biting of the tongue are hallmarks of grand mal seizures, although they do not invariably occur. Conversely, these symptoms are said to be rare in patients with NESs. Both are sometimes seen in NESs and therefore cannot provide definitive proof of an NES. Sometimes patients with NESs will give a history of some personal experience with seizures, whether as a hospital staff member having observed a seizure at some time or having observed a family member with epilepsy. In itself this means little, but such experience may have provided a template for the patient's events.

In a patient with known epilepsy, it may be found that the patient has experienced a change in seizure type, or, after a seizure-free interval, a new type of seizure has emerged. While such a change may suggest development of a new cerebral process, such as a tumor, it also is possible that NESs have intervened. In addition to a careful history, such patients require an EEG study, an imaging study, and, in doubtful cases, intensive EEG-video monitoring.

Previous sexual or physical abuse appears to be common in psychogenic NESs. In our clinic, up to 70% of patients give such a history.[12] One of the problems in assessing the relevance of these past events is the lack of data on abuse in the population with epilepsy and, indeed, in the general population. Thus, there is relatively low specificity for sexual abuse as a diagnostic aid.

It is evident that none of the above historical features in and of itself establishes a diagnosis of NES. If there is a grouping of several items, however, the possibility of NESs should be entertained. At that point, further investigations may be indicated.

Clinical Signs Suggestive of Psychogenic Nonepileptic Seizures

Certain seizures classified as NESs appear to have obvious qualities of "nonorganicity" to the professional and even to the casual observer. Thus, a patient observed to flail about with an excessive emotional reaction is usually thought to have an NES. On the other hand, seizures with subtle manifestations, such as apparent confusion or unresponsive staring, are more likely to be thought of as epileptic. A number of particular seizure phenomena suggest the possibility of NES. An NES with prominent motor characteristics often has a gradual onset with progressively increasing vigor, unlike epileptic seizures in which the onset is abrupt. Furthermore, the motor activity is frequently interrupted or discontinuous, whereas epileptic seizures usually display continuity throughout. Related to this is the apparent disjointed or "nonphysiologic" progression of symptoms in NESs. Epileptic seizures consisting primarily of motor activity have a progression of manifestations that adhere to physiologic and anatomic principles;

good examples are the progression seen in a jacksonian march and the typical sequence of generalized tonic-clonic convulsions. The motor activity of an NES is rarely so predictably organized. This is best exemplified by the chaotic, flinging, side-to-side movements often associated with NESs. Out-of-phase repetitive movements may be observed, along with intermittent dystonic posturing or pelvic thrusting.[5] Often, elements of all these phenomena coexist. Interestingly, the face is rarely involved.[13, 14] A marked emotional reaction is not unusual during or after an NES.

Duration of NESs is, on average, longer than that of epileptic seizures. In Gates' study, the NES was about 20% longer on average than true tonic-clonic convulsions.[5] Durations of up to 30 minutes or more are sometimes observed, with intermittent motor activity associated with unresponsiveness occurring throughout the event. The NES usually subsides gradually, unlike epileptic events, which usually end more abruptly. It should be noted, however, that the interface between the ictal and the postictal states in patients with complex partial seizures is often difficult to determine. Thus, in these cases, the epileptic event may appear to be prolonged with gradual cessation of symptoms.

The above signs that suggest the possibility of NESs are not specific to the diagnosis. For example, the clinical picture of seizures of frontal lobe origin is often bizarre and the motor activity chaotic.[15] The initial stages of the seizure, perhaps consisting of brief tonic posturing, are often not appreciated by an observer or seen by hospital staff members. Thus, only the striking motor phase is reported and taken to be nonepileptic in nature. Moreover, the duration of epileptic seizures may be variable, with some being of relatively long duration. Thus, duration in an individual case may not be helpful. Furthermore, intermittency in epileptic seizures may be seen if brief events occur repetitively without recovery of full awareness between events. As in the case of the history, a grouping of several clinical manifestations is required to improve specificity. Even then the diagnosis may be in doubt. Perhaps the most specific clinical sign is the ability of an examiner to provoke the patient's habitual NESs using techniques of suggestion, such as intravenous saline or application of alcohol pads.[16] Epileptic seizures are rarely provoked in this manner. The role of suggestion in confirming the diagnosis of NESs is outlined below.

PHYSIOLOGIC NONEPILEPTIC SEIZURES

There is a long list of physiologic events that mimic epileptic seizures. One of the most common is syncope—neurogenic or cardiogenic. Syncopal attacks are readily diagnosed if an accurate history is available. The characteristic premonitory symptoms, brief loss of consciousness, and lack of a postictal confusional state immediately suggest the true diagnosis. In some cases, the syncopal event is complicated by convulsive activity tonic or clonic in character.[17, 18] This motor phase is usually brief, and the patient recovers quickly. Convulsive syncope sometimes occurs when the patient does not immediately fall down. In these circumstances, the upright or sitting position prolongs the cerebral ischemic phase. The major problem lies in an observer's description wherein the event may be reported as a grand mal convulsion. Details that could confirm the syncopal nature of the attack may not be forthcoming. Such patients are often treated inappropriately with AEDs. Suspicion of syncope, however, should lead to appropriate testing, including a search for orthostatic hypotension, other forms of autonomic failure, and intermittent cardiac arrhythmias.

A variety of sleep disorders not only lead to a misdiagnosis of epilepsy but also to a misdiagnosis of psychogenic NESs. Nocturnal enuresis in children, and occasionally in adults, may raise the question of an unobserved seizure. The evidence shows, however, that unsuspected seizures are rarely the cause of nocturnal enuresis unless there are associated symptoms.[19]

Sleepwalking is a parasomnia associated with slow wave sleep.[20] The subject wanders about in an apparently confused state, reminiscent of ictal or postictal motor activity of a complex partial seizure. In this circumstance, misdiagnosis on either side of the NES-epilepsy border is possible. Akin to sleepwalking is sleep drunkenness, which occurs at the interface of sleep and wakefulness.[21] Such individuals may carry out complex motor activities in a confused state. Sleep drunkenness may occur after sleep deprivation or after consuming alcohol or taking hypnotics.[22] Narcolepsy, when symptoms are well described, is usually diagnosed without difficulty. Patients with sudden sleep episodes, however, may be wrongly diagnosed as epileptic, a problem we have encountered in our EEG-video monitoring unit. In such patients, polysomnography to confirm a sleep disorder should be carried out. An unusual parasomnia, rapid eye movement (REM) behavior disorder, has dramatic manifestations that are diagnosed as epileptic or psychiatric.[23] During REM sleep these individuals have failure of brain stem mechanisms that normally inhibit motor activity. Thus, dreams are acted out as if "real." With frightening dreams, such as those involving pursuit or struggle, the person may strike out or run, leading to injury to self or others. Deaths have even been reported as a result of jumping from a window in an apparent attempt to escape. The diagnosis may be suspected, even if the nocturnal events are not the chief complaint, if it is ascertained that a husband and wife have decided on separate bedrooms to avoid injury from kicking or striking by one of the partners during sleep. Treatment with clonazepam has been tried in such cases with some success.

Migraine, when associated with neurologic dysfunction, and especially when headache is not a prominent symptom, may be mistaken for epilepsy. A good example is a patient who presents with scintillating scotomata or other purely visual phenomena. These symptoms, common in migraine, are also seen in occipital epilepsy—the latter associated with occipital spikes and a benign prognosis.[24] EEG recordings performed during the visual symptoms of a migraine attack show only occipital slowing without epileptiform discharges.

Transient global amnesia (TGA), described by Bender in 1956,[25] amplified by Fisher and Adams in 1958,[26] and more recently reviewed by Caplan[27] presents with a confusional state that usually lasts for hours. TGA episodes may be recurrent, although a low attack frequency is the rule. During such attacks, the EEG pattern is normal.[28] If there is no opportunity to examine the patient during an attack, which is rarely possible, the question of complex partial seizures is raised. TGA often occurs in older patients with a history of cerebrovascular disease. During an attack, the patient appears to be confused although able to carry out complex activities. Because of the inability to store new information, he or she characteristically asks questions repeatedly—e.g., "What day is it?" or

"What are we doing here?" A careful history should be helpful in establishing the diagnosis in most cases.

Paroxysmal movement disorders, such as paroxysmal kinesigenic choreo-athetosis or paroxysmal dystonia, may suggest seizure activity.[29, 30] These disorders involve subcortical structures, and their etiology has been the subject of debate. Again, a careful history and observation of the attacks during EEG-video monitoring will help establish the diagnosis. These conditions sometimes respond to anticonvulsant therapy, such as carbamazepine.

Transient ischemic attacks may mimic epileptic seizures, especially if there is a dysphasic component. During such an attack the individual may appear confused and, to the casual observer, the language deficit may not be obvious. Thus, the history becomes one of episodic confusion, raising the question of complex partial seizures. In the event of associated motor deficit, or if motor-sensory deficit occurs without language impairment, the nature of the attacks is more obvious in that so-called negative motor signs (e.g., hemiparesis) are uncommon manifestations of seizures. The EEG pattern does not contain epileptiform activity but may show some lateralized slowing. Appropriate tests, including noninvasive carotid studies, should be performed in doubtful cases.

DIAGNOSTIC PROCEDURES

Diagnostic evaluation of psychogenic NESs is similar to that of epilepsy. The first step includes a routine EEG study, imaging study, and routine blood work, including AED levels, if applicable. An EEG recording after sleep deprivation or sedation should be performed if the routine record is unrevealing.[31] It is emphasized that a finding of interictal epileptiform activity on the EEG recording does not imply that the patient's spells are epileptic. On the other hand, a normal record in the context of high seizure frequency, especially seizures with apparent loss of awareness, suggests NESs.

Although the above evaluation provides useful information, EEG-video monitoring is the critical diagnostic procedure. The object is to record on videotape the behavioral aspects of the episodic event with a simultaneous EEG recording. If possible, more than one event should be recorded, preferably several, in order to look for stereotypy. Classically, epileptic seizures are stereotyped with respect to phenomenology, progression, and duration, although NESs may also reveal a stereotyped pattern. During the event, the EEG pattern is devoid of epileptiform activity. There are no premonitory spikes or amplitude depression and no postictal slowing.[32] Although the EEG record during the event may be dominated by artifact, brief windows of interpretable tracing may reveal alpha activity. The interictal record may or may not contain epileptiform discharges and cannot be considered diagnostic.

It is important to note that focal epileptiform activity underlying simple partial seizures may not be recorded with scalp electrodes.[33] Thus, a seizure recorded without any evidence of concurrent epileptiform activity is not necessarily nonepileptic in origin. A critical factor in differentiating epileptic seizures from NESs is therefore an analysis of the video-recorded behavior during the event. Every effort should be made to record several events, and, if successful, the events should be edited to a master tape and viewed one after the other. If the events are highly stereotyped in phenomenology and duration, there is a high likelihood that they are epileptic and, if more heterogeneous, nonepileptic. During monitoring, techniques of suggestion should be applied to all patients suspected of having NESs. If an event is evoked that the family recognizes as typical, even though no other events are recorded, a nonepileptic origin is likely.[16] In spite of all efforts, patients will be encountered where differentiation of NESs from epilepsy is difficult if not impossible. In these cases, another study may reveal the true diagnosis.

Ambulatory monitoring has limited usefulness in diagnosing NESs. The lack of video recording is a severe limitation, especially if seizures are of the motor type. In some cases—for example, in absence-type NESs—useful information may be obtained if the events are recorded with an event marker. Some systems are coupled with video monitoring, which may increase the usefulness of ambulatory monitoring. Still, there is currently no substitute for EEG-video monitoring with the presence of a trained observer.

Determination of prolactin levels has gained some favor in sorting out patients with NESs from those with epilepsy.[34] The most consistent finding is a marked elevation of the prolactin level after a generalized tonic-clonic convulsion in 90–100% of patients.[35] The elevation is at least twofold, often more. With complex partial seizures the elevation is variable, ranging from 43% to 100%, depending on which deep temporal structures are maximally involved.[36] Simple partial seizures raise prolactin levels only slightly, and absence attacks and NESs not at all.[37] Thus, if the differential diagnosis lies between a generalized convulsion and an NES with prominent motor activity, prolactin determination may be useful. For other seizure types, the test appears to be of lower specificity.

NEUROPSYCHOLOGICAL TESTING

Neuropsychological testing provides useful information in evaluating patients with NESs. In particular, the Minnesota Multiphasic Personality Inventory (MMPI) has been the subject of several studies and was reviewed by Dodrill et al.[38] In some cases, MMPI results in patients with NESs were compared with those in patients with epilepsy; in others, patients with coexisting NESs and epilepsy were compared with those of an epilepsy-only group. Variable results were reported, although patients with NESs tended to score higher in the hypochondriasis, depression, hysteria, and schizophrenia scales. A recent study by Dodrill compared 23 patients with NESs and 22 patients with intractable epilepsy who had undergone epilepsy surgery.[38] The four scales mentioned demonstrated elevations in patients with NESs with significant findings for hypochondriasis and hysteria. The depression scale was lower than these scales, resulting in a characteristic V-shaped profile. Dodrill et al.[38] analyzed four studies [38–41] that compared patients with "pure" NESs to patients with epilepsy.

MMPI configurational rules, devised by Wilkus et al.,[39] classified epilepsy correctly in 78% of patients, whereas the figure for NES was 65%. It was pointed out, however, that the error rate of 22% for epileptic and 35% for nonepileptic patients was significant, thus diminishing the specificity of this test.

MMPI may have other applications in the evaluation of NES. Dodrill et al.[38] found that patients with NESs with prominent affectual and minimal motor manifestations showed differences on the hypochondriasis, hysteria, and schizophrenia scales compared with epileptic patients. On the other hand, those with marked motor and minimal affectual manifestations showed no such differences. This lends support to the concept that a multiaxial classification system would be likely to provide greater insight into the mechanisms of NESs than a classification based on phenomenology alone.

PSYCHIATRIC CONSIDERATIONS

Roy conducted an early study of NES and its psychiatric concomitants.[42, 43] He used standard scales of depression and anxiety in a comparative study of NES and epilepsy and found significantly higher scores for both in patients with NESs. NES was regarded, not as a conversion of anxiety into a physical symptom, but rather as a "signal of distress." Roy considered the symptom to be a ticket of admission into the health care system for a patient with a psychiatric disorder.

In the end, NES falls under the rubric of the somatoform disorders in DSM-IV and includes conversion disorder, somatization disorder, and somatoform disorder not otherwise specified. *Conversion disorder* is the successor to the term *conversion,* which, as used by Freud, suggested that psychic energy was converted into somatic symptoms. Today, conversion is thought to be precipitated by psychic stress and continued as a result of secondary gain. Underlying psychiatric illness has been emphasized. Ford and Folks[44] noted that conversion should be viewed as a symptom, not a diagnosis.

Somatization disorder is the successor to the term *hysteria.* It is also referred to as Briquet's syndrome, after Pierre Briquet who, in 1859, reported on 430 patients with hysteria.[45] Briquet's syndrome is used to describe multiple unexplained somatic symptoms, and specific criteria for this diagnosis, which requires at least 13 unexplained medical symptoms, have been set forth in DSM-IV. NES is considered one of the possible features of this disorder. *Somatization disorder not otherwise specified* is a broad category that can include patients with medical disease who have symptoms not explained by the illness but who do not meet the criteria for somatization disorder. This may be appropriate for patients with coexisting epilepsy and NESs. Such patients have difficulty coping with stress and may use NESs as a way to continue the role of illness as a coping mechanism.

TREATMENT AND PROGNOSIS

Too often, after a diagnosis of NES is made, the patient is cast into a sort of limbo. Neurologists, having completed their work, believe they have little to contribute to future management. This problem is compounded by psychiatrists, who often are reluctant to take on these patients because of lack of experience with NESs or a lack of interest in somatoform disorders. Nonetheless, if the patient has evidence of depression or anxiety, psychiatrists may be willing to provide appropriate care, working closely with the referring neurologist.

Because psychiatric backgrounds of patients with NESs are diverse, the approach to management must be individualized. Some patients will require psychotropic medication, others short-term psychotherapy, and still others psychiatric support with a view toward coping with the symptom. Probably ideal is a multidisciplinary approach to management. Some epilepsy centers have programs to diagnose and manage the psychiatric problems of patients with NESs. Examples are Minnesota Comprehensive Epilepsy Program (MINCEP) Epilepsy Care in Minneapolis and the Minnesota Epilepsy Group in St. Paul. These groups provide a team approach to therapy, using the services of neurologists, psychiatrists, psychologists, social workers, and other personnel.[46] Team meetings comprise the forum for discussion and planning and are conducted while the patient is hospitalized at the center. After the diagnosis is presented and the patient begun on an individualized therapy program, outpatient followup is arranged with a therapist in the community.

Inpatient evaluation is costly, and many patients do not have access to such centers. Outpatient management, also using a team approach, has been shown to be an alternative.[12, 47] In this model, patients are diagnosed with NESs by EEG-video monitoring. The videotape is reviewed with a significant other to ensure that the recorded event is the same as the patient's habitual seizures. The diagnosis is then presented to the patient in a positive light; emphasis is placed on the concept that NESs are as disabling as epilepsy, that a specialized clinic deals with this particular problem, and that the outlook is optimistic. During the first NES clinic visit, the patient meets with the NES team, at which time the history is reviewed and general therapeutic goals outlined. Appointments are then made with the psychiatrist, psychologist, and social worker. After interviews are completed, a therapeutic plan is formulated and presented to the NES team. The plan depends on the specific psychiatric problem and may include pharmacotherapy, supportive therapy, and short-term psychotherapy. The patient's progress is monitored by the NES team. If the patient has seen a psychiatrist outside the clinic, the team works with that psychiatrist and supplements ongoing therapy. In all cases, continued participation by the neurologist is considered an important element in providing continuity of care and contributing to the authenticity of the treatment plan.

Overall, the prognosis for patients with NESs is favorable. Various studies report remission between 50% and 70% or marked improvement in attack frequency.[48–51] Even in the absence of formal psychiatric intervention, patients tend to improve over time. Factors considered less favorable for outcome include long duration of NESs and a true somatoform disorder. Those patients developing acute stress-related NESs of relatively short duration appear to have a more favorable outlook.

In conclusion, misdiagnosing NESs as epileptic seizures leads to continuing disability, puts the patient at risk for the adverse effects of unneeded antiepileptic medication, promotes contact with multiple physicians, and results in frustration for physician and patient alike. On the other hand, a correct diagnosis of NESs leads to exploration of the underlying psychiatric problem, allows discontinuation of AEDs with elimination of any side effects, and makes possible the application of specific treatment.

REFERENCES

1. Massey EW, McHenry LC. Hysteroepilepsy in the nineteenth century: Charcot and Gowers. Neurology 1986;36:65.
2. Liske E, Forster FM. Pseudoseizures: a problem in the diagnosis and management of epileptic patients. Neurology 1964;14:41.
3. Muxfeldt M, Price HE, Dane SH, et al. Non-epileptic seizures: characteristics and proposed classification. Epilepsia 1995;36:159.
4. Scott DF. Recognition and Diagnostic Aspects of Non-Epileptic Seizures. In TL Riley, A Roy (eds), Pseudoseizures. Baltimore: Williams & Wilkins, 1982;21.
5. Gates JR, Ramani V, Whalen SM. Ictal characteristics of pseudoseizures. Arch Neurol 1985;42:1183.
6. Desai BT, Porter RJ, Penry JF. Psychogenic seizures: a study of 42 attacks in sick patients, with intensive monitoring. Arch Neurol 1982;39:202.
7. Lesser RP. Psychogenic Seizures. In TA Pedley, BS Meldrum (eds), Recent Advances in Epilepsy (Vol 2). Edinburgh: Churchill Livingstone, 1985;273.
8. International League Against Epilepsy. Proposal for revised clinical and electroencephalographic classification of epileptic seizures. Epilepsia 1981;22:489.
9. Gates JR, Erdahl P. Classification of Non-Epileptic Events. In AJ Rowan, JR Gates (eds), Non-Epileptic Seizures. Boston: Butterworth–Heinemann, 1993;21.
10. American Psychiatric Association. Diagnostic and Statistical Manual of Mental Disorders (4th ed). Washington, DC: American Psychiatric Press, 1995.
11. Novelly RA. Cerebral Dysfunction and Cognitive Impairment in Non-Epileptic Seizure Disorders. In AJ Rowan, JR Gates (eds), Non-Epileptic Seizures. Boston, Butterworth–Heinemann, 1993;233.
12. Snyder S, Rosenbaum DH, Rowan AJ, Strain JJ. SCID diagnosis of panic disorder in psychogenic seizure patients. J Neuropsychiatry Clin Neurosci 1994;6:261.
13. Kanner AM, French JA, Rosenbaum DH, Rowan AJ. Ictal phenomena as discriminators in the diagnosis of epileptic vs. psychogenic seizures. Epilepsia 1987;28:613.
14. Kanner AM, Morris HH, Lueders H, et al. Supplementary motor area seizures mimicking pseudoseizures: some clinical differences. Neurology 1990;40:1404.
15. Williamson PD, Spencer DD, Spencer SS, et al. Complex partial seizures of frontal lobe origin. Ann Neurol 1985;18:497.
16. French JA. The Use of Suggestion as a Provocative Test in the Diagnosis of Psychogenic NES. In AJ Rowan, JR Gates (eds), Non-Epileptic Seizures. Boston: Butterworth–Heinemann, 1993;111.
17. Dohrmann MML, Cheitlin MD. Cardiogenic syncope: seizure versus syncope. Neurol Clin 1986;4:549.
18. Aminoff MJ, Scheinman MM, Griffin JC, Herre JM. Electrocerebral accompaniments of syncope associated with malignant ventricular arrhythmias. Ann Intern Med 1988;108:791.
19. Pedley TA. Differential diagnosis of episodic syndromes. Epilepsia 1983;24(Suppl 1):S31.
20. Guilleminault C, Phillips R, Dement WC. A syndrome of hypersomnia with automatic behavior. Electroencephalogr Clin Neurophysiol 1975;h38:403.
21. Thorpy MJ, Glovinsky PB. Parasomnias. Psychol Clin North Am 1987;10:623.
22. Roth B, Nevsimalova S, Rechtschaffen A. Hypersomnia with "sleep drunkenness." Arch Gen Psychiatry 1972;26:377.
23. Mahowald MW, Schenck CH. REM Sleep Behavior Disorder. In MH Kryger, T Roth, WC Dement (eds), Principles of Sleep Medicine. Philadelphia: Saunders, 1989;389.
24. Gastaut H. Benign Epilepsy of Childhood with Occipital Paroxysms. In J Roger, C Dravet, M Bureau, et al. (eds), Epileptic Syndromes in Infancy, Childhood and Adolescence. London: Hohn Libbey Eurotext, 1985;159.
25. Bender, MB. Syndrome of isolated episode of confusion with amnesia. J Hillside Hosp 1956;5:12.
26. Fisher CM, Adams RD. Transient global amnesia. Trans Am Neurol Assoc 1958;83:143.
27. Caplan LR. Transient Global Amnesia. In P Vinken, G Bruyn, H Klawans (eds), Handbook of Clinical Neurology. Amsterdam: Elsevier, 1985;205.
28. Cole AJ, Gloor P, Kaplan R. Transient global amnesia: the electroencephalogram at onset. Ann Neurol 1987;22:771.
29. Kertesz A. Paroxysmal kinesigenic choreoathetosis: an entity within the paroxysmal choreoathetosis syndrome. Description of 10 cases including 1 autopsied. Neurology 1967;17:680.
30. Lance JW. Familial paroxysmal dystonic choreoathetosis and its differentiation from related syndromes. Ann Neurol 1977;2:285.

31. Rowan AJ, Veldhuisen RJ, Nagelkerke NJD. Comparative evaluation of sleep deprivation and sedated sleep EEGs as diagnostic aids in epilepsy. Electroencephalogr Clin Neurophysiol 1982;54:357.
32. Mattson RH. Electroencephalographic (Polygraphic) Studies in the Diagnosis of Non-Epileptic Seizures. In AJ Rowan, JR Gates (eds), Non-Epileptic Seizures. Boston: Butterworth–Heinemann, 1993;85.
33. Devinsky O, Nadi SN, Theodore WH, Porter RJ. Electroencephalographic studies of simple partial seizures with subdural electrode recordings. Neurology 1989;39:527.
34. Trimble M. Serum prolactin in epilepsy and hysteria. BMJ 1978;2:1682.
35. Prichard PB, Wannamaker BB, Sagel J, Daniel C. Serum prolactin and cortisol levels in evaluation of pseudoepileptic seizures. Ann Neurol 1985;18:87.
36. Sperling MR, Pritchard PB, Engel J, et al. Prolactin in partial epilepsy: an indicator of limbic seizures. Ann Neurol 1986;20:716.
37. Bercovic S. Clinical and experimental aspects of complex partial seizures. Doctor of Medicine Thesis, University of Melbourne. Quoted in J Laidlaw, A Richens, J Oxley (eds), A Textbook of Epilepsy (3rd ed). New York: Churchill Livingstone, 1988.
38. Dodrill CB, Wilkus RJ, Batzel LW. The MMPI as a Diagnostic Tool in Non-Epileptic Seizures. In AJ Rowan, JR Gates (eds), Non-Epileptic Seizures. Boston: Butterworth–Heinemann, 1993;211.
39. Wilkus RJ, Dodrill BV, Thompson PM. Intensive EEG monitoring and psychological studies of patients with pseudoepileptic seizures. Epilepsia 1984;25:100.
40. Vanderzant CW, Giordani B, Berent S, et al. Personality of patients with pseudoseizures. Neurology 1986;36:664.
41. Henrichs TF, Tucker DM, Farha J, et al. MMPI indices in the identification of patients evidencing pseudoseizures. Epilepsia 1988;29:184.
42. Roy A. Hysterical seizures previously diagnosed as epilepsy. Psychol Med 1977;7:271.
43. Roy A. Hysterical seizures. Arch Neurol 1979;36:447.
44. Ford CV, Folks DG. Conversion disorders: an overview. Psychosomatics 1985;6:371.
45. Mai FM, Merskey H. Briquet's treatise on hysteria: a synopsis and commentary. Arch Gen Psychiatry 1980;37:1404.
46. Gumnit RJ. Inpatient Multidisciplinary Management of Non-Epileptic Seizures. In AJ Rowan, JR Gates (eds), Non-Epileptic Seizures. Boston: Butterworth–Heinemann, 1993;269.
47. Rosenbaum DH, Snyder S, Rowan AJ, et al. Outpatient Management of Non-Epileptic Seizures. In AJ Rowan, JR Gates (eds), Non-Epileptic Seizures. Boston: Butterworth–Heinemann, 1993;279.
48. Ramani V, Gumnit RJ. Management of hysterical seizures in epileptic patients. Arch Neurol 1982;39:78.
49. Williams DT, Gold AP, Shrout P, et al. The impact of psychiatric intervention on patients with uncontrolled seizures. J Nerv Ment Dis 1979;167:626.
50. French JA, Rosenbaum DH, Rowan AJ. Outcome in 55 patients with documented psychogenic seizures: clinical and EEG correlates. Epilepsia 1988;29:653.
51. Lesser RP, Lueders H, Dinner DS. Evidence for epilepsy is rare in patients with psychogenic seizures. Neurology 1983;33:502.

11
Vigabatrin and Lamotrigine

Alan Richens

In 1989, the first new antiepileptic drug (AED) to be approved in 16 years was licensed in the United Kingdom. Vigabatrin (VGB) was developed by Merrell Dow as an inhibitor of the enzyme gamma-aminobutyric acid (GABA)-transaminase, and proved to be effective in treating partial seizures. It has not yet been approved for use in the United States.

A second new drug, lamotrigine (LTG), was licensed two years later, in 1991, in the United Kingdom. Developed by Wellcome Research Laboratories, it was found to be effective in treating a wide range of seizure types. It was approved by the U.S. Food and Drug Administration (FDA) in 1994. This chapter will deal with each of these drugs in turn.

VIGABATRIN

Structure

VGB (γ-vinyl GABA; 4-amino-hex-5-enoic acid) was first synthesized in the laboratories of Merrell Dow in Strasbourg, France, in an attempt to develop a specific inhibitor of the enzyme gamma-aminobutyric acid alpha-oxoglutarate transaminase (GABA-T).[1] Its structure is shown in Figure 11.1 and is compared with that of GABA, the naturally occurring inhibitory transmitter. It can be seen that the two molecules are identical apart from a vinyl function on the carbon bearing the amine group, but this small difference confers on it a number of pharmacologic and pharmacokinetic properties that set it apart from GABA. The pure substance is freely soluble in water and exists as a racemic mixture of two enantiomers. Only the S(+)-enantiomer is active pharmacologically. In theory, it would be preferable to administer only this enantiomer in the treatment of epilepsy, but separation from the R(−)-enantiomer in commercial production is impractical.

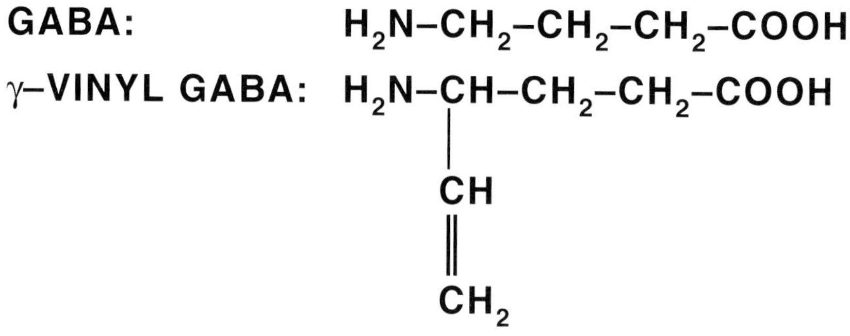

GABA: $H_2N-CH_2-CH_2-CH_2-COOH$

γ–VINYL GABA: $H_2N-CH-CH_2-CH_2-COOH$

                                           |

                                        CH

                                          ‖

                                       CH$_2$

Figure 11.1   Structure of gamma-aminobutyric acid (GABA) and vigabatrin (γ-vinyl GABA).

Mechanism of Action

GABA is the major inhibitory transmitter in the central nervous system. By activating $GABA_A$ receptors, it opens up chloride channels in the postsynaptic membrane, resulting in hyperpolarization and inhibition of neuronal activity. GABA-agonist drugs or compounds that elevate the synaptic concentration of GABA mimic this transmission and cause neuronal inhibition, which is the basis of action of AEDs.

GABA is synthesized from glutamate by the activity of glutamic acid decarboxylase (GAD) in presynaptic nerve terminals. The GABA released during neurotransmission is taken up by glial cells and also re-enters the presynaptic terminal by an active transport mechanism. It is then converted by GABA-T into glutamate and succinic semialdehyde (Figure 11.2). This mechanism is responsible for controlling the amount of GABA available for neurotransmitter action at the synapse.

VGB is also a substrate for GABA-T, but the additional vinyl group causes it to inhibit the activity of the enzyme.[1] It is thought to bind covalently to the active site as it undergoes catalytic conversion, probably forming a Schiff base with pyridoxal phosphate. A stable adduct is formed with a nucleophilic residue in the enzyme active site, resulting in irreversible inhibition. VGB is therefore said to be an enzyme-activated, irreversible inhibitor of GABA-T. The inhibition results in accumulation of GABA at the synapse and neuronal inhibition. VGB does not inhibit GAD or aspartate transaminase, but alanine aminotransferase (ALA-T) is slowly inhibited.[1, 2]

Intraperitoneal injection into mice causes a rapid decrease in GABA-T activity to about 20% of control activity within 3–4 hours.[1] Recovery to control levels takes several days because new enzyme has to be synthesized. The whole brain GABA concentration increases with a similar time course, and repeated dosing causes a more profound and sustained elevation of GABA concentration. In humans, the concentration of GABA in cerebrospinal fluid (CSF) is elevated by single doses of VGB,[3] and nuclear magnetic resonance spectroscopy has demonstrated an increase in cerebral GABA.[4] The activity of GABA-T in blood platelets is inhibited.[5]

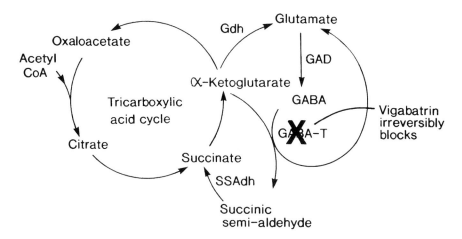

Figure 11.2   Site of action of vigabatrin on gamma-aminobutyric acid (GABA)-T in the GABA shunt.

Pharmacokinetics

A summary of the pharmacokinetic data for VGB is given in Table 11.1 and has been reviewed by Rey et al.[6]

Because VGB is freely water soluble, dissolution of the oral tablet formulation is rapid. Peak plasma concentrations of both enantiomers occur at 1–2 hours after administration and are not significantly affected by food. Peak plasma concentrations at the R(–)-enantiomer are almost double those of the pharmacological-ly active S(+)-enantiomer following administration of the racemate to healthy volunteers.[7, 8] However, the area under the concentration–time curve (AUC) is only about 30% greater for the R(–)-enantiomer. Comparison of the kinetics of the S(+)-enantiomer following administration of the racemate and of the pure substance has shown that the R(–)-enantiomer does not interfere with the S(+)-enantiomer. Furthermore, no R(–)-enantiomer is found in plasma following ingestion of the S(+)-enantiomer, indicating that chiral inversion in vivo does not take place.

VGB is not significantly bound to plasma proteins. It therefore would be expected that CSF concentration would match the plasma concentration, but in fact the former was found to be only about 10% of the latter.[3]

The terminal half-lives of the two enantiomers in plasma are similar—5–7 hours. VGB is eliminated largely by renal excretion of the unchanged drug. About 50% of an oral dose of the S(+)-enantiomer is excreted in the first 48 hours in subjects with normal renal function, but the proportion of the R(–)-enantiomer is higher—65%. Renal clearance of VGB is closely correlated with creatinine clearance. When used in elderly patients or in patients with renal failure, the maintenance dose may need to be reduced.

Renal clearance of the R(–)-enantiomer is more rapid in young children than in adults, possibly reflecting immature tubular reabsorption, but the kinetics of

Table 11.1   Summary of pharmacokinetic data for vigabatrin in adults

Absolute bioavailability*	100%
T_{max}	1–2 hours
V_d	0.8 l/kg
Percentage bound to plasma proteins	Negligible
$t_{1/2}$	5–7 hours
Cl	1.6–1.8 ml/min/kg

*In dogs. Human data not available.

T_{max} = time of maximal concentration; V_d = apparent volume of distribution; $t_{1/2}$ = elimination half-time; Cl = clearance.

the active S(+)-enantiomer were not found to differ and therefore dosage adjustment does not appear to be necessary in children 1 month old or older.[8]

Plasma concentrations of VGB fluctuate widely throughout a 24-hour period as a result of the short plasma half-life. In view of its mode of action, however, the pharmacologic effect in humans is relatively stable. Irreversible inhibition of GABA-T requires the resynthesis of new enzyme, and the half-life for this process in rats has been estimated at 3.5 days.[9] The recovery of enzyme activity in human platelets is also slow,[5] and it would not be expected that a close relationship would exist between the plasma concentration and pharmacologic effect. In view of this, plasma level monitoring would not be expected to be of value, and this line of research has not therefore been pursued.

In view of the uncomplicated pharmacokinetics of VGB, its elimination by renal excretion, and its lack of binding to plasma proteins, it would not be expected to interact to any degree with other drugs. This has proved to be correct apart from a minor interaction with phenytoin (PHT) described later.

Clinical Efficacy

Short-Term Studies

The first clinical trials of VGB were undertaken in the early 1980s in Europe. Six small, placebo-controlled, add-on, crossover studies showed clear evidence of efficacy in managing partial secondary generalized tonic clonic seizures in adults.[10–15] Administration of 2–4 g daily for 7–12 weeks in 98 patients with refractory seizures resulted in a 50% or greater reduction in seizure frequency in almost one-half of the patients.

Subsequent trials have amply confirmed these early results. A response-dependent (enrichment) study in which apparent responders in an open trial were recruited into a double-blind crossover trial showed that the patients continuing on VGB maintained a 58% reduction in seizure frequency, whereas in the placebo group there was a 22% increase.[16]

An additional, small, double-blind, add-on study has shown a significant reduction in partial seizures at a daily dose of 2 g but not at 3 g, suggesting that there might be a dose ceiling with the pharmacologic action of the drug.[17] Early trials in the United States were halted because of fears about possible neurotoxicity (microvac-

Table 11.2   A selection of long-term efficacy studies of vigabatrin in partial seizures
with or without secondary generalization

Reference	Number of patients	Treatment duration (months)	Dose (g/day)	Number (%) maintaining benefit
Pederson et al. (1985)[19]	36	Mean 9.3	Mean 2.6	20 (55)
Cocito et al. (1989)[20]	16	Range 13–15	Mean 3.0	12 (75)
Remy and Beaumont(1989)[21]	254	Mean 22.7	Mean 3.2	228 (90)
Sander et al. (1990)[22]	128	Mean 7.5	Mean 3.1	41 (32)
Reynolds et al. (1991)[23]	33	Range 14–16	Mean 2.8	17 (52)
Browne et al. (1991)[24]	66	Median 43	Median 3.2	29 (44)
Tartara et al. (1992)[25]	25	Range 52–78	47 mg/kg	15 (60)
Ylinen et al. (1992)[26]	75	Mean 72	1.5 or 3	20 (27)

uolation had been seen in the brains of rodents in preclinical studies; see below).
However, a multicenter dose-response study in adults with partial epilepsy showed
that daily doses of 3 and 6 g, but not 1 g daily, significantly reduced seizure frequency, although moving up to the higher dose added little to the drug's efficacy.[18]

Long-Term Studies

A number of trials looking at the benefit of VGB in long-term use in partial
seizures have been published (Table 11.2). These studies show that, on average,
about 60% of patients who had an initial response were continuing to benefit
from VGB. In general, the more intractable the epilepsy, the smaller the
response.[21] Furthermore, the longer the followup, the fewer the number of
patients who maintained a response.[24–26] Whether this is the result of tolerance
to the drug, random fluctuation in seizure frequency, or the natural history of the
epilepsy is a matter for conjecture. With other AEDs there is a paucity of long-
term efficacy data, and therefore it cannot be said whether VGB is better or
worse in maintaining its efficacy.

A study of mixed seizure types in mentally handicapped patients showed that
less than one-fourth of the patients continued to benefit at the end of 5 years.[27]

Monotherapy Studies

Few studies have been published assessing the efficacy of VGB in monotherapy.
One trial, in which 100 patients with newly diagnosed epilepsy were randomized
to treatment with VGB or carbamazepine (CBZ), showed no difference in efficacy. In both groups, 60% of patients were successfully treated over 1 year, and
most of those who were followed to 5 years maintained their initial good
response.[28] Although VGB caused fewer intolerable adverse effects, it had to be
withdrawn more frequently because of lack of efficacy. Other multicenter
monotherapy studies are in progress, but until the results are available, it is not
possible to state the position of VGB in monotherapy or as a first-line drug.

Studies in Children

Early results from an open, add-on study in children with refractory epilepsy indicated good efficacy, particularly in those with partial seizures, although no clear dose–response relationship was demonstrated.[29] Subsequent single-blind, placebo-controlled trials have confirmed that VGB is most effective in treating partial seizures, the response of secondary generalized tonic-clonic seizures (GTCSs) being less.[30, 31] Particularly impressive results have been observed in infants with West syndrome (infantile spasms). In an open, add-on study of refractory infantile spasms, a good response—i.e., a 50% or greater reduction in spasms—was seen in two-thirds of the patients, with more than 40% becoming seizure-free during the evaluation period of 3.2 months.[32] Those with symptomatic spasms associated with tuberous sclerosis responded best. These results have been recently confirmed, most of the responders showing an improvement within 72 hours.[33] It was suggested that VGB should be the preferred drug in the management of infantile spasms and that if there is no response within 4–5 days, it should be replaced.

Generalized Seizures

A consistent view emerges from published studies that VGB is less effective in treating generalized seizures than in treating partial seizures, and there may be a worsening of myoclonic and absence seizures.[29, 31, 34] However, some benefit has been shown in children with Lennox-Gastaut syndrome[31] and other generalized epilepsies.[35]

Dose Response

Studies in adults have used doses of up to 6 g daily, but mostly in the range of 2–4 g. A summary of these studies indicates that the optimum dose is between 2 and 3 g daily, but some patients may benefit from an increase to 4 g daily.[36] In children, the optimum range appears to be 40–80 mg/kg per day, but in infantile spasms higher doses have been used, particularly in infants.

How to Use Vigabatrin

VGB is a simple drug to use. Its pharmacokinetics are uncomplicated, it shows no important drug interactions, it has a long duration of action, and plasma drug levels do not need to be monitored. The only patients in whom a reduction in dose may be necessary are those with impaired renal function.

Starting Dose

VGB is formulated as 500-mg tablets or sachets, the latter being dissolved in water before being ingested. The powder in the sachets is freely soluble and tasteless, but it can be added to a soft drink if preferred. Because the elimination of

VGB is not affected by background therapy, the dose in monotherapy is the same as the add-on dose.

In adults, the starting dose originally recommended by the manufacturers was 2 g daily, but experience has indicated that a smaller dose is preferable because the likelihood of adverse reactions is minimized. In my practice, I start with 500 mg daily, increasing by increments of 500 mg daily every 2–4 weeks until an effective dose has been reached.

In children, a starting dose of 10–20 mg/kg per day is suggested, but in infants with infantile spasms a higher starting dose and a more aggressive escalation will allow an early assessment of the drug's efficacy so that alternative treatment can be initiated if necessary.

Maintenance Dose

The dose of VGB should be titrated until an acceptable response is seen. As discussed earlier, an optimum therapeutic response in partial seizures in adults is usually observed at doses of 2–3 g daily. An increase to 4 g daily is justified if an adequate response is not seen at a lower dose, but little benefit seems to be gained by increasing it further. In elderly patients or in those with renal impairment, there is a good theoretical reason for reducing the dose because the clearance of VGB is proportional to the creatinine clearance, although there have been no reports of specific problems occurring in these groups.

In children, the optimum maintenance dose recommended by many pediatricians is 40–80 mg/kg per day, but in infantile spasms doses of 100 mg/kg per day or more are regularly being used without harmful effects.

Plasma Level Monitoring

The "hit-and-run" type of action discussed earlier results in an absence of correlation between plasma VGB level and effect. Monitoring of levels is only helpful in detecting noncompliance, but even in this respect it is unreliable because of the short plasma half-life of the drug. It is not necessary to separate the enantiomers.

Adverse Effects

Dose Related

The adverse effects profile of VGB is similar to that of other AEDs. The most common adverse effects are drowsiness, fatigue, irritability, and dizziness. These are dose-related and can be minimized by cautious introduction of VGB and careful titration of the maintenance dose. These effects seldom require discontinuation of the drug.

Gastrointestinal adverse effects are uncommon apart from weight gain. The increase in body weight varies from 5% to 16% and is seen in 40% of adult patients in the first 3–6 months of therapy.[37]

In children, the adverse effects profile is similar to that seen in adults, although the risk of hyperactivity is also present in this age group. In one study, 17 of 66 children (26%) were reported to show hyperkinesia,[30] but this symptom necessitated discontinuation of VGB in only two children. All those experiencing this problem had mental handicap or previous psychiatric problems. Sedation (11%) and increased appetite (17%) were the most common adverse effects seen in a recent study of partial seizures.[31]

Studies of cognitive function in adult patients treated with VGB in doses of 2–3 g daily have shown variable results. Small changes in some measures of a test battery have been shown in some studies [38, 39] but not others.[40, 41] In the studies in the United States in which doses of 1, 3, and 6 g daily were used, little impact on cognitive function or quality of life was observed.[41]

Idiosyncratic Adverse Effects

Depression and other mood disturbances have been reported in adult patients receiving up to 4 g of VGB daily,[12, 43] but formal testing of mood has failed to demonstrate a drug-induced effect.[38, 39, 41] A previous history of depression is a major risk factor.[44] Psychosis has also been reported,[45] but the authors of this study treated institutionalized patients with refractory epilepsy, a population known to be particularly susceptible to psychiatric complications. A detailed analysis of a large database (JP Mumford, personal written communication, 1995) has revealed a slight increase in the incidence of psychosis in VGB-treated patients compared with a placebo-treated group and a positive relationship to the starting and maintenance dose. The incidence has been estimated at 3–6%.[46] In some patients, effective control of seizures appeared to be associated with the appearance of the psychosis, suggesting a "forced-normalization" effect.[44] In others, a sudden flurry of seizures after a period of good control seemed to be responsible, resulting in an ictal psychosis. In yet others, the psychosis appeared to be a random event. A previous history of psychosis has not been shown to be a clear risk factor[47] but trends have emerged,[44] and the drug should be used with caution in these patients, although it is not absolutely contraindicated.

When clinical trials were at an early stage, microvacuolation in the cerebral white matter of rodents and dogs was observed, and concern that this might occur in humans constrained the development program. However, there is now good evidence that this toxic effect is not seen in humans. No histologic changes have been shown in surgical and postmortem specimens,[48] and no changes are seen in VGB-treated patients with quantitative magnetic resonance relaxometry.[49]

No other idiosyncratic adverse effects have been identified with VGB. Skin rashes do not occur.

Laboratory Tests

A reduction in plasma alanine aminotransferase activity occurs with VGB as a result of in vivo inhibition of this enzyme.[2] This could possibly confound a diagnosis of hepatic disease. A slight reduction in blood hemoglobin also occurs by an unknown mechanism, but it is not of clinical significance.

Teratogenic Effects

In high doses in rabbits, VGB caused a low incidence of cleft palate (studies on file, Marion Merrell Dow). No evidence of teratogenic effects in human pregnancy have so far emerged, but the data are limited to little more than 100 pregnancies (JF Mumford, personal written communication, 1995).

Drug Interactions

Because VGB is renally excreted and is not bound to plasma proteins, interactions with other drugs would not be expected. In practice, however, a small (25%) reduction in plasma PHT levels is seen when VGB is added to PHT therapy, but the mechanism by which this occurs is unknown.[50] There is no evidence that VGB interferes with other concurrently administered medication, including oral contraceptives.

Discontinuation of Vigabatrin Treatment

There is no clear evidence of withdrawal effects on stopping VGB therapy. The pharmacodynamic half-life is long (see above) and therefore the pharmacologic effect would be expected to wear off gradually over 1–2 weeks. However, it is wise to withdraw the drug slowly, reducing it by 500 mg every week or two.

Conclusion

VGB has been shown to be an effective drug in treating adults and children with partial and secondarily GTCSs when added to existing therapy. Insufficient evidence is available on the use of VGB as monotherapy as well as on its relative efficacy compared with established anticonvulsants. It should be used as adjunctive therapy until this information is available.

Different seizure types and epilepsy syndromes respond to VGB, with the exception of myoclonic and absence seizures, which may be worsened. It therefore resembles CBZ and PHT in its spectrum of activity.

VGB has not been directly compared in clinical trials with other newer anticonvulsants such as LTG and gabapentin. Hence, it is not possible to put these drugs in an order of preference in their role as adjunctive therapy in epilepsy.

The simple pharmacokinetics, lack of clinically important drug interactions, and long duration of action of VGB make it a simple drug to use in clinical practice. Plasma concentrations of VGB do not need to be monitored. Its safety profile is good apart from a low incidence of depression and psychosis, and its use is best avoided in patients with a previous history of psychiatric disorders.

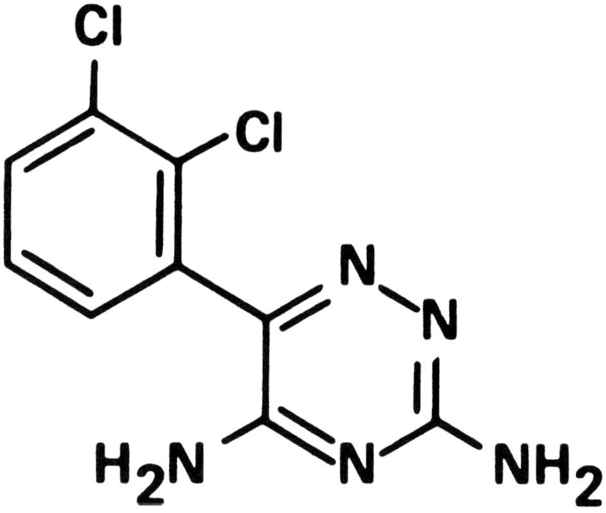

Figure 11.3   Structure of lamotrigine.

LAMOTRIGINE

Structure

LTG (3,5-diamino-6-(2,3-dichlorophenyl)-1,2,4-triazine) was first synthesized by Wellcome Research Laboratories in a search for folate antagonists that might be useful in treating epilepsy. Its structure is shown in Figure 11.3. It is a chemically stable, tasteless, odorless white powder that is poorly soluble (<1 in 1,000) in water. It has no optical activity.

Mechanism of Action

In the 1960s, it was realized that the standard AEDs available at that time, predominantly phenobarbitone and PHT, could lower serum folate levels and occasionally cause macrocytosis. Following their observations that folic acid supplements could worsen seizures, Reynolds et al.[51] put forward the hypothesis that AEDs might reduce seizures by an antifolate action. Although controlled trials have failed to support this hypothesis, a search among antifolate triazines and pyrimidines in the Wellcome Laboratories identified LTG as having anticonvulsant activity in animal models unrelated to its antifolate action.

Subsequent studies[52] revealed that LTG blocks veratrine-induced glutamate and aspartate release from rat brain slices, but not the release evoked by high levels of K^+. This selective action suggested that it might act by inhibiting fast sodium channels. Whole cell or patch-clamp recordings in cultured neurones show that LTG blocks sustained repetitive firing induced by a current pulse, and as

Table 11.3   Summary of pharmacokinetic data for lamotrigine in adults

Absolute bioavailability	98%
T_{max}	1–2 hours
V_d	1.2l/kg
Percentage bound to plasma proteins	55%
$t_{1/2}$ monotherapy*	30 hours
enzyme induced	15 hours
valproate treated	60 hours
Cl monotherapy	0.4 ml/min/kg

*$t_{1/2}$ depends upon background therapy: see text.

T_{max} = time of maximal concentration; V_d = apparent volume of distribution; $t_{1/2}$ = elimination half-time; Cl = clearance.

with PHT and CBZ, this action is voltage- and use-dependent.[53, 54] This effect was presumed to be a result of inactivation of the voltage-dependent sodium channel. Inhibition of nitric oxide synthesis is one consequence of this action, a property shared by the noncompetitive *N*-methyl-D-aspartate (NMDA)-glutamate receptor antagonist MK801, and may account partly for the pharmacologic effect of LTG.[55]

Pharmacokinetics

A summary of the pharmacokinetic data for LTG is given in Table 11.3 and has been reviewed by Rambeck and Wolf.[56]

Following oral administration, LTG is rapidly and completely absorbed with no presystemic metabolism. Food delays its absorption but does not influence its bioavailability. It rapidly distributes to body tissues and is moderately bound to plasma proteins. The pharmacokinetics of LTG are described by a one-compartment model[57] and are linear at therapeutic doses.

In healthy drug-free volunteers, the plasma elimination half-life is around 30 hours,[58] but in the presence of hepatic enzyme–inducing drugs (PHT, CBZ, phenobarbitone, and primidone) it is shortened to a degree depending on the doses of these drugs. Conversely, valproic acid inhibits the metabolism of LTG, doubling its half-life in adults[59] and children.[60] A combination of inducers and valproic acid brings the half-life back to a normal value.[61] It is essential that the dose of LTG be tailored to the background therapy. Children metabolize LTG more rapidly than adults,[60] as would be expected. In elderly patients, the clearance is reduced by about one-third.[58]

LTG is conjugated in the liver by uridine diphosphate glucuronosyltransferase to a 2-N-glucuronide conjugate, which accounts for 75–90% of the drug in urine. In patients with a conjugation defect—i.e., Gilbert syndrome—the formation of this metabolite is reduced.[62] The remainder of the drug in urine is as the parent compound together with a small amount of a 5-*N*-glucuronide. Renal impairment reduces the elimination of LTG and the glucuronide, and therefore reduced doses should be given to patients with renal disease.[63]

Table 11.4   Controlled add-on trials of lamotrigine in partial seizures in adults

Reference	Number of patients	Percentage with 50% reduction in seizure frequency	Statistical significance
Binnie et al. (1989)[64]	30	7	< 0.02
Jawad et al. (1989)[65]	21	67	< 0.002
Sander et al. (1990)[66]	18	11	ns
Loiseau et al. (1990)[60]	23	30	< 0.05
Schapel et al. (1993)[68]	41	22	< 0.001
Smith et al. (1993)[69]	62	18	< 0.0001
Schmidt et al. (1993)[70]	21	29	< 0.05
Messenheimer et al. (1994)[71]	88	20	< 0.001
Stolarek et al. (1994)[72]	22	45	< 0.01
Total/mean	326	24	—

Note: All trials were cross-over in design and recruited patients with intractable seizures.

In clinical practice, use of LTG is complicated by the effect that background therapy has on the rate of metabolism of the drug. It is thought, but so far unproved, that the therapeutic effect is proportional to the plasma concentration, and therefore the size and frequency of the dose should be matched to the elimination half-life. In general, once or twice daily dosing is satisfactory. Recommended doses are discussed below.

Clinical Efficacy

Short-Term Studies in Partial Seizures

The first clinical trials of LTG were undertaken in the mid-1980s in Europe. Four small placebo-controlled, add-on, crossover trials[64–67] gave clear evidence of efficacy in partial seizures (Table 11.4). Five additional crossover studies[68–72] confirmed these findings, with a mean of 24% of patients achieving a 50% or greater reduction in seizure frequency over the 8- to 18-week treatment period. The patients recruited into these trials had partial seizures that had proved resistant to other drugs—including some of the newer agents—and therefore the modest number of responders is not surprising. The poorest responses were obtained in patients in residential centers,[64, 66] presumably reflecting the severity of their epilepsy.

In these trials, secondary GTCSs were reduced in frequency as well. Smith et al.[69] assessed quality of life in addition to seizure frequency and found a significant improvement in two measures—mastery and happiness—with LTG compared with placebo, raising the possibility of a positive psychotropic effect of the drug. This had been noted anecdotally in earlier trials.

An analysis of the outcome of treatment in 677 patients recruited in open trials in a number of centers indicated that 30% of patients with partial seizures and

40% of those with tonic-clonic seizures (mainly secondary generalized) responded to LTG.[73]

Long-Term Studies in Partial Seizures

In an add-on, placebo-controlled, parallel group study lasting 6 months, a U.S. trial group[74] found that one-third of patients on 500 g daily and one-fifth of those on 300 g daily had a 50% or greater reduction in seizure frequency. Median seizure frequency dropped by 36% and 20%, respectively, compared with 8% with the placebo. Long-term open studies have shown a continuing benefit in many of the short-term responders.[75–77]

An analysis of the long-term response in the first 199 patients who received LTG for more than 1 year is given by Binnie.[73] No loss of control was apparent with treatment periods of up to 3 years.

Monotherapy Studies

The first trial of LTG monotherapy in newly diagnosed epilepsy[78] included 260 adult patients with partial or generalized seizures. They were randomized to LTG (median dose, 150 mg daily) or CBZ (median dose, 600 mg daily) and followed for 48 weeks. No difference in efficacy was detected, but LTG was better tolerated; significantly more patients remained on this drug than on CBZ. Of those started on LTG, 15% withdrew because of adverse events compared with 27% of those started on CBZ. Seizures presenting with a focal onset responded less well to either drug than did primary generalized seizures, but both types responded equally well to the two drugs. A similar outcome has been observed in a smaller comparative study against PHT.[79] If these results are confirmed in subsequent studies, LTG might be considered as a drug of first choice in managing newly diagnosed epilepsy.

Generalized Seizures and Studies in Children

An early analysis of a number of open studies[80] suggested that LTG might be effective in treating idiopathic generalized epilepsies as well as partial epilepsies, but this finding was based on a small number of patients. The monotherapy studies described above also indicate that LTG may be effective in managing primary GTCSs in adults, bearing in mind that at the time of diagnosis there may be some uncertainty about the seizure classification. In a well-defined group of adults with juvenile myoclonic epilepsy, however, a good effect of LTG was observed; it was indistinguishable from that of sodium valproate (VPA).[81] LTG may be a valuable substitute for sodium VPA in this syndrome when the latter is poorly tolerated.[82]

Several studies in children have shown that LTG is effective in various generalized seizure types and syndromes: typical and atypical absences,[82–85] myoclonic absences,[83, 86] eyelid myoclonia with absences,[87] other nonprogressive myoclonic epilepsies,[83, 84] Lennox-Gastaut syndrome[82, 83, 88] and Rett syndrome.[89] West syndrome (infantile spasms) has also been shown to respond.[83] Partial seizures in children appear to respond less well than generalized seizures.[82, 83] In general, refractory epilepsies in children benefit from addition of LTG.[90]

Combination of Lamotrigine and Sodium Valproate

A combination of LTG and sodium VPA has been found to be particularly effective in treating intractable myoclonic epilepsy,[91] intractable typical absence seizures,[92] West syndrome,[93] and complex partial seizures.[94] It is thought that this interaction is more than pharmacokinetic (i.e., inhibition of the metabolism of LTG by valproic acid, resulting in a higher plasma concentration of LTG). A pharmacodynamic interaction in the brain is considered likely, and this hypothesis receives support from animal studies in which LTG enhanced the GABA release associated with sodium VPA.[95]

How to Use Lamotrigine

On current evidence, LTG can be chosen for any type of epilepsy and in any age group excepting that the evidence from trials is very limited in some areas. Nevertheless, there are clear signs that LTG has a broad spectrum of activity. Although initial testing was in partial seizures, as is usual for a new drug, its activity is probably more suited to generalized seizures, and in this way it is more comparable with sodium VPA than with PHT or CBZ.

Starting Dose

Adding LTG on to existing therapy is complicated by the fact that a higher dose is required in patients on hepatic enzyme inducers, whereas a smaller dose is necessary in patients on sodium VPA compared with those on no background treatment and those on a combination of inducers and VPA. A further complication is that the incidence of hypersensitivity skin rashes correlates with the size of the starting dose; a cautious approach will therefore lessen the risk of this adverse event. No reduction in dose in elderly patients is necessary because the effect of age on the metabolism of LTG is small. Recommended starting doses are given in Table 11.5.

Maintenance Dose

As with the starting dose, the maintenance dose depends on background therapy (see Table 11.5). It should be remembered, however, that the dose of LTG may need to be changed if the background therapy is altered; e.g., removal or addition of sodium VPA. Failure to do this may result in loss of effect or toxicity. The relatively low toxicity of LTG on the central nervous system allows the dose to be increased up to higher levels than were initially recommended. Maintenance

Table 11.5 Recommended starting and maintenance doses of lamotrigine

	Weeks 1 and 2	Weeks 3 and 4	Maintenance dose
Adults and children over 12 years (total daily dose in mg/day)			
Monotherapy	25 (once a day)	50 (once a day)	100–200 (once a day or in two divided doses)
Add-on to:			
Inducers	50 (once a day)	100 (two divided doses)	200–400 (two divided doses)
Valproate	25 (on alternate days)	25 (once a day)	100–200 (once a day or in two divided doses)
Children aged 2–12 years (total daily dose in mg/kg)			
Add-on to:			
Inducers	2 (two divided doses)	5 (two divided doses)	5–15 (two divided doses)
Valproate	0.2 (once a day)	0.5 (once a day)	1–5 (once a day or in two divided doses)

Note: No recommendations are given for monotherapy in children aged 2–12 years or in children younger than 2 years because insufficient experience is available.

doses of up to 500–800 mg daily are regularly being used in enzyme-induced adults, but in patients on sodium VPA only as co-medication, the dose should be restricted to 200–300 mg daily.

Once-daily dosing is possible with monotherapy or when LTG is added to sodium VPA, but in enzyme-induced subjects twice-daily dosing is necessary.

Plasma Level Monitoring

Initial clinical trials were designed to dose LTG to a target plasma concentration range of 1–3 mg/liter.[64, 65] Although efficacy was demonstrated at these levels, it has been realized that higher concentrations can be achieved with better effect but without toxicity. A later study demonstrated efficacy within the range of 1–4 mg/liter.[71] A recent study in children[90] with refractory epilepsy obtained best results at plasma concentrations of 0.5–5.4 mg/liter. However, no clear relationship between plasma level and therapeutic efficacy has been demonstrated.[96]

Adverse Effects

The safety and tolerability of LTG have been reviewed by Srinivasan and Richens.[97]

Dose Related

An analysis of the pooled results of the first four clinical trials[98] showed that, compared with placebo, the most common adverse events were asthenia, diplopia, headache, somnolence, and ataxia. Only with the last of these was the difference on the borderline of significance. Subsequent studies have added dizziness,[68, 71] nausea, vomiting, and insomnia[69] to this list. Dizziness and diplopia seem to be particularly prominent in patients on CBZ (see below).

A similar spectrum of adverse events was seen in a monotherapy study in patients with newly diagnosed epilepsy,[78] but fewer patients withdrew from LTG therapy than from CBZ because of intolerance. This could have been predicted from early studies in healthy volunteers[99] in which CBZ impaired saccadic eye movements and adaptive tracking and increased body sway, whereas LTG had no effect.

These adverse events with LTG are usually mild and generally require dose adjustment only, rather than drug withdrawal. Furthermore, it has been observed by many investigators that some patients seem much brighter and more responsive when on LTG. Most of these reports are anecdotal, but Smith et al.[69] included a health-related quality of life measure in their placebo-controlled study and found a significant improvement in the subscales for happiness and mastery. More patients elected to continue LTG than appeared to receive benefit in terms of improved seizure control, suggesting that other factors influenced their decision. Banks and Beran[100] applied a neuropsychological test battery and found that LTG does not impair cognitive or mnemonic function.

Idiosyncratic Adverse Effects

Type IV (delayed hypersensitivity) skin rashes occur with LTG. These are typically maculopapular in nature, appear within the first 4 weeks of treatment, and resolve rapidly when the drug is withdrawn.[97] Rarely, it may be more severe and lead to mucosal involvement and desquamation, resulting in a Stevens-Johnson–like syndrome. Surprisingly, the incidence of skin rash depends on the starting dose, being much higher with a large dose or when added to sodium VPA therapy. Overall, an incidence of 2.3% has been quoted.[98] Brodie et al.[78] in their monotherapy study found that skin rashes occurred less commonly with LTG than with CBZ. Sometimes LTG can be reintroduced cautiously after a rash has resolved and the patient remains rash-free.

Weight gain, which is seen with some of the other AEDs, has not been associated with LTG. Early concerns about the incidence of sudden death[101] and disseminated intravascular coagulation have proved to be unfounded.[102]

Laboratory Tests

Although LTG comes from a family of folate antagonists, it does not affect folate metabolism in epileptic patients.[103] No clinically significant change in hepatic or renal function test results occurs.[97]

Teratogenic Effects

In preclinical studies, no teratogenic effect of LTG was seen. To date, insufficient evidence has accumulated in patients to assess whether teratogenic effects will occur, but in the manufacturer's database of almost 100 patients, no clear evidence of such a risk is discernible (AWC Yuen, personal written communication, 1995).

Drug Interactions

The effects of concurrent AED therapy on the metabolism of LTG have been described above. The acute inhibitory effect of sodium VPA on LTG metabolism has been clearly demonstrated.[104] A small increase in the clearance of LTG occurs with paracetamol administration.[105]

Although LTG appears to induce its own metabolism to a small degree, it does not induce the metabolism of other drugs.[106] There is also no evidence that it has an inhibitory action.

In terms of pharmacodynamic interactions, LTG and CBZ when combined appear to cause a much higher incidence of adverse effects in the central nervous system than when given alone. Earlier suggestions that this was the result of elevation of CBZ epoxide levels by LTG have not been sustained, and it is now thought that it is caused by a pharmacodynamic interaction.[107] A combination of LTG and sodium VPA results in a higher incidence of tremor than with sodium VPA alone.[108]

Discontinuation of Lamotrigine Treatment

The elimination half-life of LTG is relatively long (except in induced patients), and therefore the plasma level will fall gradually over several days after abrupt cessation of treatment. However, this is not recommended even though there is no clear evidence of withdrawal effects occurring. Gradual discontinuation over 3–6 weeks, depending on the starting dose, will avoid potential problems.

Conclusion

LTG has been shown to have a broad spectrum of therapeutic effect in epilepsy and should probably be positioned as an alternative agent to sodium VPA. Generalized seizures appear to respond better than do partial seizures.

The marked effect of background therapy complicates its use as an add-on drug, and therefore its use in monotherapy should be considered. The first monotherapy trials in adults indicate that it is as effective as CBZ and PHT in partial and generalized seizures and is better tolerated. It could be argued that it should therefore be a first-line drug in all seizure types. The publication of additional monotherapy trials should be awaited before this recommendation is justified. Publication of the results of comparative monotherapy trials against sodium VPA, which have been completed, are eagerly awaited.

LTG's adverse reaction profile is good provided that a small starting dose is used to minimize the risk of a skin rash. Its central nervous system effects are mild and rarely require the drug to be stopped. If evidence of a positive psychotropic effect is substantiated in future studies, this will give it a substantial advantage over those drugs that have a negative effect on mood and cognitive function.

REFERENCES

1. Yung MJ, Lippert B, Metcalf MW, et al. γ-Vinyl GABA (4-amino-hex-5-enoic acid), a new selective irreversible inhibitor of GABA-T effects on brain GABA metabolism in mice. J Neurochem 1977;29:797.
2. Foletti GB, Delisle M-C, Bachmann C. Reduction of plasma alanine aminotransferase during vigabatrin treatment. Epilepsia 1995;36:804.
3. Ben-Menachem E, Persson L, Schechter PJ, et al. Effects of single doses of vigabatrin on CSF concentrations of GABA, homocarnosine, homovanillic acid, 5-hydroxyindoleacetic acid in patients with complex partial epilepsy. Epilepsy Res 1988;2:96.
4. Petroff OAC, Rothman DL, Behar KL, et al. Initial observations on effect of vigabatrin on in vivo ¹H spectroscopic measurements of aminobutyric acid, glutamate, and glutamine in human brain. Epilepsia 1995;36:457.
5. Rimmer E, Kongola G, Richens A. Inhibition of the enzyme, GABA-aminotransferase, in human platelets by vigabatrin, a potential antiepileptic drug. Br J Clin Pharmacol 1988;25:251.
6. Rey E, Pons G, Olive G. Vigabatrin: clinical pharmacokinetics. Clin Pharmacokinet 1992;23:267.
7. Haegele KD, Schechter PJ. Kinetics of the enantiomers of vigabatrin after an oral dose of the racemate or the active S-enantiomer. Clin Pharmacol Ther 1986;40:581.
8. Rey E, Pons G, Richard MO, et al. Pharmacokinetics of the individual enantiomers of vigabatrin (γ-vinyl GABA) in epileptic children. Br J Clin Pharmacol 1990;30:253.
9. Jung MJ, Palfreyman MG. Vigabatrin. Mechanism of Action. In RH Levy, RH Mattson, BS Meldrum (eds), Antiepileptic Drugs (4th ed). New York: Raven, 1995
10. Rimmer EM, Richens A. Double-blind study of gamma-vinyl GABA in patients with refractory epilepsy. Lancet 1984;1:189.
11. Gram L, Klosterskov-Jensen P, Dam M. Gamma-vinyl GABA. A double-blind placebo-controlled trial in partial epilepsy. Clin Neurol 1985;17:262.
12. Loiseau P, Hardenberg JP, Pestre J. Double-blind placebo-controlled study of vigabatrin (γ-vinyl GABA) in drug resistant epilepsy. Epilepsia 1986;27:115.
13. Tartara A, Manni R, Galimberti CA, et al. Vigabatrin in the treatment of epilepsy: a double-blind placebo-controlled study. Epilepsia 1986;27:717.
14. Remy C, Favel P, Tell G, et al. Etude en double aveugle contre placebo en permutations croisées du vigabatrin dans l'épilepsie de l'adulte résistant a la thérapeutique. Boll Lega Ital Epil 1986;54/55:241.
15. Tassinari CO, Michelucci R, Ambrosetto G, et al. Double-blind study of vigabatrin in the treatment of drug-resistant epilepsy. Arch Neurol 1987;44:907.
16. Ring HA, Heller AJ, Farr IN, et al. Vigabatrin: rational treatment for chronic epilepsy. J Neurol Neurosurg Psychiatry 1990;53:1051.
17. McKee PJ, Blacklaw J, Friel E, et al. Adjuvant vigabatrin in refractory epilepsy: a ceiling to effective dosage in individual patients? Epilepsia 1993;34:937.
18. Penry JK, Wilder BJ, Sachdeo RC, et al. Multicentre dose response study of vigabatrin in adults with focal (partial) epilepsy. Epilepsia 1993;34(Suppl 6):S67.
19. Pedersen SA, Klosterskov-Jensen P, Gram L, et al. Long-term study of gamma-vinyl GABA in the treatment of epilepsy. Acta Neurol Scand 1985;72:295.
20. Cocito L, Maffini M, Perfumo P, et al. Vigabatrin in complex partial seizures: a long term study. Epilepsy Res 1989;3:160.
21. Remy C, Beaumont D. Efficacy and safety of vigabatrin in the long term treatment of refractory epilepsy. Br J Clin Pharmacol 1989;27:125S.
22. Sander JWAS, Trevisol-Bittencourt PC, Hart YM, et al. Evaluation of vigabatrin as an add-on drug in the management of severe epilepsy. J Neurol Neurosurg Psychiatry 1990;53:1008.
23. Reynolds EH, Ring HA, Farr IN, et al. Open, double-blind and long term study of vigabatrin in chronic epilepsy. Epilepsia 1991;32:530.
24. Browne TR, Mattson RH, Penry JK, et al. Multicentre long-term safety and efficacy study of vigabatrin for refractory complex partial seizures: an update. Neurology 1991;41:363.
25. Tartara A, Manni R, Galimberti CA, et al. Six year follow-up study on the efficacy and safety of vigabatrin in patients with epilepsy. Acta Neurol Scand 1992;86:247.
26. Ylinen A, Sivenius J, Pitkänen A, et al. Gamma-vinyl GABA (vigabatrin) in epilepsy: clinical, neurochemical and neurophysiologic monitoring in epileptic patients. Epilepsia 1992;33:917.
27. Pitkänen A, Ylinen A, Matilainen R, et al. Long-term antiepileptic efficacy of vigabatrin in mentally-retarded patients. A 5-year follow-up study. Arch Neurol 1993;50:24.

28. Kälviäinen R, Äikiä M, Mervaala E, et al. Vigabatrin versus carbamazepine monotherapy in newly diagnosed patients with epilepsy. Arch Neurol 1995;52:989.
29. Livingston JH, Beaumont D, Arzimanoglou A, et al. Vigabatrin in the treatment of epilepsy in children. Br J Clin Pharmacol 1989;27:109.
30. Dulac O, Chiron C, Luna D, et al. Vigabatrin in childhood epilepsy. J Child Neurol 1991;6(Suppl 2):30.
31. Bernadina BD, Fontana E, Vigerano F, et al. Efficacy and tolerability of vigabatrin in children with refractory partial seizures: a single blind, dose-increasing study. Epilepsia 1995;36:687.
32. Chiron C, Dulac O, Beaumont D. Therapeutic trial of vigabatrin in refractory infantile spasms. J Child Neurol 1991;6(Suppl 2):52.
33. Appleton RE, Montiel-Viesca F. Vigabatrin in infantile spasms—why add-on? Lancet 1993;341:962.
34. Mervaala E, Partanen J, Nousianen U, et al. Electrophysiologic effects of γ-vinyl GABA and carbamazepine. Epilepsia 1989;30:189.
35. Gram L, Sabers A, Dulac O. Treatment of paediatric epilepsies with gamma-vinyl GABA (vigabatrin). Epilepsia 1992;33(Suppl 5):S26.
36. Kälviäinen R, Mervaala E, Sivenius J, et al. Vigabatrin. Clinical Use. In RH Levy, RH Mattson, BS Meldrum (eds), Antiepileptic Drugs (4th ed). New York: Raven, 1995;925.
37. Tartara A, Manni R, Galimberti CA, et al. Vigabatrin in the treatment of epilepsy: a long term follow-up study. J Neurol Neurosurg Psychiatry 1989;52:467.
38. Grunewald RA, Thompson PJ, Corcoran R, et al. Effects of vigabatrin on partial seizures and cognitive function. J Neurol Neurosurg Psychiatry 1994;57:1057.
39. McGuire AM, Duncan JS, Trimble MR. Effects of vigabatrin on cognitive function and mood when used as add on therapy in patients with intractable epilepsy. Epilepsia 1992;33:128.
40. Gilham RA, Blacklaw J, McKee PJ, et al. Effect of vigabatrin on sedation and cognitive function in patients with refractory epilepsy. J Neurol Neurosurg Psychiatry 1993;56:1271.
41. Dodrill CB, Arnett JL, Sommerville KW, et al. Effects of differing doses of vigabatrin (Sabril) on cognitive abilities and quality of life in epilepsy. Epilepsia 1995;36:164.
42. Ring HA, Crellin R, Kirker S, et al. Vigabatrin and depression. J Neurol Neurosurg Psychiatry 1993;56:925.
43. Aldenkamp AP, Vermeulen J, Mulder OG, et al. Gamma-vinyl GABA (vigabatrin) and mood disturbances. Epilepsia 1994;35:999.
44. Thomas L, Trimble M, Schmitz B, et al. Vigabatrin and behaviour disorders: a retrospective survey. Epilepsy Res 1996;25:21.
45. Sander JW, Hart YM, Trimble MR, et al. Vigabatrin and psychosis. J Neurol Neurosurg Psychiatry 1991;54:435.
46. Sabers A, Gram L. Pharmacology of vigabatrin. Pharmacol Toxicol 1992;70:237.
47. Wong ICK. Retrospective study of vigabatrin and psychiatric behavioural disturbances. Epilepsy Res 1995;21:227.
48. Cannon DJ, Butler WH, Mumford JP, et al. Neuropathologic findings in patients receiving long-term vigabatrin therapy for chronic intractable epilepsy. J Child Neurol 1991;6 (Suppl 2):17.
49. Jackson GD, Grunewald RA, Connelly A, et al. Quantitative MR relaxometry study of effects of vigabatrin on the brains of patients with epilepsy. Epilepsy Res 1994;18:127.
50. Gatti G, Bartoli A, Marchiselli R, et al. Vigabatrin-induced decrease in serum phenytoin concentration does not involve a change in phenytoin bioavailability. Br J Clin Pharmacol 1993;36:603.
51. Reynolds EH, Milner G, Matthews DM, et al. Anticonvulsant therapy, megaloblastic haemopoeisis and folic acid metabolism. QJM 1966;35:521.
52. Leach MJ, Marden CM, Miller AA. Pharmacological studies on lamotrigine, a novel potential antiepileptic drug. II. Neurochemical studies on the mechanism of action. Epilepsia 1986;27:490.
53. Lang DG, Wang CM, Cooper BR. Lamotrigine, phenytoin and carbamazepine interactions on the sodium current present in N4TG1 mouse neuroblastoma cells. J Pharmacol Exp Ther 1993;255:829.
54. Lees G, Leach MJ. Studies on the mechanism of action of the novel anticonvulsant lamotrigine (Lamictal) using primary neurological cultures from rat cortex. Brain Res 1993;612:190.
55. Lizasoain I, Knowles RG, Moncada S. Inhibition by lamotrigine of the generation of nitric oxide in rat forebrain slices. J Neurochem 1995;64:636.
56. Rambeck B, Wolf P. Lamotrigine clinical pharmacokinetics. Clin Pharmacokinet 1993;25:433.
57. Ramsay RE, Pellock JM, Garnett WR, et al. Pharmacokinetics and safety of lamotrigine (Lamictal) in patients with epilepsy. Epilepsy Res 1991;10:191.
58. Posner J, Holdich T, Crome P. Comparison of lamotrigine pharmacokinetics in young and healthy volunteers. J Pharmaceut Med 1991;1:121.

59. Binnie CD, Van Emde Boas W, Kasteleijn-Nolste Trenité DGA, et al. Acute effects of lamotrigine (BW430C) in persons with epilepsy. Epilepsia 1986;27:248.
60. Vauzelle-Kervroëdan F, Rey E, Cieuta C, et al. Influence of the concurrent antiepileptic medication on the pharmacokinetics of lamotrigine as add-on therapy in epileptic children. Br J Clin Pharmacol 1996;41:325.
61. Jawad S, Oxley J, Yuen WC, et al. Lamotrigine: single dose pharmacokinetics and initial 1 week experience in refractory epilepsy. Epilepsy Res 1987;1:194.
62. Posner J, Cohen AF, Land G, et al. The pharmacokinetics of lamotrigine (BW430C) in healthy subjects with unconjugated hyperbilirubinaemia (Gilbert's syndrome). Br J Clin Pharmacol 1989;28:117.
63. Fillastre JP, Taburet AM, Fialaire A, et al. Pharmacokinetics of lamotrigine in patients with renal impairment: influence of haemodialysis. Drugs Exp Clin Res 1993;19:25.
64. Binnie CD, Debets RMC, Engelsman M, et al. Double-blind crossover trial of lamotrigine (Lamictal) as add-on therapy in intractable epilepsy. Epilepsy Res 1989;4:222.
65. Jawad S, Richens A, Goodwin G, et al. Controlled trial of lamotrigine (Lamictal) as add-on therapy for refractory partial seizures. Epilepsia 1989;30:356.
66. Sander JWAS, Patsalos PN, Oxley JR, et al. A randomized, double-blind, placebo-controlled, add-on trial of lamotrigine in patients with severe epilepsy. Epilepsy Res 1990;6:221.
67. Loiseau P, Yuen WC, Duché B, et al. A randomized, double-blind, placebo-controlled, crossover add-on trial of lamotrigine in patients with treatment-resistant partial seizures. Epilepsy Res 1990;7:136.
68. Schapel GJ, Beran RG, Vajda FJ, et al. Double-blind, placebo-controlled, crossover study of lamotrigine in treatment resistant partial seizures. J Neurol Neurosurg Psychiatry 1993;56:448.
69. Smith D, Baker G, Davies G, et al. Outcomes of add-on treatment with lamotrigine in partial epilepsy. Epilepsia 1993;34:312.
70. Schmidt D, Ried S, Rapp P. Add-on treatment with lamotrigine for intractable partial epilepsy. Epilepsia 1993;34(Suppl 2):66.
71. Messenheimer J, Ramsay RE, Willmore LJ, et al. Lamotrigine therapy for partial seizures: a multicentre, placebo-controlled, double-blind, crossover trial. Epilepsia 1994;35:113.
72. Stolarek I, Blacklaw J, Forrest G, et al. Vigabatrin and lamotrigine in refractory epilepsy. J Neurol Neurosurg Psychiatry 1994;57:921.
73. Binnie CD. The efficacy of lamotrigine. Rev Contemp Pharmacother 1994;5:115.
74. Matsuo F, Bergen D, Faught E, et al. Placebo-controlled study of the efficacy and safety of lamotrigine in patients with partial seizures. US Lamotrigine Protocol 0.5 Clinical Trial Group. Neurology 1993;43:2284.
75. Pisani F, Russo M, Trio R, et al. Lamotrigine in refractory epilepsy: a long-term open study. Epilepsy Res Suppl 1991;(Suppl 3):187.
76. Cocito L, Maffini M, Loeb C. Long-term observations on the clinical use of lamotrigine as add-on drug in patients with epilepsy. Epilepsy Res 1994;19:123.
77. Sander JWAS, Trevisol-Bittencourt PC, Hart YM, et al. The efficacy and long-term tolerability of lamotrigine in the treatment of severe epilepsy. Epilepsy Res 1990;7:226.
78. Brodie MJ, Richens A, Yuen AW. Double-blind comparison of lamotrigine and carbamazepine in newly diagnosed epilepsy. UK Lamotrigine/Carbamazepine Monotherapy Trial Group. Lancet 1995;345:476.
79. Steiner TJ, Yuen AWC. Comparison of lamotrigine and phenytoin monotherapy in newly diagnosed epilepsy. Epilepsia 1994;35(Suppl 8):31.
80. Richens A, Yuen AWC. Overview of the clinical efficacy of lamotrigine. Epilepsia 1991;32(Suppl 2):S13.
81. Timmings PL, Richens A. Lamotrigine in primary generalized epilepsy. Lancet 1992;339:1300.
82. Buchanan N. Lamotrigine: clinical experience in 93 patients with epilepsy. Acta Neurol Scand 1995;92:28.
83. Schlumberger E, Chavez F, Palacios L, et al. Lamotrigine in treatment of 120 children with epilepsy. Epilepsia 1994;35:359.
84. Gibbs J, Appleton RE, Rosenbloom L, et al. Lamotrigine for intractable childhood epilepsy: a preliminary communication. Dev Med Child Neurol 1992;34:368.
85. Ferrie CD, Robinson RO, Knott C, et al. Lamotrigine as an add-on drug in typical absence seizures. Acta Neurol Scand 1995;91:200.
86. Manonmani V, Wallace SJ. Epilepsy with myoclonic absences. Arch Dis Child 1994;70:288.
87. Richens A. Treatment of Eyelid Myoclonia with Absences. In J Duncan, CP Panayiotopoulos (eds), Eyelid Myoclonia with Absences. London: John Libbey, 1996;117.

88. Timmings PL, Richens A. Lamotrigine as an add-on drug in the management of Lennox-Gastaut syndrome. Eur Neurol 1992;32:305.
89. Uldall P, Hansen FJ, Tonnby B. Lamotrigine in Rett syndrome. Neuropediatrics 1993;24:339.
90. Battino D, Buti D, Croci D, et al. Lamotrigine in resistant childhood epilepsy. Neuropediatrics 1994;24:332.
91. Ferrie CD, Panayiotopoulos CP. Therapeutic interaction of lamotrigine and sodium valproate in intractable myoclonic epilepsy. Seizure 1994;3:157.
92. Panayiotopoulos CP, Ferrie CD, Knott C, et al. Interaction of lamotrigine with sodium valproate. Lancet 1993;341:445.
93. Veggiotti P, Cieuta C, Rey E, et al. Lamotrigine in infantile spasms. Lancet 1994;344:1375.
94. Pisani F, Di Perri R, Pcrucca E, et al. Interaction of lamotrigine with sodium valproate. Lancet 1993;341:1224.
95. Ahmad S, Fowler LJ, Leach MJ, et al. The effects of lamotrigine and sodium valproate (VPA) co-administration on veratridine-evoked glutamate and GABA release in the rat ventral hippocampus in vivo. Br J Pharmacol 1996;117:302.
96. Kilpatrick ES, Forrest G, Brodie MJ. Concentration-effect-toxicity relationships with lamotrigine—a prospective study. Epilepsia 1996;37:534.
97. Srinivasan J, Richens A. The safety and tolerability of lamotrigine. Rev Contemp Pharmacother 1994;5:147.
98. Betts T, Goodwin G, Withers RM, et al. Human safety of lamotrigine. Epilepsia 1991;32(Suppl 2):S17.
99. Hamilton MJ, Cohen AF, Yuen AWC, et al. Carbamazepine and lamotrigine in healthy volunteers: relevance to early tolerance and clinical trial dosage. Epilepsia 1993;34:166.
100. Banks GK, Beran RG. Neuropsychological assessment in lamotrigine treated epileptic patients. Clin Exp Neurol 1991;28:230.
101. Brodie MJ. Lamotrigine. Lancet 1992;339:1397.
102. Yuen AWC, Bihari DJ. Multiorgan failure with disseminated intravascular coagulation in severe convulsive seizures. Lancet 1992;340:618.
103. Sander JW, Patsalos PN. An assessment of serum and red blood cell folate concentrations in patients with epilepsy on lamotrigine therapy. Epilepsy Res 1992;13:89.
104. Yuen AWC, Land G, Weatherley BC, et al. Sodium valproate acutely inhibits lamotrigine metabolism. Br J Clin Pharmacol 1992;33:511.
105. Depot M, Powell JR, Messenheimer JA, et al. Kinetic effects of multiple oral doses of acetaminophen on a single oral dose of lamotrigine. Clin Pharmacol Ther 1990;48:346.
106. Posner J, Webster H, Yuen AWC. Investigations of the ability of lamotrigine, a novel antiepileptic drug, to induce mixed function oxygenase enzymes. Br J Clin Pharmacol 1991;32:658P.
107. Schapel GJ, Wollman W, Beran RG, et al. No effect of lamotrigine on carbamazepine and carbamazepine epoxide concentrations. Epilepsia 1991;32:58.
108. Reutens DC, Duncan JS, Patsalos PN. Disabling tremor after lamotrigine with sodium valproate. Lancet 1993;342:185.

.

12
Gabapentin and Felbamate

R. Eugene Ramsay and John DeToledo

Maximal electroshock (MES), first used in 1937 to identify phenytoin (PHT), and pentylenetetrazol tests have been the cornerstones for screening drugs for potential anticonvulsant activity. Many compounds tested were selected in a somewhat arbitrary fashion, with many being derivatives of an existing drug line known to have some effect in the central nervous system (CNS). Development of new antiepileptic drugs (AEDs) changed enormously as new insights were gained into the pathogenesis of epilepsy and knowledge expanded on the role of excitatory and inhibitory mechanisms in epilepsy. The change was largely the result of studies in the early 1980s reporting that valproic acid (VPA) resulted in a net increase in gamma-aminobutyric acid (GABA) concentrations in the CNS. This was the first strong association between a clinically effective drug and a specific neurotransmitter effect. This success led to efforts to identify substances that may affect GABA metabolism or GABA receptors in an attempt to produce more effective AEDs.

GABAPENTIN

Background

Gabapentin (GPN, Neurontin) was designed as a GABA analog (Figure 12.1) and is structurally unrelated to any other anticonvulsants. GPN is an amino acid molecule, 1-(aminomethyl) cyclohexane acetic acid, synthesized by Godecke, a division of Parke-Davis Laboratories in Freiburg, Germany. Because systemically administered GABA does not cross the blood–brain barrier, a lipophilic cyclohexane ring was attached to the GABA molecule, increasing its penetration into the CNS. In the standard animal models of epilepsy used to screen for anticonvulsant potential, GPN was effective primarily in MES seizures. This suggested a potential role in the treatment of partial and tonic-clonic seizures. In toxicology studies, a very favorable profile was found along

223

GABA   Gabapentin

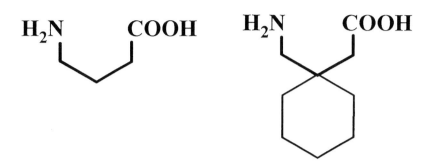

Figure 12.1   The molecular structures of gamma-aminobutyric acid (GABA) and gabapentin.

with a high therapeutic index. (The therapeutic index is the ratio of the median effective dose [ED_{50}] to the median lethal dose [LD_{50}]. The LD_{50} is the dose that is lethal to 50% of animals. The dose that prevents 50% of animals from developing seizures is defined as the ED_{50}. The higher the ratio, the better the safety profile of the drug.)

Mechanism of Action

Naturally occurring amino acids are ionized at physiologic hydrogen ion concentration (pH) and have poor lipid solubility and very little permeability to cell membranes. The passage of amino acids across cell membranes is facilitated by several classes of specialized membrane-bound proteins. GPN is an artificial amino acid with three-dimensional similarities to L-leucine.[1, 2] It has limited permeability across cell membranes without facilitated transport by one of the endogenous transport systems. GPN appears to be transported across the intestinal membrane via the non–sodium-dependent neutral amino acid transporter, the L-system transporter.[3] The transport of [^{14}C]-GPN and [^{3}H]-L-phenylalanine at the L-system transporter are mutually inhibitory and concentration dependent, and the affinity of the transporter for L-leucine and GPN appears to be very similar.[1] The L-transporter is likely involved in the rapid permeation of GPN across the blood–brain barrier and the membrane of synaptosomes and astrocytes, leading to rapid accumulation of GPN in the cytosol of brain tissue.[1, 4] Autoradiographic studies with [^{3}H]GPN demonstrated a novel high-affinity binding site in the CNS,[5, 6] and different GPN derivatives displace binding at the binding site with a potency that is correlated with the anticonvulsant activity.[7] The highest densities of specific binding sites are in layers I and II of the rat neocortex and dendritic CA1, CA2, and CA3 layers of the hippocampus[5, 6] and have a similar distribution to glutanergic neurons.

Because of the molecular similarity, GPN was expected to mimic the action of GABA at inhibitory synapses. Its mechanism of action, although not entirely defined, appears to be a novel one because its spectrum of activity is distinct from those of marketed AEDs. The early research suggested that GPN indeed acted on GABAergic neurotransmitter sites.[8] It soon became apparent, however, that despite its configurational similarity to GABA, GPN did not affect the neuronal content of GABA or bind to its receptors.[2, 9, 10] The putative GABA mimetic action of GPN was studied on a series of ligand-binding and GABA-turnover experiments using mostly valproate or tritiated ligands but failed to elucidate the mechanism of action.[11] GPN increased GABA turnover (the apparent rate of GABA synthesis) in various regions of the brain in rats, but the duration of changes in GABA synthesis did not correlate well with the duration of anticonvulsant effects.[12, 13] GPN also increased the release of GABA from rat brain slices in vitro but only over a relatively narrow range of concentrations (0.1–1.0 µmol/L) with no effect at 10 µmol/L.[13] From the early in vitro studies, the narrow range of active concentrations suggested that direct increase of GABA release was not relevant for the anticonvulsant actions of GPN. Some inhibition of GABA-T by GPN was demonstrated[2] and seemed an attractive hypothesis. However, the concentrations of GPN needed to inhibit GABA-T were higher than those encountered in vivo,[14] making it an unlikely candidate. Despite the inability of those studies to establish a correlation between the antiseizure activity of GPN and GABAergic neurotransmitter systems, the hypothesis that the two were somehow related was supported by studies demonstrating the efficacy of GPN in preventing seizures elicited by drugs that inhibit GABA.[8, 10] At therapeutic concentrations, GPN does not interact with $GABA_A$, $GABA_B$, glutamate, glycine, or dopamine receptors.[2] Electrophysiologic data indicate that GPN modulates sustained repetitive firing of action potentials in cultured neurons.[15] However, this may be an indirect action at sodium channels, since the effect requires many hours of tissue incubation to become apparent.[16] GPN is not a substrate for branched chain amino acid aminotransferase (BCAA-T), but it exhibits a potent, competitive inhibition of cytosolic and mitochondrial forms of brain BCAA-T. The K_i values (0.8–1.4 µmol/L) for inhibition of transamination by GPN were close to the apparent K_m values for the branched-chain amino acids L-leucine, L-isoleucine, and L-valine (0.6–1.2 µmol/L). This suggests GPN may significantly reduce synthesis of glutamate by acting on BCAA-T.[17] In addition, GPN was found to enhance the nonsynaptic release of GABA in a use-dependent fashion.[18] The effect is maximal in rapidly firing neurons, at which time GABA-mediated inhibition would be increased. Thus, there is evidence that GPN reduces excitation and increases inhibition.

Pharmacokinetics

GPN is not bound to plasma protein, does not undergo hepatic metabolism, and is eliminated through the kidneys by passive filtration as unchanged drug. Time to maximum plasma concentration (T_{max}) with oral dosing was 2–3 hours and the plasma half-life ranges from 5 to 9 hours.[14, 19–24] GPN has a linear relationship of dose and maximal plasma concentration (C_{max}) up to dosages of 600 mg, and the bioavailability is approximately 60% (Parke-Davis, data on file). Single- and multiple-dose proportionality studies showed that the mean area under the plasma level–time curve (AUC) and C_{max} increase with dose. Although the change is not linear, increases in both these measures are evident for doses ranging from 1,200 to 4,800 mg per day (Parke-Davis, data on file). GPN elimination and terminal half-life ($T_{1/2}$) are directly related to renal function as measured by creatinine clearance. Elimination rate is not inducible, as the plasma half-life did not change after repeated dosing and was independent of dose. As would be expected from a compound that is not metabolized in the liver, GPN does not effect antipyrine clearance, nor does it induce or inhibit the mixed function oxidase enzymes. Since protein bindings and hepatic function are not affected, GPN does not change the pharmacokinetics of any other drug or drug metabolite.[25-28] The absence of drug to drug interactions makes GPN attractive for use in patients with renal or hepatic disease, human immunodeficiency virus (HIV) infection, porphyria, or organ transplants and in elderly patients.

Dosage and Administration

With the relatively short half-life of 5–9 hours, the total daily dose should be administered three times a day. The duration of brain effect does not mirror the plasma concentration. In animal studies, the peak brain levels occur at 45 minutes after GPN administration, whereas maximal protection against MES is evident 2 hours later when the plasma level and brain levels are falling (Figure 12.2). The clinical implications of this have not been formally tested, although some patients have successfully converted to twice-a-day dosing. This is unlikely to be applicable in patients taking higher doses of GPN.

Initiation of GPN therapy with 300 mg once on day 1, 300 mg twice on day 2, and 300 mg three times on day 3 has been recommended. More rapid introduction can be used, and an initial dose of 3,600 mg per day was well tolerated in the inpatient monotherapy study.[29] In long-term, open-label clinical trials, doses of 2,400–3,600 mg per day have been well tolerated.[30] The initial dose should be increased as necessary for seizure control, and doses of 900–1,800 mg per day are often effective. However, patients with medically refractory seizures likely will require 3,600–4,800 mg per day before control is realized. The maximum useful and effective dose has not been determined, although use of 6,000 mg per day has been anecdotally reported[31] (also, RF Ramsay, J DeToledo, unpublished observations, 1996). Dosage should be adjusted down based on renal function,[32, 33] because GPN clearance is directly related to creatinine clearance. There have been no reports of withdrawal effects when GPN is discontinued. Therefore, rapid tapering of GPN over a week or less may be safely accomplished.[34]

Most patients tolerate 300 mg three times a day as the starting dose. However, significant side effects are encountered infrequently when GPN is started in patients taking maximally tolerated doses of another AED, particularly carbamazepine (CBZ). The side effect is often typical of the initial drug (e.g., visual blurring and downbeat nystagmus on lateral gaze with CBZ) and can be eliminated by reduction of the existing AED. This is a pharmacokinetic interaction with enhancement of the effect within the brain, since GPN does not alter the metabolism or protein binding of any medication.

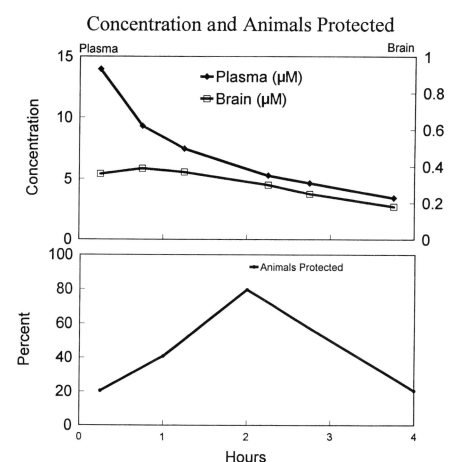

Figure 12.2 Plasma and brain concentrations of gabapentin in rodents after intravenous administration. The bottom graph shows the percentage of animals protected against maximal electroshock seizures. The greatest anticonvulsant activity occurs at 2 hours post dosing, which is well after the highest concentrations are found in the blood and brain.

Efficacy

Dose-Ranging Studies

Initial clinical trials of GPN were performed as dose-ranging studies in patients with epilepsy without regard to seizure type. In a three-way, double-blind, crossover study involving 25 patients, 900 mg per day resulted in a 45% (p <0.001) decrease in seizure frequency,[35] while 9 of 21 patients experienced at least a 50% decrease in seizure frequency. Bauer et al.[36] studied 52 patients with at least four seizures per month with simple or complex partial seizures (n = 29), primarily or secon-

Table 12.1   Summary of gabapentin efficacy data from three placebo-controlled clinical trials as add-on therapy in patients with refractory partial seizures

Reference	Total number of patients (number evaluable)	Mean adjusted response ratio[a]	Responder rate (%)	Mean change in seizure frequency (%)
UK Study 1990[38]	127 (113)	—	—	—
GPN 1,200 mg	61 (52)	−0.192[b]	25.0	−29.2
Placebo	66 (61)	−0.060	9.8	−12.5
US Study 1993[41]	306 (287)	—	—	—
GPN 600 mg	53 (49)	−0.151	18.4	−24.3
GPN 1,200 mg	101 (91)	−0.118[c]	17.6	−20.0
GPN 1,800 mg	54 (53)	−0.233[d]	26.4	−31.9
Placebo	98 (95)	−0.025[b]	8.4	−5.9
International study[34, 40, 42]	272 (245)	—	—	—
GPN 900 mg	111 (96)	−0.139[d]	22.9	−21.8
GPN 1,200 mg	52 (50)	−0.157[b]	28.0	−17.8
Placebo	109 (99)	−0.024	10.1	−0.3

[a]Response ratio = $(T - B)/(T + B)$, where T is the number of seizures per 28 days during treatment and B is the number of seizures per 28 days during the baseline period.
[b]$p < 0.005$ level of significance.
[c]$p < 0.01$ level of significance.
[d]$p < 0.001$ level of significance.
GPN = gabapentin.

darily generalized tonic-clonic seizures (n = 20), and absence seizures (n = 10). AED therapy was kept stable during a 3-month baseline period, followed by GPN, which was added and titrated up until seizure control was attained or a maximum dosage of 1,800 mg per day was reached. Over the next 2 months, a 50% seizure reduction occurred in 28% of patients, and some decrease was found in 71% of patients. In a double-blind study, patients with medically resistant partial seizures were randomized to have GPN at 900 mg per day (n = 16), GPN at 1,200 mg per day (n = 9), or a placebo (n = 18) added to their existing AED regimen after a 3-month baseline period.[37] The decrease in seizure frequency from the baseline value was 6.5% and 13.0% in patients receiving 900 mg per day (*p* = 0.42) and 1,200 mg per day (*p* = 0.01), respectively. Although the number of patients was small, this study suggested that dosages of 1,200 mg per day resulted in improved seizure control compared with dosages of 900 mg per day or placebo.

Placebo-Controlled Trials

Randomized, multicenter, double-blind, placebo-controlled, parallel-group efficacy trials have been completed in patients with refractory partial seizures (Table 12.1).[38–41] The design and methods for each of these trials were similar. Patients stabilized on one or two conventional AEDs and experiencing at least four partial seizures per month for 3 months baseline were enrolled. Individuals with seizure-free intervals of 28 days or more were excluded. After a 12-week prospective baseline period, patients were randomized to receive one of four doses of GPN (doses used varied between the three studies) or a placebo for 12 weeks. Concomitant AEDs were maintained at stable doses during the entire study.

Patient demographics were similar across the studies and between patients in the GPN versus placebo treatment arms. The mean age was 33 years, median seizure frequency was 10 per month, mean duration of the epilepsy was 21 years, and 34% were on more than one AED on entry into the studies. Efficacy was measured by three methods: (1) responder rate, which is the percentage of patients in whom the number of seizures decreased by at least 50% from baseline; (2) response ratio (RR), which normalizes the data so parametric statistical analysis can be used; and (3) percentage change in seizure frequency. The RR is equal to $(T - B)/(T + B)$, where T is the number of seizures per 28 days during treatment and B is the number of seizures per 28 days during the baseline period. The RR ranges from -1 to 1, with negative values indicating a decrease in seizure frequency. A RR of -0.33 corresponds to a 50% decrease in the number of seizures.

In the UK Gabapentin Study, 127 patients were enrolled (113 evaluable for efficacy)[38] (see Table 12.1). Patients in the GPN arm were started on 600 mg per day for 2 weeks and then increased to 1,200 mg per day. The responder rate was 25% for patients taking GPN (n = 61) compared with 9.8% for patients receiving the placebo (n = 66, $p < 0.043$). The mean adjusted RR was -0.192 for patients receiving GPN and -0.060 for those receiving the placebo ($p = 0.0056$). By both measures, the seizure reduction was significant. The antiepileptic activity of GPN occurred within the first 2 weeks of the trial and was maintained throughout the 12-week study period. The results of the U.S. Gabapentin Study Group[41] were similar (see Table 12.1). Patients were randomized to receive GPN, 600 mg per day (n = 53), GPN, 1,200 mg per day (n = 101), GPN, 1,800 mg per day (n = 54), or a placebo (n = 98) for 12 weeks. The RR ranged from -0.118 to -0.233 for evaluable patients receiving GPN (n = 193) compared with -0.025 for patients receiving the placebo (n = 95). Responder rates for patients treated with GPN ranged from 17.6% to 26.4% versus 8.4% for patients receiving the placebo. The median percentage decrease in seizure frequency in GPN-treated patients ranged from 20.0% to 31.9% compared with 5.9% for placebo-treated patients. The most effective dosage regimen was 1,800 mg per day (RR = -0.233, responder rate = 26.4%, decrease in seizure frequency = 31.9%) and a statistically significant dose-response effect was found. GPN reduced the frequency of all partial seizures and was particularly effective in controlling secondarily generalized seizures.

A third international study compared the response of GPN, 900 mg per day (n = 111) and 1,200 mg per day (n = 52) with a placebo (n = 109)[34, 40, 42] (see Table 12.1). Primary efficacy was a comparison of the group receiving 900 mg per day GPN with the placebo group. The group receiving GPN at 1,200 mg/day was included to obtain additional dose-response information. By all three measures of efficacy, a significant improvement occurred in patients receiving GPN (see Table 12.1).

The combined results of these three large clinical trials clearly demonstrate the efficacy of GPN in patients with refractory partial seizures (see Table 12.1) with a dose-response effect evident for simple partial, complex partial, and secondarily generalized tonic-clonic seizures.[42] Patients of both sexes responded to GPN, with women exhibiting a slightly better response.[42]

Open-Label Follow-Up Trials

In open-label follow-up studies, GPN has been maintained for 2 months to as long as 5 years (Table 12.2). Dosages ranged from 100 mg per day to 3,600 mg per day. In all studies, efficacy was maintained or improved.[31, 38, 40, 41, 43–50] These data strongly suggest that tolerance does not occur and that long-term control of partial seizures can be maintained.

Gabapentin Monotherapy

Two monotherapy trials have been completed with GPN. Eighty-two patients with medically refractory seizures undergoing evaluation for epilepsy surgery were enrolled. The presurgical assessment included tapering and discontinuation of AEDs while undergoing continuous electroencephalogram-video monitoring. When the evaluation was completed, patients could enter the study if all AEDs had been stopped and they had experienced a requisite number of seizures: (1) at least three seizures in the prior 72 hours, or (2) at least four seizures in 5 days. After randomization, patients were treated in a double-blind fashion for 8 days with 300 or 3,600 mg per day of GPN. The two primary outcome measures were the time to the fourth seizure and the number of patients who completed 8 days without experiencing four seizures. By both measures, the group treated with 3,600 mg per day GPN did statistically better. The high-dose group was started on day 1 with 3,600 mg per day, which was tolerated very well. The incidence of side effects was higher in this group but no patient was dropped from the trial for this reason. The second trial was conducted in patients with medically refractory seizures taking stable doses of one or two AEDs. After an 8-week baseline period, patients were randomly assigned to receive 600 (n = 93), 1,200 (n = 90), or 2,400 (n = 91) mg per day of GPN. Conversion of GPN monotherapy comprised a 2-week add-on GPN followed by an 8-week taper of the concurrent AED or AEDs. The blinded monotherapy treatment phase lasted 16 weeks. To be randomized to the double-blind treatment, patients had to have had in the 8-week baseline period a minimum of four complex partial seizures/generalized tonic-clonic seizures with no less than two seizures in either 4-week baseline period, no more than five complex partial seizures/generalized tonic-clonic seizures in 1 day, or no more than 28 seizure-free days. Criteria for treatment failure included the occurrence of status epilepticus in the double-blind phase; a secondarily generalized tonic-clonic seizure if one had not been experienced within 2 years of study entry; a twofold or more increase in seizure frequency in the 28-day period compared with the maximum 28-day seizure rate during the baseline period; and a 2-day seizure rate that was more than two times the maximum 2-day study seizures rate during the baseline period. Initial analysis failed to show any difference in outcome between the three dosage groups. Further evaluation of the data revealed that patients taking CBZ at the time they entered the trial were more

Table 12.2 Summary of data from long-term studies using gabapentin as add-on or monotherapy in patients with all seizure types

Reference	Number of patients	Follow-up (months)	Dose (mg/day)	Response ratio[a]	Responder rate[b]	Reduction in seizure frequency	Other (response)
Handforth et al. 1989[43]	9	NR	LD 1,000–1,200 HD>1,600	NR	2/9 4/9	NR 51.2%	8/9 patients reported improved well-being, stamina, initiative, and emotional vivacity
Abou-Khalil et al. 1990[44]	36	2–9	NR	NR	36%	NR	Improved cognitive, affect, and social functions; 3 patients became seizure-free
Sivenius et al. 1990[45]	25	10–27	1,200–1,800	NR	48%	9/25 (36%)	12/25 discontinued for lack of efficacy
Wiener et al. 1990[46]	23	3–24	NR	NR	8/23	6/23	14/23 (61%) seizures less disabling, increase of seizure-free days; 9/23 little or no response or increased seizure frequency
Schear et al. 1991[47]	23	5–37	≤2,400	NR	3/23	8/23	16/23 (70%) improved; 4/23 no change; 3/7 had increased seizures
Abou-Khalil et al. 1992[31]	US 217	≤24	100–3,600	−0.129 to −0.379	PS 50%; AS 38%	NR	—
	Int 63	—	—	NR	PS 39%		—
Leppik et al. 1992[48]	US 240	≤60	600–2,400	−0.226 to −0.429	36–61%	NR	—
	Int 203	—	—	−0.254	36%	NR	—
Ojemann et al. 1992[49]	35	24	1,200–2,400	NR	NR	NR 25%	Patients reported increased concentration, memory, mood, and perception; 5 achieved monotherapy with 1 seizure-free

Table 12.2   (continued)

Reference	Number of patients	Follow-up (months)	Dose (mg/day)	Response ratio[a]	Responder rate[b]	Reduction in seizure frequency	Other (response)
Browne et al. 1993[50]	774	≤18	NR	NR	NR	46% (12 mos); 45% (18 mos)	Dropped for lack of efficacy: 14.9% (12 mos); 19.1% (18 mos)

[a]Response ratio = (T–B)/(T+B) where T is the number of seizures per 28 days during treatment and B is the number of seizures per 28 days during the baseline period.
[b]Responder rate = the percentage of patients in whom the number of seizures decreased by ≥50% from baseline.
NR = not reported; LD = low dose; HD = high dose; AS = all seizure types; PS = partial seizures; US = patients from studies conducted in the United States; Int = patients from studies conducted internationally.

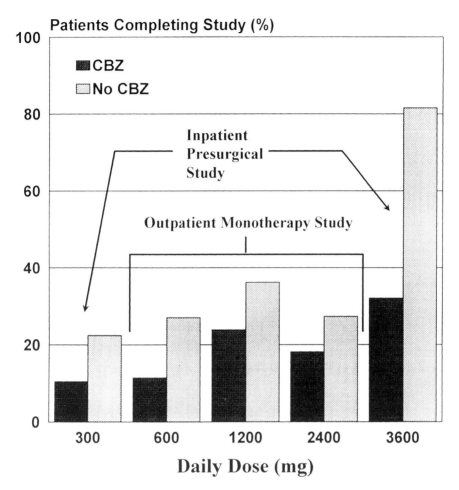

Figure 12.3 The percentage of patients who completed the blinded treatment phase is graphed. Results are included for both of the gabapentin monotherapy trials that have been completed, displaying results by the daily dose received. In each group, patients were less likely to successfully convert to gabapentin monotherapy if carbamazepine (CBZ) was being discontinued (dark bars) compared to the removal of other antiepileptic drugs (light bars), such as phenytoin or valproic acid. (Reprinted with permission from RH Fuerst, NM Graves, IE Leppik, et al. Felbamate increases phenytoin but decreases carbamazepine concentrations. Epilepsia 1988;29[4]:488.)

likely to fail. Similar results were found in the inpatient presurgical trial. Looking at the results from both studies and all doses used, patients taking CBZ were less likely to successfully complete the study (Figure 12.3). A withdrawal effect from CBZ complicated the outcome of the outpatient trial. The doses used in the inpatient trial (300 and 3,600 mg/day) produced a fivefold difference in blood levels between the two treatment groups. Only a threefold difference in plasma levels occurred between the low- (600 mg/day) and high-dose (2,400 mg/day) groups

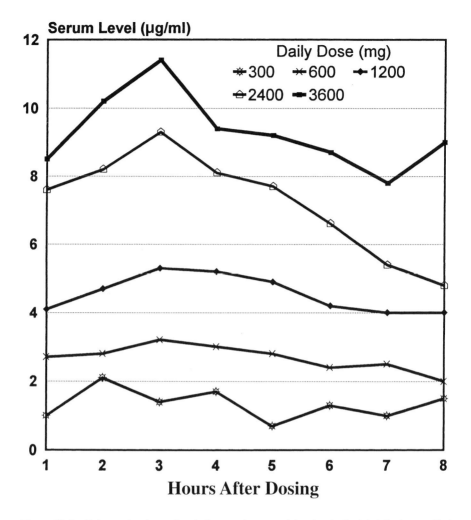

Figure 12.4   Gabapentin plasma levels from patients participating in double-blind controlled trials. Blood samples were drawn at various times postdose, which provides information at different time intervals after dosing of the drug.

in the outpatient trial (Figure 12.4) and was not sufficient to overcome the CBZ withdrawal effect. Patients tolerated all doses well; only 7% of patients were dropped from the trial because of adverse effects. The side-effect profile was similar to that reported in prior trials.[28]

Comparative Trials with Currently Available Antiepileptic Drugs

GPN has been compared with CBZ in the treatment of patients with active epilepsy attempting to achieve seizure control with a single AED.[51] As part of a randomized, double-blind, three-way crossover study, patients were treated with GPN 1,200 mg per day, CBZ 1,200 mg per day, or both AEDs. Median monthly seizure frequency was 10 with GPN monotherapy, 4.9 with CBZ monotherapy, and 4.6 during treatment with both AEDs (p <0.01 for GPN versus CBZ). Side effects were more common with CBZ than with GPN monotherapy. The dosage of GPN used in this study was, perhaps, inadequate to improve seizure control.

Pediatric Efficacy

Clinical trial results in children have been very limited with GPN, although open use has grown. A small trial in petit mal seizures failed to demonstrate efficacy, but the dose of GPN used was much less than the dose found effective in adult partial seizure trials. Mikati et al.[52] reported in open clinical experience in refractory partial seizures with GPN that 34.4% of patients had a seizure reduction of less than 50% using a mean dosage of 26.7 mg/kg. These results are similar to or better than those reported for adult patients with refractory partial seizures. Two large, double-blind, controlled clinical trials have been started to demonstrate efficacy, including monotherapy use. These involve (1) GPN versus a placebo in patients with new onset benign rolandic epilepsy of childhood, and (2) add-on of GPN versus a placebo in children with refractory partial seizures. GPN appears likely to be important in treatment of partial seizures, and the overall spectrum of activity in childhood seizures remains to be defined.

Adverse Events and Safety

All available AEDs have a significant adverse effects profile, which plays a major role in the tolerability and acceptance of an AED in treating a given seizure type.[53–55] Forty percent or more of patients experience side effects, which often limits the use of the drugs. The adverse event profile of GPN compiled from clinical trials and long-term follow-up studies is shown in Table 12.3. Because GPN was studied mainly as add-on therapy, a causal relationship with specific adverse events was not established. Although side effects were reported more often in the GPN-treated groups, a clear dose-effect relationship was not always evident. Somnolence was more common in the placebo-treated group than the group treated with 900 mg per day GPN, whereas the incidence of dizziness was higher in the group treated with 900 mg per day than in the group treated with 1,800 mg per day GPN[34, 42] (data on file, Parke-Davis). The majority of adverse effects were of mild to moderate severity. The most common adverse events reported were those affecting the CNS and included somnolence (24.4%), dizziness (20.3%), and ataxia (17.4%) (see Table 12.3).[42] Patients reported onset of CNS symptoms within a median of 3 days of initiating GPN treatment, in contrast to a 14-day median onset of CNS symptoms in the placebo-treated group (data on file, Parke-Davis). In both groups, the median duration of adverse effects was the same—14 days. Long-term therapy with GPN did not result in the appearance of new adverse events or a rise in the number of

Table 12.3   Summary of most frequent adverse events in patients receiving gabapentin

| | Controlled studies | | | | All studies | |
| | Placebo | | Gabapentin | | Gabapentin | |
	(*n = 307*)		(*n = 485*)		(*n = 1,160*)	
Number (%) of patients with ≥1 adverse effect	174	(56.7)	369	(76.1)	944	(81.4)
Adverse events:						
Somnolence	30	(9.8)	98	(20.2)	283	(24.4)
Dizziness	24	(7.8)	87	(17.9)	235	(20.3)
Ataxia	16	(5.2)	64	(13.2)	202	(17.4)
Fatigue	15	(4.9)	54	(11.1)	171	(14.7)
Nystagmus	15	(4.9)	45	(9.3)	174	(15.0)
Headache	28	(9.1)	42	(8.7)	176	(15.2)
Tremor	12	(3.9)	35	(7.2)	174	(15.0)
Diplopia	6	(2.0)	31	(6.4)	124	(10.7)
Nausea and/or vomiting	23	(7.5)	29	(6.0)	108	(9.3)
Rhinitis	12	(3.0)	22	(4.5)	101	(8.7)

Source: Adapted from TR Browne. Efficacy and Safety of Gabapentin. In D Chadwick (ed), New Trends in Epilepsy Management: The Role of Gabapentin. London: Royal Society of Medicine Services, 1993;47.

events.[42] The use of GPN in 59 patients 65 years old or older showed no increased frequency of adverse events in this age group compared with younger patients.[33]

Few patients withdrew from the GPN clinical trials because of adverse events (GPN, 7%, versus placebo, 3%).[33, 34, 38, 41] Very few potentially serious adverse events requiring discontinuation of GPN therapy were reported with more than 2,000 patient exposures during clinical trials. These include rash (0.54%), decreased white blood cell (WBC) count to less than 3,000/mm^3 (0.19%), increased blood urea nitrogen level (0.09%), decreased platelet count (0.09%), and angina or electrocardiographic changes (0.04%).[33] The low incidence of rash compares favorably with an average 5–10% incidence of rash requiring discontinuation of therapy with other AEDs.[56] Low WBC counts were noted in 8% of GPN-treated and 7% of placebo-treated groups (data on file, Parke-Davis). Finally, no changes in liver function were observed that required discontinuation of GPN therapy (data on file, Parke-Davis). By March 1996, more than 160,000 patients worldwide had been exposed to GPN with no reported drug-induced fatalities to date.

These data indicate that the rate of adverse events with GPN is similar to or better than that of other currently available AEDs. The transient nature of the symptoms and the lack of serious adverse events are also desirable properties. Other than baseline laboratory studies, clinical trials with GPN indicate that routine laboratory monitoring is not necessary.[33]

Cognition and Affect

Anecdotally, patients receiving GPN have reported a sense of well being.[35, 43, 44, 49, 57] This could be related to factors such as improved seizure control rather than a direct effect on affect. However, in 10 healthy volunteers, improved performance in alphabetical reaction test, memory, and concentration were found with 200-mg doses with additional improvement noted after a 400-mg dose.[57] In the double-blind, outpatient monotherapy trial, formal neuropsychological testing and quality of life measures were obtained during baseline period and after monotherapy was obtained.[58] Statistically significant improvement was found in 18 of 37 measures obtained and was not limited to patients with a reduction in seizures. In a study comparing cognitive effects of GPN with those of CBZ, 15 patients with partial seizures were randomized into a double-blind, three-way crossover study.[58] Patients received GPN alone, CBZ alone, or both combined for 4–8 months. Neuropsychological, mood, and psychosocial effects were tested at the end of each phase. The results suggested that GPN has only limited or no effect on cognitive function and may be associated with improved performance on measures of intelligence, memory, and attention. Further study is warranted in this area, as GPN appears to provide improved seizure control without negatively influencing cognitive abilities and may be associated with improved performance on measures of intelligence, memory, and attention.[58]

Weight Gain

Weight gain was not reported with the earlier GPN studies that used doses of GPN up to 1,800 mg per day. Because doses of GPN higher than 3,000 mg per day were used on a more systematic basis, an increasing number of patients experienced problems with weight gain. The weight trends were reviewed in 44 patients in our clinic treated with GPN for 12 months or longer.[59] Thirty-one patients were receiving GPN doses above 3,600 mg per day. Thirteen patients gained between 3% and 9% of baseline body weight (25%). Significant weight gain of 10% or more from the baseline value occurred in 10 of 44 patients (23%). Weight increase started by the second month of drug treatment in most patients. In 8 of 10 patients who gained more than 10% of basal body weight, weight gain tended to stabilize after 6–9 months of treatment, even though GPN doses remained unchanged. Higher daily doses of GPN were associated with a higher risk for weight gain. Weight gain occurred in patients taking GPN in combination with each of the major AEDs, including felbamate (Felbatol, FBM), and also occurred when GPN was used in monotherapy. No correlation was found between improved seizure control, decreased AED toxicity, or mood changes and change in weight. GPN and VPA may induce weight gain, but it appears that the mechanisms involved do not entirely overlap. Patients with a history of previous excessive weight gain with VPA were successfully treated with GPN without recurrence of the weight problems. VPA seems to be more often associated with decreased sense of satiation (unpublished observation), whereas patients on GPN tend to eat several times a day.

Teratogenesis and Tissue Toxicology

Although there are no studies of GPN in pregnant women, there was no evidence of fetal harm or teratogenic effects in reproduction studies in mice receiving up to 62 times the human dosage or in rats and rabbits receiving up to 31 times the human dosage of 2,400 mg per day.[33] These data suggest a lack of teratogenic potential, but clinical experience is needed to confirm this impression. Evidence from preclinical studies in animals indicates that GPN has low systemic toxicity and is neither teratogenic nor genotoxic. GPN was not mutagenic in standard bacterial plate incorporation assays at concentrations up to 10,000 mg per plate. GPN concentrations up to 10,000 mg/ml in cultured mammalian cells did not induce forward mutations nor increase the frequency of structural chromosome aberration. GPN administered to hamsters at doses up to 400 mg/kg did not increase the frequency of chromosome aberrations or micronuclei in bone marrow.[60] In animal toxicology studies, an increase in pancreatic acinar cell tumors was found, but only in male rats. Results in female rats and mice of both sexes were negative. After a single dose of [^{14}C]GPN, the radioactivity concentrated in the pancreas of rodents but not in the pancreas of monkeys, suggesting that the distribution of GPN is species specific. Carcinogens usually result first in an increase in hyperplastic cells, then the appearance of carcinoma in situ; invasive carcinoma is the last change to become evident. With GPN, all three stages appeared at the same time and very late in the lives of the animals. Despite the presence of the tumors, the animals treated with high-dose GPN survived longer than did the controls. The relevance of these tumors to the carcinogenic risk in humans is questionable, as the rat is not a generally accepted model for human pancreatic cancer.[50] In September 1991, an advisory council convened by the National Institutes of Health (NIH) reviewed the results and concluded the pancreatic tumor finding in male rats did not indicate or predict carcinogenesis in humans.

Non-Antiepileptic Use of Gabapentin

One proposed mechanism of action for GPN is reduction in glutamate synthesis. Amyotrophic lateral sclerosis (ALS) is a neurodegenerative disease characterized by progressive loss of spinal and cortical motor neurons. The etiopathologic features are incompletely defined, but evidence is mounting that glutamate excitotoxicity is important in the progression of the disease. In a model of motor neuron degeneration using cultured sections of postnatal rat spinal cord, GPN was found to be neuroprotective.[61] Familial human ALS has been linked to a deficiency in Zn, Cu superoxide dismutase (SOD) enzyme activity. A neuroprotective effect of GPN has also been demonstrated in a transgenic mouse strain with deficient SOD activity.[62] These findings led to a double-blind clinical trial in which 152 patients with ALS were randomized to receive GPN (1,800 mg/day) or a placebo. Primary outcome was a global score of forearm muscle testing. GPN-treated patients had an improved clinical course, but the difference was not statistically significant ($p = 0.056$).[63]

Soon after GPN was first marketed, efficacy in pain syndromes was described and several anecdotal reports were published. This was followed by reports of small series employing open treatment in patients with central (tic douloureux and poststroke) and peripheral (reflex sympathetic dystrophy, painful diabetic neuropathy, postherpetic neuropathy, and compression neuropathy) types of pain.[64–66] Although controlled trials have not been completed, more than 30% of the prescribed use of GPN is for pain control. Because of the very favorable outcome in open clinical use, double-blind controlled trials have been initiated in painful diabetic neuropathy, acquired immunodeficiency syndrome (AIDS) neuropathy, trigeminal neuralgia, and reflex sympathetic dystrophy.

Pain sensation is conducted through the dorsal horn into the spinal cord by small unmyelinated A and C fibers. The initial synaptic terminal in laminae I and II of the dorsal horn is thought to be mediated by glutamate, producing a postsynaptic excitatory effect. Incoming pain signals stimulate the dendrites of cells lying in lamina III, which then project rostrally via the lateral spinothalamic tract to the medial thalamus and the cortex. The A fibers mediate quick-onset sharp pain and the C fibers mediate dull, burning, deep, diffuse, long-duration pain. Short interneurons in lamina II are also activated by the incoming dorsal roots sensory fibers and modulate the activity of neurons in lamina II and III by the release of GABA. The proposed mechanism of GPN would affect both components of this neuronal circuit responsible for sensation and pain by reducing the availability of glutamate and also enhancing the use-dependent release of GABA. Case reports and small clinical series have also been reported on the effectiveness of GPN in a number of other neurologic disorders, including restless leg syndrome,[67] essential tremor,[68] migraine headache,[69] panic disorder,[65] and episodic dyscontrol.[70] Based on these reports, controlled clinical trials have been initiated in each of these areas. GPN shows promise to be effective in the treatment of a number of neurologic disorders in addition to epilepsy.

Conclusions

GPN shows significant potential for the treatment of various types of seizures. The efficacy and safety of GPN for the treatment of partial and secondarily generalized seizures have been established in several large randomized, double-blind, placebo-controlled clinical trials. Many patients with partial seizures that were inadequately controlled were successfully treated with the addition of GPN to their AED regimen. Data on long-term use of GPN, including data on patients who have received the drug for as long as 5 years, is accumulating. Patients have maintained a decrease in seizure frequency compared with baseline values during long-term use. Some patients have had their concurrent AEDs tapered and discontinued and maintained seizure control with GPN monotherapy. Controlled clinical trials to evaluate its effectiveness as monotherapy are ongoing. GPN is very well tolerated. Adverse events, when present, were mild and transient. GPN may be of particular value because of its lack of drug interactions with other AEDs and with other commonly used drugs.[34, 38, 41] This is especially important in the treatment of epilepsy because a significant number of patients require therapy with multiple AEDs and other drugs for coexisting conditions. Because of its many desirable qualities, GPN is a valuable therapeutic option in patients with partial seizures. The results from monotherapy studies and wider clinical use are awaited with interest.

FELBAMATE

Development

FBM (2-phenyl-1,3-propanediol dicarbamate; Felbatol) was synthesized by Wallace Laboratories, Cranbury, NJ, as a derivative of meprobamate. Based on structural and initial pharmacologic data, it was submitted for anticonvulsant testing to the Anticonvulsant Drug Testing Program at the NIH. FBM has been shown to be effective in MES, pentylenetetrazol (PTZ), and picrotoxin models of epilepsy but confers no protection in bicuculline and strychnine-induced seizures. From this, a broader spectrum of AED activity has been proposed for FBM than for CBZ or PHT.[71] However, so far FBM has been shown in controlled clinical trials to be effective predominantly in partial seizures.

Mechanism of Action

Several possible mechanisms of action have been investigated. FBM blocks sustained repetitive firing of neurons by affecting voltage-dependent sodium channels. It also blocks convulsions secondary to the voltage-dependent K^+-channel antagonist, 4-aminopyridine. FBM inhibits N-methyl-D-aspartate (NMDA)- and quisqualate-induced seizures. Binding studies failed to demonstrate any effect on the GABA or BZP receptors, and no alteration in adenosine uptake or carbonic anhydrase was found. Tolerance was not encountered against MES-induced seizures with chronic FBM administration. The principal mechanism by which FBM exerts its anticonvulsant action has not been determined.

Pharmacokinetics

FBM is well absorbed from the gastrointestinal (GI) tract and the plasma T_{max} occurs 2–4 hours after dosing. More than 90% of the administered dose can be recovered in urine, of which 40–49% occurs as unmetabolized drug. The absorption and elimination is linear in the doses used clinically. In animal studies, doses above 240 mg/kg did not produce proportional increases in the plasma concentration. The highest dose used in clinical studies has been 3,600 mg per day. Protein-binding is relatively low (25–35%), and thus binding interactions with other AEDs unlikely to occur. Volume of distribution (V_d) is approximately 0.8 liter/kg. The mean plasma $T_{1/2}$ after a single dose in volunteers was 20 hours and did not change with chronic administration. Closure (Cl), or clearance, of FBM, which is the total rate of elimination of the drug from the body, is 0.8 ml/min/kg. An increase in Cl results in a decrease in the plasma level. FBM is metabolized by the hepatic P450 enzyme system, with significant interactions occurring with the major AEDs.[72–74] The co-administration of CBZ induces the metabolism of FMB and increases Cl by approximately 20%. The metabolism is further induced by 16% (total mean increase of 36%) with the co-administration of CBZ and PHT.[75] VPA has the opposite effect. The metabolism of FBM is inhibited, Cl is reduced, and the plasma levels are 75–85% higher when FBM and VPA are used together. Conversely, FBM significantly affects Cl of the major

AEDs. PHT doses must be reduced 10–30% when FBM is added to maintain stable plasma levels.[76] VPA clearance is also reduced by FBM. VPA levels increase by 28% and 54% with the addition of FBM in doses of 1,200 and 2,400 mg per day, respectively.[75] The effect on CBZ elimination is more complex. FBM will lower CBZ levels by 10–40%, whereas the epoxide metabolite increases by approximately 30%. Although the diol metabolite level of CBZ did not change, the epoxide/CBZ and epoxide/diol ratios increased with the addition of FBM. The mechanism appears to be similar to that seen with VPA—epoxide hydrolase activity is inhibited and CBZ hydrolase activity is induced. When FBM is discontinued, CBZ epoxide levels return to baseline levels after 2–3 weeks.

Efficacy

The first controlled trial with FBM was a two-site NIH-sponsored study. A standard double-blind, placebo-controlled, cross-over design was employed. Patients with medically refractory partial seizures on stable doses of CBZ and PHT were enrolled. Because of expected drug interactions, doses of CBZ and PHT were adjusted by an unblinded pharmacist during the blinded treatment phase to maintain plasma levels within 20–25% of those found in the baseline period. Initially, the highest dose used was 3,000 mg per day, but this was reduced to 2,600 mg per day because of reports of nausea and vomiting. A small but statistically significant reduction in seizure frequency was observed ($p = 0.046$) during the FBM treatment phase. At the same time, a three-period, cross-over, double-blind, placebo-controlled study in patients with medically refractory seizures on CBZ was conducted. The design was employed to control for carry-over effect between treatment phases and reduce interpatient variability. The initial results from the 28 patients failed to show a significant effect of FBM. However, the CBZ levels had fallen by an average of 24%. When the reanalysis took this into consideration, a significant effect was found ($p = 0.002$), suggesting that the seizure frequency would have decreased by one-half if the CBZ levels had been maintained at the baseline level.

Two additional studies with unique designs have been conducted. In the first design, patients were studied while they were undergoing inpatient presurgical evaluations. AEDs were discontinued as part of the routine clinical evaluation. After the evaluation was completed, FBM or a placebo was added to the patient's regimen. The endpoint was (1) the time to the fourth seizure and (2) the number of patients completing 28 days of therapy. Fifteen of 28 patients on FBM compared with 4 of 33 patients on the placebo completed the 28 days,[77] showing a significant anticonvulsant effect of FBM. The other unique design compared FBM with an active control. In this double-blind, randomized, parallel design, FBM at 3,600 mg per day was compared with 15 mg/kg VPA in monotherapy.[78, 79] During the first 28 days of blinded treatment, the concurrent AEDs were tapered while FBM or VPA was started. The escape criteria was a worsening of the patient's seizures. This study biases against FBM for side effects but against VPA for seizure control. By all measures, high-dose FBM was found to be superior to the beginning dose of VPA ($p < 0.001$).

The only other controlled study has been in Lennox-Gastaut syndrome. Seventy-four patients were entered into this double-blind, placebo-controlled, parallel add-on trial. Doses were increased from 15 up to 45 mg/kg per day over a 2-week period. Significant improvement was found only in atonic seizures and the parental global evaluation and total seizure count.[80] Of 13 patients followed for more than 28 days, four experienced a 75–100% reduction in seizures. These results in this very difficult seizure syndrome are very encouraging.

Safety

One apparent advantage of FBM was its low toxicity in animal studies. Single doses of 3 g/kg and chronic dosing of 1 g per day were given without side effects except crystalluria. Because of the high-tolerated dose in rats, a LD_{50} could not be calculated.[76] In clinical trials involving more than 2,000 patients, the most frequently reported adverse effects have been anorexia, headache, nausea, dyspepsia, vomiting, dizziness, and somnolence.[81] In the trial comparing high-dose FBM to low-dose VPA, the relative incidence of side effects was the same for both groups. Mild weight loss was documented with FBM monotherapy in the controlled studies. With chronic dosing, headaches, weight loss, and insomnia have been observed with increasing frequency.

FBM was approved July 1993 in the United States and March 1994 in Europe. As of September 1994, 27 cases of aplastic anemia and 11 cases of drug-induced hepatic toxicity had been reported to the manufacturer.[81] Outcome was fatal in 4 of the 11 experiencing hepatotoxicity and 8 of the 27 with aplastic anemia. A thorough risk-benefit assessment has been completed and FBM-induced aplastic anemia has been estimated at 1 in 4,000–6,000 patients treated. The incidence of fatality is placed at 1 in 20,000 exposures. The incidence of fatal hepatotoxicity was estimated to be similar to that with VPA. Because of the significantly increased risk of fatalities from aplastic anemia and hepatotoxicity, the use of FBM should only be considered in those patients with severe epilepsy who have failed to respond all other appropriate AEDs.

Conclusions

FBM is effective in a broad spectrum of epilepsies, including some of the childhood syndromes for which we have few therapeutic options. With chronic dosing, significant side effects (predominantly anorexia, weight loss, insomnia, and headaches) occurred that often required the dose to be reduced or the drug to be discontinued. The high mortality from hepatic failure and aplastic anemia markedly limits the usefulness of FBM. However, in patients with frequent atonic or tonic-clonic seizures, the risk of serious injury or demise is sufficiently high that a trial with FBM may be warranted.

REFERENCES

1. Taylor CP. Emerging perspectives on the mechanisms of action of gabapentin. Neurology 1994;44(Suppl 5):S10.

2. Bartoszky GD, Meyerson N, Reinmann W, et al. Gabapentin. In B Meldrum, R Porter (eds), New Anticonvulsant Drugs. London: John Libbey, 1986;147.
3. Stewart BH, Kugler AR, Thompson PR, et al. A saturable transport mechanism in the intestinal absorption of gabapentin is the underlying cause of lack of proportionality between increasing dose and drug level in plasma. Pharm Res 1993;10:276.
4. Welty DF, Schielke GP, Vartanian MG, et al. Gabapentin anticonvulsant action in rats: disequilibrium with peak drug concentration in plasma and brain micrordialysate. Epilepsy Res 1993;16:175.
5. Hill DR, Suaman-Chauhan J, Woodruff GN. Localization of [^{3}H]-gabapentin to a novel site in rat brain: autoradiographic studies. Eur J Pharmacol Mol Pharmacol 1993;244:303.
6. Suaman-Chauhan N, Webdale L, Hill DR, et al. Characterization of [^{3}H]-gabapentin binding to a novel site in rat brain: homogenate binding studies. Eur J Pharmacol Mol Pharmacol 1993;244:293.
7. Taylor CP, Vartanian MG, Yuen PW, et al. Potent and stereospecific anticonvulsant activity of 3-isobutyl GABA relates to in vitro binding at a novel site labeled by tritiated gabapentin. Epilepsy Res 1992;14:11.
8. Bartoszyk GD, Fritschi E, Herrmann M, et al. Indications for an involvement of the GABA system in the mechanism of action of gabapentin [abstract]. Naunyn Schmiedebergs Arch Pharmacol 1983;22(Suppl):R94.
9. Haas HL, Wieser HG. Gabapentin: action on hippocampal slices of the rat and effects in human epileptics. In Proceedings of the Golden Jubilee Conference, North European Epilepsy Meeting, York, September, 1986.
10. Taylor CP. Mechanisms of Action of New Antiepileptic Drugs. In D Chadwick (ed), New Trends in Epilepsy Management: The Role of Gabapentin. London: Royal Society of Medicine Services, 1993;3.
11. Schmidt B. Potential Antiepileptic Drugs: Gabapentin. In R Levy, R Mattson, B Meldrum, et al. (eds), Antiepileptic Drugs (3rd ed). New York: Raven, 1989;925.
12. Loscher W, Honack D, Taylor CP. Gabapentin increases aminooxyacetic acid-induced GABA accumulation in regions of the rat brain. Neurosci Lett 1991;128:150.
13. Gotz E, Feuerstein TJ, Lais A, Meyer DK. Effects of gabapentin on release of γ-aminobutyric acid from slices of rat neostriatum. Arzneimforsch Drug Res 1993;43:636.
14. Vollmer KO, von Hodenberg A, Kolle EU. Pharmacokinetics of gabapentin in rat, dog, and man. Arzneimittelforschung 1986;36:8309.
15. Wamil AW, Taylor CP, McLean MJ. Effects of gabapentin on repetitive firing of action potentials and GABA responses of mouse central neurons in cell culture [abstract]. Epilepsia 1991;32(Suppl 3):20.
16. Wamil AW, McLean MJ. Limitation by gabapentin of high frequency action potential firing by mouse central neurons in cell culture, Epilepsy Res 1994;17:1.
17. Goldlust A, Su TZ, Welty DF, et al. Effects of anticonvulsant drug gabapentin on the enzymes in metabolic pathways of glutamate and GABA. Epilepsy Res 1995;22:1.
18. Honmou O, Kocsis JD, Richerson GB. Gabapentin potentiates the conductance increase induced by nipocotic acid in CA1 pyramidal neurons in vitro. Epilepsy Res 1995;20:193.
19. Anhut H, Leppik I, Schmidt B, Thomann P. Drug interaction study of the new anticonvulsant gabapentin with phenytoin in epileptic patients [abstract]. Naunyn Schmiedebergs Arch Pharmacol 1988;337(Suppl):R127.
20. Ben-Menachem E, Persson LI, Hedner T. Selected CSF biochemistry and gabapentin concentrations in the CSF and plasma in patients with partial seizures after a single oral dose of gabapentin. Epilepsy Res 1992;11:45.
21. Comstock TJ, Sica DA, Bockbrader HN, et al. Gabapentin pharmacokinetics in subjects with various degrees of renal function [abstract]. J Clin Pharmacol 1990;30:862.
22. Graves NM, Holmes GB, Leppik IE, et al. Pharmacokinetics of gabapentin in patients treated with phenytoin [abstract]. Pharmacotherapy 1989;9:196.
23. Hooper WD, Kavanagh MC, Herkes GK, Eadie MJ. Lack of a pharmacokinetic interaction between phenobarbitone and gabapentin. Br J Clin Pharmacol 1991;31:171.
24. Richens A. Clinical Pharmacokinetics of Gabapentin. In D Chadwick (ed), New Trends in Epilepsy Management: The Role of Gabapentin. London: Royal Society of Medicine Services, 1993;41.
25. Graves NM, Holmes GB, Fuerst RH, Leppik IE. Effect of felbamate and carbamazepine serum concentrations. Epilepsia 1989;30:225.
26. Richens A. Clinical Pharmacokinetics of Gabapentin. In D Chadwick (ed), New Trends in Epilepsy Management: The Role of Gabapentin. London: Royal Society of Medicine Services, 1993;41.
27. Eldon MA, Underwood BA, Randinitis EJ, et al. Lack of effect of gabapentin on the pharmacokinetics of a norethindrone acetate/ethinyl estradiol-containing oral contraceptive [abstract]. Neurology 1993;43:A307.

28. Ramsay RE. Clinical efficacy and safety of gabapentin. Neurology 1994;44(Suppl 5):S23.
29. Bergey GK, Crockett JG, Leiderman DB, et al. U.S. GBP Study Group 088/89. Multicenter, double-blind study of gabapentin (GBP; Neurontin) monotherapy in patients with medically refractory partial seizures. Epilepsia 1995;36(Suppl 4):68.
30. Garofalo EA, Hayes AG, Greeley CA, et al. U.S. GBP Study Group 088/89. An open label extension study of gabapentin (GBP; Neurontin) monotherapy in patients with medically refractory partial seizures. Epilepsia 1985;36(Suppl 4):68.
31. Abou-Khalil B, Shellenberger MK, Anhut H. Two open-label, multicenter studies of the safety and efficacy of gabapentin in patients with refractory epilepsy [abstract]. Epilepsia 1992;33(Suppl 3):77.
32. McClean MJ. Clinical pharmacokinetics of gabapentin. Neurology 1994;44(Suppl 5):S17.
33. Parke Davis. Investigator's Brochure—Gabapentin (CI-945), Research Report No: RR-X 720-03092, May 21, 1992.
34. Goa KL, Sorkin EM. Gabapentin: a review of its pharmacological properties and clinical potential in epilepsy. Drugs 1993;46:409.
35. Crawford P, Ghadiali E, Lane R, et al. Gabapentin as an antiepileptic drug in man. J Neurol Neurosurg Psychiatry 1987;50:682.
36. Bauer G, Bechinger D, Castell M, et al. Gabapentin in the Treatment of Drug-Resistant Epileptic Patients. In J Manelis et al. (eds), Advances in Epileptology (Vol 17). New York: Raven, 1989;219.
37. Sivenius J, Kalviainen R, Ylinen A, Riekkinen P. Double-blind study of gabapentin in the treatment of partial seizures. Epilepsia 1991;32:539.
38. U.K. Gabapentin Study Group. Gabapentin in partial epilepsy. Lancet 1990;335:1114.
39. Ramsay RE, Wallace J, Shellenberger K, Wibberg M. Efficacy and safety of gabapentin (Neurontin) as add-on therapy in patients with uncontrolled partial seizures. Neurology 1991;41(Suppl 1):330.
40. Bruni J, Saunders M, Anhut H, Sauermann W. Efficacy and safety of gabapentin (Neurontin): a multicenter, placebo-controlled, double-blind study [abstract]. Neurology 1991;41(Suppl 1):330.
41. U.S. Gabapentin Study Group No. 5. Gabapentin as add-on therapy in refractory partial epilepsy: a double-blind, placebo-controlled, parallel-group study. Neurology 1993;43:2292.
42. Browne TR. Efficacy and Safety of Gabapentin. In D Chadwick (ed), New Trends in Epilepsy Management: The Role of Gabapentin. London: Royal Society of Medicine Services, 1993;47.
43. Handforth A, Treiman DM, Norton LC. Effect of gabapentin on complex partial seizure frequency [abstract]. Neurology 1989;39(Suppl 1):114.
44. Abou-Khalil B, McLean M, Castro O, Courville K. Gabapentin in the treatment of refractory partial seizures [abstract]. Epilepsia 1990;31:644.
45. Sivenius J, Kälviäinen R, Ylinen A, Riekkinen P. Efficacy of gabapentin in long-term therapy in partial seizures [abstract]. Epilepsia 1990;31:644.
46. Wiener JA, Schear MJ, Rowan AJ, Wallace JD. Safety and effectiveness of gabapentin in the treatment of partial seizures [abstract]. Epilepsia 1990;31:644.
47. Schear MJ, Wiener JA, Rowan AJ. Long-term efficacy of gabapentin in the treatment of partial seizures [abstract]. Epilepsia 1991;32(Suppl 3):6.
48. Leppik IE, Shellenberger MK, Anhut H. Two open-label, multicenter studies of the safety and efficacy of gabapentin as add-on therapy in patients with refractory partial seizures [abstract]. Epilepsia 1992;33(Suppl 3):117.
49. Ojemann LM, Wilensky AJ, Temkin NR, et al. Long-term treatment with gabapentin for partial epilepsy. Epilepsy Res 1992;13:159.
50. Browne TR, and the United States, International, and Parke-Davis Gabapentin Study Groups. Long-term efficacy and toxicity of gabapentin [abstract]. Neurology 1993;43:A307.
51. Temkin NR, Ojemann LM, Ricker B, et al. Gabapentin and carbamazepine as monotherapy and combined: a pilot study. Epilepsia 1992;33(Suppl 3):77.
52. Mikati M, Kjurana D, Riviello J, et al. Efficacy of gabapentin in children with refractory partial seizures. Neurology 1995;45(Suppl 4):A201.
53. Homan RW, Miller B, and the Veterans Administration Epilepsy Cooperative Study Group. Causes of treatment failure with antiepileptic drugs vary over time. Neurology 1987;37:1620.
54. Mattson RH, Cramer JA, Collins JF, et al. Comparison of carbamazepine, phenobarbital, phenytoin, and primidone in partial and secondarily generalized tonic-clonic seizures. N Engl J Med 1985;313:145.
55. Smith DB, Mattson RH, Cramer JA, et al. Results of a nationwide Veterans Administration Cooperative Study comparing the efficacy and toxicity of carbamazepine, phenobarbital, phenytoin, and primidone. Epilepsia 1987;28(Suppl 3):S50.
56. Mattson RH, Cramer JA, Collins JF, and the Department of Veterans Affairs Epilepsy Cooperative Study No. 264 Group. A comparison of valproate with carbamazepine for the treatment of complex

partial seizures and secondarily generalized tonic-clonic seizures in adults. N Engl J Med 1992;327:765.

57. Saletu B, Grunberger J, Linzmayer L. Evaluation of encephalotropic and psychotropic properties of gabapentin in man by pharmacy-EEG and psychometry. Int J Clin Pharmacol Ther Toxicol 1986;24:362.

58. Dodrill CB, Wilensky AJ, Ojemann LM, et al. Neuropsychological, mood, and psychosocial effects of gabapentin [abstract]. Epilepsia 1992;33(Suppl 3):117.

59. DeToledo J, Toledo C, DeCerce J, Ramsay RE. Changes in body weight with chronic, high dose gabapentin therapy. Ther Drug Monit (in press).

60. Food and Drug Administration. Gabapentin: Summary Basis for Approval. Washington, DC, January 20, 1993.

61. Rothstein JD, Kunel RW. Neuroprotective strategies in a model of chronic glutamate-mediated motor neuron toxicity. J Neurochem 1995;65:643.

62. Gurney ME, Cutting FB, Zhai P, et al. Benefit of vitamin E, riluzole, and gabapentin in a transgenic model of familial amyotrophic lateral sclerosis. Ann Neurol 1996;39:147.

63. Miller RG, Gelinas D, Moore D, et al. A placebo-controlled trial of gabapentin in amyotrophic lateral sclerosis. Neurology 1996;46(2):A469.

64. Mellick GA, Mellick LB. Gabapentin in the management of reflex sympathetic dystrophy. Am J Pain Manag 1995;10:265.

65. Mellick GA, Seng ML. The use of gabapentin in the treatment of reflex sympathetic dystrophy and a phobic disorder. J Pain Symptom Manag 1995;5:7.

66. Segal AZ, Rordorf G. Gabapentin as a novel treatment for postherpetic neuralgia. Neurology 1966;26(4):1075.

67. Mellick GA, Mellick LB. Successful treatment of restless leg syndrome with gabapentin. Neurology 1995;45(Suppl 4):A285.

68. Burrows GT, King RB. Gabapentin in essential tremor. Neurology 1995;45(Suppl 4):A187.

69. Mathew NT, Lucker C. Gabapentin in migraine prophylaxis: a preliminary open label study. Neurology 1996;46:A286.

70. Ryback R, Ryback L. Gabapentin for behavioral dyscontrol. Am J Psychiatry 1995;152:1399.

71. Swinyard EA, Sofia RD, Kupferberg HJ. Comparative anticonvulsant activity and neurotoxicity of felbamate and four prototype antiepileptic drugs in mice and rats. Epilepsia 1987;27:27.

72. Albani F, Theodore WH, Washington P, et al. Effect of felbamate on plasma levels of carbamazepine and its metabolites. Epilepsia 1991;32:130.

73. Graves NM, Holmes GB, Fuerst RH, Leppik IE. Effect of felbamate and carbamazepine serum concentrations. Epilepsia 1989;30(2):225.

74. Fuerst RH, Graves NM, Leppik IE, et al. Felbamate increases phenytoin but decreases carbamazepine concentrations. Epilepsia 1988;29(4):488.

75. Wagner ML, Graves NM, Marienau K, et al. Discontinuation of phenytoin and carbamazepine in patients receiving felbamate. Epilepsia 1991;32(3):398.

76. Graves NM. Pharmacokinetics and interactions of antiepileptic drugs. Am J Hosp Pharm 1993;50(Suppl 5):S23.

77. Bourgeois BFD, Leppik IE, Sackellares JC, et al. Felbamate double-blind efficacy trial following presurgical monitoring. Epilepsia 1991;32(Suppl 3):18.

78. Faught RE, Sachdeo RC, Remler MP, et al. Felbamate monotherapy for partial onset seizures: an active-control trial. Neurology 1993;43:688.

79. Sachdeo R, Kramer LD, Rosenberg A, Sachdeo S. Felbamate monotherapy: controlled trial in patients with partial onset seizures. Ann Neurol 1992;32:386.

80. Ritter F, Dreifuss FE, Sackellares JC, et al. Double-blind trial of felbamate in Lennox-Gastaut syndrome. Epilepsia 1991;32(Suppl 3):8.

81. Stables JP, Bialer M, Johannessen SI, et al. Progress report on new antiepileptic drugs: a summary of the Second Eliat Conference. Epilepsy Res 1995;22:235.

13
Rational Drug Therapy of Epilepsy

David Chadwick

At a time when there is a sudden and dramatic increase in the number and choice of drugs to treat epilepsy, it is perhaps important to consider some broad principles that need to be applied to treatment.

1.   The diagnosis of seizures or epilepsy should be secure. There is no place for a therapeutic trial when the diagnosis is uncertain. Furthermore, the diagnostic process for every patient should include not only the differentiation of epileptic seizures from nonepileptic attacks, but, wherever possible, a satisfactory classification of seizures and epilepsy syndromes.[1, 2] Acute symptomatic seizures must be differentiated from seizures occurring spontaneously as a part of epilepsy. Acute symptomatic seizures will rarely need anything other than acute treatment together with treatment of the underlying cause (e.g., alcohol withdrawal, acute metabolic disorders). An adequate classification of seizures and epilepsy syndromes will also lead to the necessary consideration of the etiology of epilepsy, which may also require specific treatment in addition to the prescription of antiepileptic drugs (AEDs) (for example, treatment of cerebral tumors, arteriovenous malformations, etc.).

2.   An initiation or change in AED therapy needs a full and adequate discussion with the patient. He or she needs to be fully aware of the aims of treatment, the benefits, and the potential adverse effects. Many of the decisions to be made in the treatment of epilepsy are not of a black-and-white nature but are varying shades of grey. The individual's personal circumstances and views therefore become enormously important in ensuring compliance with regimes. In many circumstances, the physician should be a provider of relevant information rather than a decision-maker. Compliance is a major issue in the long-term management of epilepsy, and poor compliance does not identify the "bad" patient, it identifies a poor doctor-patient relationship and an inadequately informed patient.

3.   The ultimate aim of treatment of epilepsy will be no seizures and no drugs. This may not be readily achievable for many patients with epilepsy who have a chronic disorder. The first step in treating epilepsy will always be to choose the

minimum effective dose of an appropriate AED. In practice, this means initiating treatment usually at a low dose of an AED and slowly increasing this dose if and when further seizures occur. This approach, using a single AED (monotherapy) will usually be successful in 50–80% of new patients with epilepsy. Alternative monotherapies or combined treatments (polytherapy) will only be necessary in the minority with more severe epilepsies. In this group of patients, a law of diminishing returns will apply. Briefly stated, the longer seizures remain poorly controlled, the less likely a drug-induced (or spontaneous) remission of epilepsy.[3, 4] This has two logical consequences. The first is that some agreement will often need to be reached with the patient regarding an acceptable compromise between a reduced seizure frequency and severity and unwanted side effects of AEDs. The second is that nonpharmacologic treatments may demand serious consideration at a relatively early stage (see Chapter 17).

4.   In choosing between different drugs, a number of issues will demand careful consideration. These include judgments about the efficacy of the drug for an individual patient and its tolerability (the risk of adverse effects). Both of these factors will contribute to the overall effectiveness of an AED (barbiturate coma may be highly efficacious in preventing seizures, but it is not an acceptable management policy other than in the short-term). In the current age of "evidence-based medicine," it is implicit that comparative judgments of efficacy, tolerability, and effectiveness be based on the results of appropriate randomized clinical trials.[5] In addition to these fundamental principles, it is helpful if AEDs are simple for patients to use, needing no more than twice-daily dosing and not requiring troublesome blood level monitoring. It is also helpful for health care systems if AEDs are inexpensive.

There is now very good evidence from many studies (see below) that the chief factor determining relative effectiveness is likely to be the spectrum of adverse effects of AEDs. Thus, it has proved difficult to detect significant differences in efficacy outcomes in comparative monotherapy studies, but differences often are apparent in the proportion of patients who withdraw from studies because of adverse effects.[6–8] AEDs possess dose-related, largely central nervous system (CNS) adverse effects and idiosyncratic side effects. In addition, because of the long periods for which they may be taken, these drugs have also been associated with chronic toxicity as well as teratogenicity, as they may be taken by women through childbearing years. All these issues need to be taken into account in choosing drug treatment (see below).

STARTING THERAPY

Antiepileptic treatment has, in the past, been advocated before seizures occur. Such prophylactic treatment has been undertaken in patients with a high prospective risk of epilepsy after head injury[9] and craniotomy for various neurosurgical conditions.[10] Because no clear evidence exists that antiepileptic treatment is effective in preventing late epilepsy,[9, 11] it seems better to delay treatment until seizures have occurred rather than to adopt a policy of treatment of all those at risk, particularly because there may be a high incidence of side effects with prophylactic treatment[12] and therefore poor compliance.[13]

When two or more unprovoked seizures have occurred within a short interval, antiepileptic therapy is usually indicated. Problems do arise, however, in defining a short interval. Most would include periods of 6 months to 1 year within the definition. Even where seizures occur in a close temporal relationship, the identification of specific precipitating factors may make it more important to counsel patients than to commence drug therapy. The most common examples are febrile convulsions in children and alcohol-withdrawal seizures in adults. Less commonly, seizures may be precipitated in photosensitive subjects by television, visual display units (VDUs), or other photic stimuli.

CHOICE OF DRUG

There is now considerable evidence[14] that patients with newly diagnosed epilepsy should be treated with a single drug. While many clinicians have been persuaded that one is likely to be most effective against particular seizure types and epileptic syndromes, it is difficult to identify satisfactory clinical trials that support this contention.[15]

The key issue in the choice of a first drug at diagnosis is an accurate and adequate diagnosis of seizure type and, if possible, epilepsy syndrome. By no means are all drugs effective against all seizure types. The spectrum of efficacy of drugs is represented graphically in Figure 13.1. It is particularly important to avoid the use of drugs that may exacerbate seizures. Hence, there is evidence that carbamazepine (CBZ) and vigabatrin (VGB)[16] may exacerbate absence and myoclonic seizures in the generalized epilepsy syndromes. It is perhaps here that syndromic classification of epilepsy becomes most important, because a drug should be chosen that would be effective against all seizure types known to occur in that syndrome rather than only those seizures that have occurred in a patient at one point in time.

Improvements in clinical classification of seizures and epilepsy syndromes in the last 20 years have also occurred at a time when we have developed a clearer understanding of the mechanism of action of AEDs. It is now becoming possible to associate particular antiepileptic mechanisms with effects against seizure types and associate them with different spectra of adverse effects. Inevitably, many AEDs, particularly valproate (VPA), lamotrigine (LTG), and topiramate (TPM), may have multiple mechanisms of action, some of which are not fully understood. Table 13.1 summarizes different mechanisms of action for AEDs. Several drugs modify ionic sodium conduction across membranes, binding to ion channels in order to keep them in an inactivated state, thereby blocking repetitive neuronal firing. Drugs that possess this property include phenytoin (PHT), CBZ, LTG, TPM, and VPA.[17] All these drugs are effective in preventing partial seizures and generalized and secondarily generalized tonic-clonic seizures. Most of these drugs (with the exception of VPA) can be associated with dose-related neurotoxicity syndromes that include ataxia, nystagmus, and diplopia. The second direct membrane effect is displayed by drugs such as ethosuximide and possibly VPA, which modify slow or T-calcium currents in the thalamus. This mechanism seems particularly relevant to spike-wave (SW) epilepsies and absence seizures. These same calcium conductances can be enhanced by gamma-

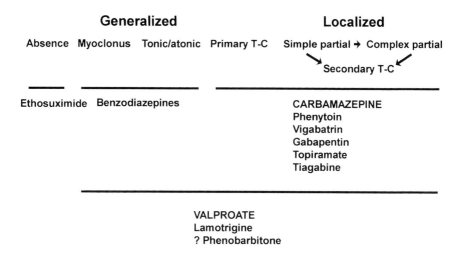

Figure 13.1   Spectrum of efficacy of antiepileptic drugs (AEDs) by seizure type.

aminobutyric acid (GABA)ergic inputs to the thalamus via $GABA_B$ receptors,[18] a factor that may explain the exacerbation of absences by VGB and possibly by other GABAergic drugs (tiagabine [TGB]). A number of AEDs seem to exert their properties through modulation of the $GABA_A$ receptor/chloride ionophore. Thus, benzodiazepines (BZDs) and barbiturates bind close to this site to increase chloride conductance and maintain membrane hyperpolarization. Newer drugs, such as VGB and TGB, may have more direct effects in prolonging the synaptic action of GABA. Evidence suggests that these drugs are effective against partial and secondary generalized seizures but may exacerbate SW epilepsies. They are less likely to cause sedation and ataxia but may have a higher risk of psychiatric disorder, including depression.[19] Drugs that interfere with excitatory neurotransmission via glutamate and aspartate receptors may yet prove valuable AEDs. Some of the antiepileptic properties of felbamate (FBM) may be a result of its ability to interfere with the action of glycine in facilitating glutaminergic activity, and a number of drugs with potential glutaminergic activity have entered clinical trial programs with varying success.

Actions, common side effects, and indications for use are briefly summarized in Table 13.2; a detailed discussion is beyond the scope of this chapter. Further details of the pharmacokinetics of these drugs are presented later in the chapter.

Partial (Localization-Related) Epilepsies

Issues concerning the necessity or otherwise of drug treatment in benign childhood partial epilepsies are discussed in Chapter 9. Currently, a large number of drugs can be considered for treating patients with cryptogenic partial epilepsies.

Table 13.1 Mode of action of antiepileptic drugs

Drug	Slow Ca²⁺ currents	Voltage-sensitive Na⁺ channels	GABAergic	Glutaminergic
Phenobarbitone	—	?	+	—
Phenytoin	—	+	—	—
Carbamazepine	—	+	—	—
Lamotrigine	—	+	—	—
Valproate	?	+	?	?
Ethosuximide	+	—	—	—
Vigabatrin	—	—	+	—
Gabapentin	—	—	—	—
Topiramate	—	+	+	?+

GABA = gamma-aminobutyric acid.

These include older and newer drugs, including those with a spectrum of efficacy limited to the partial epilepsies and those with broader spectrum effects (see Figure 13.1). There are an increasing number of studies available that have compared individual drugs in monotherapy regimes. There would currently be a consensus that CBZ is probably the drug of first choice in treating these epilepsies. None of the larger monotherapy studies have demonstrated a drug with greater efficacy,[6, 20] and the Second Veterans Administration Cooperative Study[7] showed some small advantages in efficacy over VPA in some reported measures of efficacy. Mattson et al.[6] showed that PHT and CBZ were better tolerated than barbiturate AEDs (phenobarbitone and primidone). A study by Brodie ct al.[8] comparing the first of the newer AEDs to be studied in a monotherapy design showed that LTG at doses used in this study were better tolerated than CBZ. Two other studies comparing LTG with PHT and CBZ, however, failed to differentiate between efficacy or effectiveness.[21, 22]

In our clinic, PHT is no longer considered a first-line AED in partial epilepsy because of its complex pharmacokinetics, which demand blood level monitoring, its untoward cosmetic chronic side effects, its enzyme-inducing properties that result in drug-drug interactions, and its teratogenicity. Clinicians in the United States may, however, take a different view.

The place of new AEDs other than LTG requires further definition with comparative monotherapy studies against CBZ.

Generalized Epilepsies

Management and treatment of the cryptogenic/symptomatic generalized epilepsies are dealt with in Chapter 8 and will not be discussed further here. The choice of drug therapy in idiopathic generalized epilepsies is, however, a major issue because collectively these may represent between 20% and 30% of all human epilepsies. There is a general consensus that VPA is the drug of choice for treating these epilepsies; it possesses a broad spectrum of activity that includes all the seizure types occurring in these syndromes. The possible exception to this would

Table 13.2   The mode of action, spectrum of efficacy, and toxicity of antiepileptic drugs

Drug	Mode of action	Indications
Clobazam	Allosteric enhancement of GABA-mediated inhibition	Occasional use: tonic-clonic and partial seizures particularly perimenstrual; (value is limited by development of tolerance)
Carbamazepine	Limits repetitive firing of Na^+-dependent action potentials	Drug of choice: complex partial seizures (particularly if complicated by psychiatric disturbance), tonic-clonic, and simple partial seizures
Clonazepam	Allosteric enhancement of GABA-mediated inhibition	Effective in: status epilepticus Effective in: absence, myoclonus Occasional use: slowly increasing doses tonic-clonic and partial seizures; (value greatly limited by development of tolerance)
Diazepam	Allosteric enhancement of GABA-mediated inhibition	Effective in: status epilepticus; occasional use: absence, myoclonus; (value limited by development of tolerance)
Ethosuximide	Reduce low-threshold calcium current	Drug of choice: simple absence
Phenobarbitone	Enhancement of GABA-mediated inhibition	Effective in: tonic, clonic and partial seizures; occasional use: status epilepticus, absence, myoclonus
Lamotrigine	Has carbamazepine and phenytoin-like effect on repetitive firing	Refractory partial and secondary generalized seizures. Probably also effective in generalized epilepsy
Phenytoin	Inhibits sustained repetitive firing effects on Na^+-dependent voltage channels	Effective in: tonic-clonic, simple and complex partial seizures
Primidone	As phenobarbitone	Occasional use: tonic-clonic and partial seizures
Sodium valproate	? Enhancement of GABA-mediated inhibition Limits sustained repetitive firing ? Reduces effects of excitatory neurotransmitters	Drug of choice: idiopathic generalized epilepsies, partial and secondary generalized seizures
Vigabatrin	Enzyme-activated suicidal inhibitor of GABA aminotransaminase	Treatment of partial epilepsy not satisfactorily controlled by other drugs
Gabapentin	May increase GABA release. Binds to unique receptor nature of which is uncertain	Refractory partial and secondarily generalized tonic-clonic seizures
Topiramate	Inactivates voltage-sensitive sodium channels. May bind to GABA receptors and have an action at glutaminergic receptors	Refractory partial and secondarily generalized tonic-clonic seizures

NB = note well; GABA = gamma-aminobutyric acid.

Dose	
Adults	*Children*
Up to 30 mg daily in 2 or 3 doses	>3 yr; half adult dose (maximum)
300–1,600 mg daily; initial dose low with slow increments (NB auto-induction of metabolism)	<1 yr 100–200 mg; 1–5 yr 200–400 mg; 5–10 yr 400–600 mg; 10–15 yr 0.6–1 g; *or* commence on 10 mg/kg/day for 5–7 days; then 20–40 mg/kg/day thereafter
Orally: 0.5–4 mg 3 times daily in slowly increasing doses	<1 yr 0.5–1 mg/day; 1–5 yr 1–3 mg/day; 6–12 yr 3–6 mg/day; *or* 0.1–0.2 mg/kg/day and usually commence on 0.02 mg/kg/day
Intravenous; rectal administration may be of value when venous access difficult; little effect orally	0.3–0.4 mg/kg (intravenous or rectal administration)
Up to 2 g/day in 2 or 3 doses	<6 yr 250 mg/day; >6 yr 0.5–1 g/day; *or* 20–40 mg/kg/day
Up to 200 mg/day in 2 or 3 doses	Usually 4–5 mg/kg/day
100–600 mg/day; NB enzyme-inducing drugs reduce half-life, valproate increases it	—
200–600 mg/day in 1 or 2 doses	5–8 mg/kg/day
500–1,500 mg/day in 2 or 3 doses	10–30 mg/kg in 2 or 3 doses (rarely used)
600–3,000 mg in 2 or 3 doses	20–60 mg/kg/day (usually 20–30 mg/kg/day)
2–4 g/day in 1 *or* 2 doses	3–9 yr 1 g/day; >9 yr 2 g/day; *or* 50–150 mg/kg/day in 2 or 3 divided doses
900–2,400 mg/day	No indication
200–800 mg/day	No indication

Table 13.2   (continued)

Drug	Optimal range	Dose-related
Clobazam	Not routinely measured	Drowsiness and sedation
Carbamazepine	4–10 µg/ml (but little evidence to support this)	Dizziness, double vision, unsteadiness, nausea, and vomiting
Clonazepam	Not routinely measured	Sedation and drowsiness
Diazepam	Not routinely measured	Sedation
Ethosuximide	40–80 µg/ml	Nausea, drowsiness, dizziness, unsteadiness, may exacerbate tonic-clonic seizures
Phenobarbitone	15–35 µg/ml; upper and lower limits modified by development of tolerance	Drowsiness, unsteadiness
Lamotrigine	1–3 µg/ml	Nausea and vomiting, headache, diplopia, aggression, swollen ankles
Phenytoin	10–20 µg/ml; the non-linear relationship between dose and serum concentration necessitates frequent blood-level monitoring	Drowsiness, unsteadiness, slurred speech, occasionally abnormal movement disorders
Primidone	As phenobarbitone—to which it is metabolized	Drowsiness, unsteadiness, often tolerated poorly on initiation and a slow increase in dose advisable
Sodium valproate	Uncertain: blood levels vary considerably during the day and a single specimen is unreliable	Tremor, irritability, restlessness; occasionally confusion
Vigabatrin	Unrelated to known mode of action	Drowsiness and fatigue, nervousness, irritability, depression, confusion, altered memory, mild gastrointestinal disturbance
Gabapentin	—	Drowsiness, headache, tremor
Topiramate	—	Impaired memory and cognition, drowsiness, paraesthesiae.

Side effects	
Idiosyncratic	*Chronic toxicity*
—	—
Rashes, reduced white cell count	Few known: absence of major effects on intellectual function and behavior is major benefit
Inflammation of veins	—
—	Habituation
Rashes	—
Rashes	Tolerance, habituation, withdrawal seizures; adverse effects on intellectual function and behavior
Rashes	Not yet known
Rashes, swelling of lymph glands (pseudolymphoma), hepatitis	Gingival hypertrophy, acne, coarsening of facial features, hirsutism, folate deficiency
See phenobarbitone	See phenobarbitone
Gastric intolerance, hepatotoxicity (mainly children)	Weight gain; alopecia
Psychosis	—
None known	Not yet known
None known	Renal calculi, weight loss

be that ethosuximide could be considered as an alternative first-line treatment in childhood absence epilepsy where the risk of tonic-clonic seizures is relatively low, at least during childhood and early adolescence. The place of newer AEDs in these syndromes has yet to be defined. There is suggestive evidence from open studies that LTG is effective (see Chapter 11). Because VPA use is limited by an increased incidence of weight gain[7] as well as concerns about potential teratogenicity (see Chapter 16), there is an urgent need for comparative monotherapy studies of VPA versus LTG.

Unclassified Epilepsy

Decisions about starting AED treatment often have to be made in the face of some uncertainty concerning a syndromic classification. Although the clinician may be certain that seizures have occurred, there may be insufficient information available from a relatively few poorly witnessed events to provide a definite seizure diagnosis. Common situations in which this occurs are where the patient has had witnessed tonic-clonic seizures during sleep and infrequent daytime trancelike episodes, which might represent absence or complex partial seizures. Where this uncertainty exists, it is relatively unusual for the electroencephalographic (EEG) study or other investigations to provide definitive information. In these circumstances, a broad-spectrum AED, such as VPA or LTG, would be the first choice.

ACUTE DOSE-RELATED TOXICITY

Most AEDs, including PHT, CBZ, LTG, barbiturates, and BZDs, give rise to a nonspecific encephalopathy associated with high blood concentrations. Patients exhibit sedation and nystagmus and, with increasing blood levels, ataxia, dysarthria, and ultimately confusion and drowsiness.[23] In some instances, seizure frequency may increase with high blood levels, and occasionally involuntary movements are seen, particularly with PHT.[24] PHT is especially likely to result in dose-related toxicity because of its unusual pharmacokinetics (see below). CBZ may cause similar symptoms if the dose is not built up slowly. This is probably related to autoinduction of liver microsomal enzymes. Sodium VPA does not appear to be associated with this typical syndrome of neurotoxicity, but some patients with high blood levels may exhibit restlessness and irritability (sometimes with a frank confusion state). Postural tremor is a common accompaniment.[25]

All AEDs may have adverse effects on cognitive function and behavior at therapeutic concentrations that become more apparent with polytherapy and with increasing blood concentrations. Agents such as CBZ and VPA have fewer adverse effects in this respect, and this is one argument for preferring these agents to longer-established AEDs.

Toxicity may occur because of drug interactions. Thus, VPA may potentiate the sedative effects of phenobarbitone and greatly prolong the half-life of LTG, making dosage reduction necessary during comedication.

ACUTE IDIOSYNCRATIC TOXICITY

Many AEDs, particularly PHT, CBZ, and LTG, may cause a maculopapular erythematous eruption, which, in more severe cases, may be associated with fever, lymphadenopathy, and hepatitis.[23] The incidence of allergic skin reaction with PHT may be as high as 10% and with CBZ up to 15%.[12] LTG is also associated with similar problems in up to 5% of new prescriptions.[19] It may be possible to avoid such reactions with a cautious buildup of initial doses. Marrow aplasia is a rare complication of CBZ, but is more common with FBM. Reports of fatal cases of liver failure in association with VPA therapy largely concern children under the age of 2 years who are often multiply handicapped and receiving many different AEDs. It may be that they have an underlying error of metabolism that predisposes them to liver failure.[26] VGB has been associated with behavior disorders, depression, and psychosis, particularly in patients with a previous psychiatric history.[27] The potential for rare idiosyncratic side effects of TPM and gabapentin (GBP) is currently uncertain.

CHRONIC TOXICITY

AEDs are unusual in that they may be administered to patients over long periods as treatment for chronic epilepsy. This may lead to the development of a wide variety of syndromes of chronic toxicity (Table 13.3). A number of factors seem to predispose patients to the development of these disorders (i.e., use of multiple drug therapy, dosage, and length of therapy). While it appears that sodium VPA and CBZ may have fewer chronic toxic effects than barbiturates and PHT, the length of time that elapsed before quite common chronic toxic effects were recognized with the older agents should warn us that continued vigilance is needed in the use of the newer AEDs.

TERATOGENICITY

All AEDs must be regarded as potentially teratogenic. PHT, and probably barbiturate AEDs, seem to increase the risk of major fetal malformations by two to three times: the most common malformations are harelip, cleft palate, and cardiovascular anomalies. The risks are higher with polytherapy than with monotherapy. There appears to be an association between neural tube defects and exposure to sodium VPA or CBZ. Estimates of this risk suggest it is 1–2% of pregnancies occurring while women are taking these drugs.[28, 29] Early screening for neural tube defects, using ultrasound and amniocentesis, and testing for alpha-fetoprotein, therefore seems to be indicated in women becoming pregnant while taking these drugs. It is now good practice to prescribe folate supplements to women taking AEDs who are sexually active (see Chapter 16).

   The role of newer AEDs in pregnancy has yet to be determined. TPM has been shown to possess the typical teratogenicity of carbonic anhydrase inhibitors in animal species. Other new drugs do not appear to possess animal teratogenicity, but human experience is limited (see Chapter 16).

Table 13.3   Chronic toxicity of anticonvulsants

Nervous system
  Memory and cognitive impairment
  Hyperactivity and behavioral disturbance
  Pseudodementia
  Cerebellar atrophy
  Peripheral neuropathy
Skin
  Acne
  Hirsutism
  Alopecia
  Chloasma
Liver
  Enzyme induction
Blood
  Megaloblastic anemia
  Thrombocytopenia
  Lymphoma
Immune system
  Immunoglobulin A deficiency
  Drug-induced systemic lupus erythematosus
Endocrine system
  Decrease thyroxine levels
  Increased cortisol and sex hormone metabolism
Bone
  Osteomalacia
Connective tissue
  Gum hypertrophy
  Coarsened facial features
  Dupuytren's contracture
Pregnancy
  Obstetric complications
  Teratogenicity
  Fetal hydantoin syndrome

Source: Reprinted with permission from D Chadwick, N Cartlidge, D Bates. Medical Neurology. Edinburgh: Churchill Livingstone, 1989.

LONG-TERM MANAGEMENT OF DRUG THERAPY

The great majority of patients developing epilepsy achieve a long-lasting remission soon after the start of therapy. For these patients, drug withdrawal may be considered after 2, 3, or more years (see below). Some 20% of patients developing epilepsy have a chronic disorder that is never completely controlled by drugs. In patients whose seizures are not controlled but who comply with maximal tolerated doses of a single AED, about 30% may respond to an alternative monotherapy,[30] particularly if the reason for failure is intolerance. In this same study, five of the original 100 patients with newly diagnosed epilepsy required two drugs for seizure control, compared with 28 whose seizures remained uncontrolled even after being exposed to the combination of CBZ and PHT. A policy of polytherapy, however, inevitably increases the risks of dose-related, idiosyncratic, and chronic toxicity.[31] In essence, a law of diminishing returns applies. Thus, for this group of patients an appropriate aim may not be complete remission of seizures but rather a compromise of reduced seizure frequency with less severe seizures to be achieved with one, or at most two, drugs.

Some patients may continue to have seizures but are not disabled by them; they may have very infrequent seizures or seizures that are minor in their symptomatology or confined to sleep. In such patients, assuming that a single drug has been used that is appropriate to the seizure type and epilepsy syndrome, there is usually little to be gained from alternative drugs or additional drugs.

Patients who continue to be disabled by the occurrence of seizures despite treatment with a single drug in optimal dosage demand further careful consideration. In particular, it is important to consider whether there are factors that would explain an unsatisfactory response to therapy (e.g., unidentified structural pathologic entities, the presence of complex partial seizures, poor compliance, or pseudoseizures). If this is not the case, then it is important to review the diagnosis: A common reason for failure of therapy is that the patient does not have epilepsy.

Where none of these conditions applies, it may be reasonable to try alternative drugs as monotherapy and then to undertake a trial of the addition of a second drug. However, this demands careful discussion with the patient and the understanding that the second drug will be withdrawn in the absence of a satisfactory sustained response.

REFRACTORY EPILEPSY AND RATIONAL POLYTHERAPY

We are entering an era in which the importance of polytherapy and drug combinations will need to be re-examined. In the 1970s and 1980s, a dogma of monotherapy became established with the recognition that large numbers of patients with epilepsy respond very adequately to a single AED and with the knowledge that polytherapy may, at least when used injudiciously, complicate management by increasing the frequency of adverse events and poor compliance, thereby necessitating more AED monitoring. This was seen by some as being a far greater problem than any minimal improvement in seizure control. These assumptions must be increasingly questioned, bearing in mind that they largely arose from uncontrolled "before and after" studies with little or no validity.[32]

DO COMBINATIONS POSSESS GREATER EFFICACY THAN SINGLE DRUGS?

I do not know of any randomized clinical trial that has compared alternative monotherapy with add-on therapy in groups of patients with poorly controlled epilepsy. However, Mattson et al.[6] placed 82 patients whose monotherapy had failed to control seizures on two-drug regimes. Forty percent of these patients were judged to be improved and 11% became seizure-free. Marson et al.,[19] in reviewing placebo-controlled add-on studies with new AEDs in populations of patients with refractory partial epilepsy, concluded that the odds ratios for a reduction in seizure frequency of 50% or greater were between two and five times that of the placebo for add-on treatment with all the drugs tested in this type of clinical trial. Empirically, all those experienced in treating patients with epilepsy recognize that most patients with refractory epilepsy will receive combinations of therapy and that it will be extremely difficult to reduce therapy to achieve treatment with a single drug. Thus, the weight of evidence suggests that drug combinations can possess greater efficacy in patients where monotherapy fails. What remains an issue is the degree of benefit and the extent to which it may be offset by increased risk of adverse events.

DO COMBINATIONS OF THERAPIES INCREASE THE RISK OF ADVERSE EVENTS?

There is overwhelming evidence suggesting that combinations of therapies increase the risk for most groups of adverse events.[31] Potentially, pharmacokinetic and pharmacodynamic drug-drug interactions might contribute to this phenomenon.

There are many examples of polytherapy leading to problems with dose-related neurotoxicity. Thus, the ability of sulthiame to inhibit the metabolism of PHT and that of VPA to inhibit the metabolism of LTG[33] can result in symptoms of intoxication. However, the ability of patients to tolerate particular blood levels of CBZ and LTG may be strongly influenced by whether they are taking other drugs that have actions on sodium conductances. Thus, the incidence of ataxia and diplopia in placebo-controlled add-on studies of LTG to other sodium channel drugs, such as CBZ, is strikingly higher than the incidence of these symptoms with add-on GABAergic drugs, such as VGB and TGB.[19]

Although acute idiosyncratic adverse events are not usually considered to be influenced by pharmacokinetic variables, there is considerable evidence to the contrary.[12] It does seem that VPA hepatotoxicity is much more common in polytherapy,[26] and there is considerable evidence that comedication with VPA greatly increases the risk of acute drug-related rash resulting from LTG therapy (see Chapter 11).

The impact of polytherapy on the incidence of chronic toxicity and teratogenicity in patients with epilepsy is more difficult to study for obvious reasons. There is, however, a consensus that chronic toxicity is more commonly seen in patients exposed to long-term polytherapy, and there is also evidence that the incidence of teratogenicity rises strikingly with the number of AEDs administered during pregnancy, such that pregnancies that are completed under three-drug regimes may be associated with up to a 50% incidence of teratogenicity.[34]

RATIONAL POLYTHERAPY

Consideration of the above evidence leads to two conclusions. First, there is an urgent need for pragmatic clinical trials to examine the benefits of combination

Table 13.4 Pharmacokinetics of anticonvulsants

Drug	Absorption (time to peak serum concentration [h] after oral dose)	Protein binding (%)	Active metabolites	Metabolism Half-life (h)	Doses/day
Carbamazepine	4–24	75	10,11-Epoxide	8–30	2 or 3
Ethosuximide	1–4	—	—	40–70	2 or 3
Gabapentin	2–3	0	—	5–9	—
Lamotrigine	2–3	50	—	12–48	2
Phenobarbitone	1–6	45	—	50–160	2
Phenytoin	4–12	90	—	9–140	1
Primidone	2–5	20	Phenobarbitone phenylethyl-malonamide	4–12	2
Topiramate	1.5–4.0	15	—	12–24	—
Valproate	1–4	90	—	8–20	2 or 3
Vigabatrin	1–2	—	—	5–7	1 or 2

therapy. Second, when polytherapy is used, it should satisfactorily embrace a number of principles suggested by Ferrendelli.[35]

1. It is best to combine AEDs with different mechanisms of action than to prescribe combinations of AEDs that have similar mechanisms of action. (The additional efficacy will be limited but the incidence of adverse events would be expected to be multiplied.)
2. It is best to select AEDs with relatively little potential for drug-drug interaction.
3. Patients treated with polytherapy demand more intensive monitoring, clinically and possibly for AED blood levels.

What remains at issue is, of course, the combinations of drugs that may carry with them particular benefits in effectiveness. A number of hypotheses remain to be examined. Perhaps the most pressing is the belief that combining VPA and LTG has a particular synergistic effect in control of generalized seizures and production of tremor as a side effect. Could the combination of GABAergic and glutaminergic AEDs have particular benefits? Is the best balance between efficacy and tolerability achieved through highly specific limited mechanisms of action within the nervous system or through broader, multiple mechanisms of action? It is only possible to conclude that rational polytherapy is urgently in need of rational examination.

ADMINISTERING AND MONITORING DRUG THERAPY

Pharmacokinetic data (Table 13.4) define drug absorption, distribution, metabolism, and elimination, but they do not describe the mode of action of drugs in the CNS. One clinical application of pharmacokinetics is therapeutic drug monitoring in serum or plasma, but this technique samples a physiologic pool that can be remote from the site of drug action.

PHT has a nonlinear relationship between the dose and the serum concentration[36]—a dose-related neurotoxicity. This results in a narrow therapeutic window, and monitoring is necessary to avoid neurotoxicity in patients whose dosage is being increased. The concept of the "therapeutic" or "optimal" range for PHT has been extended to other AEDs, and many laboratories now routinely estimate serum concentrations of drugs other than PHT. This is seen as an increasingly questionable practice.

A single measurement will give a good approximation of the steady-state concentration for drugs with long half-lives (PHT and phenobarbitone) but not for drugs with short half-lives. Measurements of VPA concentrations from specimens taken at random during the day are virtually uninterpretable because they may represent unpredictable peak, trough, or intermediate concentrations. Collecting early morning specimens for measuring troughs is, however, rarely practicable.

It is important to be aware of what is measured during routine estimations of blood concentrations of AEDs and, perhaps more important, what is not measured. Some drugs have metabolites that contribute to therapeutic effect but that are not routinely assayed. These include the 10,11-epoxide of CBZ and phenylethylmalonamide derived from primidone. Most laboratories in the United Kingdom determine drug concentration in whole plasma or serum. PHT, CBZ, and VPA are heavily protein-bound, but only the free drug fraction is in equilibrium with the brain and pharmacologically active. Measurement of free drug concentrations by equilibrium dialysis or ultrafiltration techniques are expensive and not readily available.

Even when concentrations of free drugs and their metabolites in the blood are known, important pharmacodynamic considerations may alter the relationship between blood concentration and therapeutic effect. Thus, for VPA the onset of action is slower and longer lasting than can be explained by the pharmacokinetics of the drug.[37] Similarly, tolerance to the neurotoxicity and therapeutic effects of BZDs and barbiturate drugs is unexplained by pharmacokinetic changes and must be the result of drug-receptor interaction.

There are further fundamental biologic reasons for doubting the value of routine monitoring of blood concentrations of AEDs. The upper limit of a therapeutic range may be defined as the concentration of the drug at which toxic effects are likely to appear. The most consistent relationship between serum concentration and toxic effect is for PHT, but even with this drug some patients may tolerate, and indeed require, serum concentrations above 20 μg/ml.[38] For VPA, phenobarbitone, and CBZ, there is wide variation in tolerance of serum concentrations.

The lower limit of the therapeutic range is even more difficult to define, and most patients have epilepsy that is controlled by antiepileptic serum concentrations well below the optimal range.[39] Unquestioning acceptance of therapeutic ranges creates problems: Patients with satisfactory control of seizures and low blood concentrations of drugs may have their doses needlessly increased, and patients who tolerate and need high blood concentrations may have their doses reduced. Treating patients is much more important than treating blood concentrations.

Routine monitoring should increasingly be restricted to certain categories of patients: First, those receiving PHT or multiple-drug treatment in whom dosage adjustment is necessary because of dose-related toxicity and poor seizure control; second, mentally retarded patients in whom the assessment of toxicity may be difficult; third, patients with renal or hepatic disease, and perhaps pregnant patients[40] in whom monitoring of free drug concentrations may be indicated; and, last, patients who may not be complying with treatment.

The place of AED monitoring in the use of new AEDs remains uncertain, although it seems of little benefit in the use of VGB and GBP.

ANTIEPILEPTIC DRUG WITHDRAWAL

The fact that AEDs have been associated with many adverse reactions is a potent argument for exploring the possibility of withdrawing drugs in patients who achieve remissions lasting 2, 3, or more years. Against this are the dangers of a recurrence of seizures, which may have important consequences for driving and employment as well as self-esteem.

Advice offered to patients on this subject varies widely. Pediatricians and pediatric neurologists suggest a trial withdrawal of AEDs in most children attaining remission, because they are concerned about the impact of drugs on cognitive function and learning and are impressed by the high expectation of success. Neurologists tend to be much more circumspect when dealing with adults, expressing concern over the possible effects of further seizures on driving and employment. In the United Kingdom, if not elsewhere, most patients attaining prolonged remission are unlikely to receive any advice from a neurologist or other physician with an interest in the treatment of epilepsy because they will have been discharged from regular follow-up. Of 122 patients with a history of epilepsy drawn from general practice, 49 had stopped treatment, most of them on their own initiative.[41]

The few studies that have been undertaken to determine the success of withdrawing drugs and the factors that identify patients likely to remain free of seizures have been reviewed.[42] Comparison of the available studies is difficult because there is often little information about patients, a lack of uniformity in the length of remission before withdrawal of AEDs, and no information about the period over which withdrawal occurred and for how long patients were subsequently followed.

One question that has not been widely considered is the relative risk of recurrence on withdrawal of AEDs compared with continued treatment. The Medical Research Council Antiepileptic Drug Withdrawal Group[43] studied this in a randomized clinical trial. The risk of relapse on continued treatment was approximately 10% per annum, but was two to three times greater in the group withdrawing from treatment for up to 2 years after commencing withdrawal.

A most detailed assessment of prognostic factors has also been undertaken in the Medical Research Council Antiepileptic Drug Withdrawal Study. Relatively few clinical factors influenced the risk of recurrence.

A Cox's proportional hazard model selected six prognostic factors for increased risk of seizures recurring in addition to whether AED treatment was continued: (1) age 16 years and older (relative risk 1.75); (2) taking more than one AED (1.83); (3) a history of seizures after starting AED treatment (1.56); (4) a history of tonic-clonic seizures (primary or secondarily generalized) (1.56); (5) a history of myoclonic seizures (1.84); and (6) abnormal EEG findings in the previous year (1.32). The risk of recurrence also declined as the period without seizures increased, but in a complex way.

Table 13.5   Factors for the calculation of the prognostic index (z) for seizure recurrence by 1 and 2 years after continued antiepileptic drug treatment or gradual withdrawal

Factor	
Starting score (all patients)–175	*Value to be added to starting score*
Age >16 years	45
Taking >one antiepileptic drug	50
Seizures occurred after start of antiepileptic drug treatment	35
History of primary or secondarily generalized tonic-clonic seizures	35
History of myoclonic seizures	50
Electroencephalographic study in past year:	
not available	15
abnormal features	20
Duration of seizure-free period (years)(t)	200/t
Total score (T)	–
$z = e^{T/100}$	

	Probability	
Treatment schedule	*by 1 year*	*by 2 years*
Continued treatment	$1-0.89^{z}$	$1-0.79^{z}$
Slow withdrawal	$1-0.69^{z}$	$1-0.60^{z}$

These factors have been used to generate a statistical model for everyday practical use (Table 13.5).[44] The index can be used to obtain estimates of the probabilities of seizures recurring within 1 and 2 years of starting slow withdrawal of AEDs or continuing treatment. The estimates can easily be calculated on a pocket calculator.

This model, derived from the only randomized study of withdrawal of AEDs from patients in remission, provides the best available information for patients considering drug withdrawal. It should be emphasized that the decisions to be made about stopping AEDs lic with the patient, because social factors, such as possession of a driver's license, are often as important or more important than the risk of seizure recurrence.

REFERENCES

1. Commission on Classification and Terminology of the International League Against Epilepsy. Proposal for revised clinical and electro-encephalographic classification of epileptic seizures. Epilepsia 1981;22:489.
2. Commission on Classification and Terminology of the International League Against Epilepsy. Proposal for revised classification of epilepsies and epileptic syndromes. Epilepsia 1989;30:389.
3. Annegers JF, Hauser WA, Elverback LR. Remission of seizures and relapse in patients with epilepsy. Epilepsia 1979;20:729.

4. Reynolds EH. Early treatment and prognosis of epilepsy. Epilepsia 1987;28:97.
5. Marson AG, Beghi E, Berg A, et al. The Cochrane Collaboration and its relevance to epilepsy. Epilepsia 1996;37:917.
6. Mattson RH, Cramer JA, Collins JF, et al. Comparison of carbamazepine, phenobarbital, phenytoin and primidone in partial and secondary generalized tonic-clonic seizures. N Engl J Med 1985;313:145.
7. Mattson RH, Cramer JA, Collins JF, et al. A comparison of valproate with carbamazepine for the treatment of complex partial seizures with secondarily generalized tonic-clonic seizures in adults. N Engl J Med 1992;327:765.
8. Brodie MJ, Richens A, Yuen AWC. Double-blind comparison of lamotrigine and carbamazepine in newly diagnosed epilepsy. Lancet 1995;345:476.
9. Temkin NR, Dikmen SS, Wilensky AJ, et al. A randomized, double-blind study of phenytoin for the prevention of post-traumatic seizures. N Engl J Med 1990;323:497.
10. Foy PM, Copeland GP, Shaw MDM. The incidence of postoperative seizures. Acta Neurochir 1981;55:253.
11. Foy PM, Chadwick DW, Rajgopalan N, et al. Do prophylactic anticonvulsant drugs alter the pattern of seizures following craniotomy? J Neurol Neurosurg Psychiatry 1992;55:753.
12. Chadwick D, Shaw MDM, Foy P, et al. Serum anticonvulsant concentrations and the risk of drug-induced skin eruptions. J Neurol Neurosurg Psychiatry 1984;47:642.
13. McQueen JK, Blackwood DH, Harris P, et al. Low risk of late post-traumatic seizures following severe head injury: implications for clinical trials of prophylaxis. J Neurol Neurosurg Psychiatry 1983;46:899.
14. Reynolds EH, Shorvon SD, Galbraith AW, et al. Phenytoin monotherapy for epilepsy: a long-term prospective study, assisted by serum level monitoring, in previously untreated patients. Epilepsia 1981;22:475.
15. Chadwick D, Turnbull EH. The comparative efficacy of antiepileptic drugs for partial and tonic-clonic seizures. J Neurol Neurosurg Psychiatry 1985;48:1073.
16. Gibbs JM, Appleton RE, Rosenbloom L. Vigabatrin in intractable childhood epilepsy: a retrospective study. Pediatr Neurol 1992;8:338.
17. McDonald RL, Meldrum BS. Principles of Antiepileptic Drug Action. In RH Levy, RH Mattson, BS Meldrum (eds), Antiepileptic Drugs (4th ed). New York: Raven, 1995;61.
18. Crunelli V, Leresche N. A role for $GABA_B$ receptors in excitation and inhibition of thalamocortical cells. Trends Neurol Sci 1991;14:16.
19. Marson AG, Kadir ZA, Hutton JL, Chadwick DW. New antiepileptic drugs; a systematic review of their efficacy and tolerability. BMJ 1996;313:1169.
20. Heller AJ, Chesterman P, Elwes RDC, et al. Phenobarbitone, phenytoin, carbamazepine or sodium valproate for newly diagnosed adult epilepsy. J Neurol Neurosurg Psychiatry 1995;58:44.
21. Reunanen M, Dam M, Yuen AWC. A randomized open multicenter comparative trial of lamotrigine and carbamazepine as monotherapy in patients with newly diagnosed or recurrent epilepsy. Epilepsy Res 1996;23:149.
22. Steiner TJ, Yuen AWC. Comparison of lamotrigine and phenytoin monotherapy in newly diagnosed epilepsy. Epilepsia 1994;35:31.
23. Schmidt D. Adverse Effects of Antiepileptic Drugs. New York: Raven, 1982.
24. Chadwick D, Reynolds EH, Marsden CD. Anticonvulsant induced dyskinesias: a comparison with dyskinesias induced by neuroleptics. J Neurol Neurosurg Psychiatry 1976;39:1210.
25. Turnbull DM, Rawlins MD, Weightman D, Chadwick DW. Plasma concentrations of sodium valproate: their clinical value. Ann Neurol 1983;14:38.
26. Dreifuss FE, Santilli N, Langer DH, et al. Valproic acid fatalities: a retrospective review. Neurology 1987;37:379.
27. Sander JWAS, Trevisol-Bittencourt PC, Hart YM, Shorvon SD. Evaluation of vigabatrin as an add-on drug in the management of severe epilepsy. J Neurol Neurosurg Psychiatry 1990;53:1008.
28. Lindhout D, Schmidt D. In-utero exposure to valproate and neural tube defects. Lancet 1986;1:1392.
29. Rosa FH. Spina bifida in maternal carbamazepine exposure cohort data. Teratology 1990;41:587.
30. Hakkarainen H. Carbamazepine vs diphenylhydantoin vs their combination in adult epilepsy [abstract]. Neurology 1980;30:354.
31. Beghi E, Di Mascio R, Tognoni G. Drug treatment of epilepsy. Outline, criticisms and perspectives. Drugs 1986;31:249.
32. Reynolds EH, Shorvon SD. Monotherapy or polytherapy for epilepsy? Epilepsia 1981;22:1.
33. Richens A, Perucca E. Clinical Pharmacology and Medical Treatment. In J Laidlaw, A Richens, D Chadwick (eds), Textbook of Epilepsy (4th ed). Edinburgh: Churchill Livingstone, 1993;495.

34. Nakane Y, Okuma T, Takashi R, et al. Multi-institutional study on the teratogenicity and fetal toxicity of antiepileptic drugs. A report of a collaborative study group in Japan. Epilepsia 1980;21:663.

35. Ferrendelli JA. Rational polypharmacy. Epilepsia 1995;36:5115.

36. Richens A, Dunlop A. Serum phenytoin levels in the management of epilepsy. Lancet 1975;2:247.

37. Rowan AJ, Binnie CD, Warfield CA, et al. The delayed effect of sodium valproate on the photo-convulsive response in man. Epilepsia 1979;20:61.

38. Gannaway DJ, Mawer GE. Serum phenytoin concentrations and clinical response in patients with epilepsy. Br J Clin Pharmacol 1981;12:833.

39. Turnbull DM, Howell D, Rawlins MD, Chadwick DW. Which drug for the adult epileptic patient: phenytoin or valproate? BMJ 1985;290:815.

40. Knott C, Williams CP, Reynolds F. Phenytoin kinetics during pregnancy and the puerperium. Br J Obstet Gynaecol 1986;93:1030.

41. Goodridge DMG, Shorvon SD. Epileptic seizures in a population of 6000: II—treatment and prognosis. BMJ 1983;287:645.

42. Berg I, Shinnar S. Relapse following discontinuation of antiepileptic drugs: a meta-analysis. Neurology 1994;44:601.

43. Medical Research Council Antiepileptic Drug Withdrawal Study Group (D Chadwick, Clinical Co-ordinator). Randomized study of antiepileptic drug withdrawal in patients in remission. Lancet 1991;337:1175.

44. Medical Research Council Antiepileptic Drug Withdrawal Study Group (D Chadwick, Clinical Co-ordinator). Prognostic index for recurrence of seizures after remission of epilepsy. BMJ 1993;306:1374.

14
Status Epilepticus

John M. Pellock and Robert J. DeLorenzo

Status epilepticus (SE) is a medical and neurologic emergency associated with significant morbidity and mortality.[1–4] Since Babylonian times, it has been identified as a prolonged and malignant form of seizure.[5] SE occurs in children and adults and may be the accompaniment of an acute insult to the brain or a manifestation of already existing epilepsy, as the initial symptom or as a prolonged exacerbation of the seizures.[6–8] The definition and classification of SE have been changed numerous times over the years. This term refers to seizures that do not stop after a limited, short duration. Rather, some fundamental mechanism allows the single seizure to occur repetitively or to persist for an extended period.[9] Recent studies suggest that SE frequently goes unrecognized, and its occurrence has been underestimated in the general population.[8] This chapter reviews the definition, classification, epidemiology, etiology, treatment, and prognosis of SE. The morbidity and mortality of SE are considerable and are directly dependent on the prompt and appropriate recognition, medical therapy, and etiology of the episode.

DEFINITION

The International Classification of Epileptic Seizures defines SE as a seizure lasting for more than 30 minutes or intermittent seizures lasting for more than 30 minutes from which the patient does not regain consciousness. The International League Against Epilepsy and the World Health Organization previously defined SE as "a condition characterized by an epileptic seizure that is so frequently repeated or so prolonged as to create a fixed and lasting condition."[10, 11] Lack of recovery for a fixed period, possible frequent repetition, prolongation, and possible propagation of further seizures are inherent in the definition. Prior definitions used a period of 1 hour to define SE, but more recent studies following the International Classification of Epileptic Seizures have used 30 minutes.

Table 14.1   International classification of status epilepticus

International	Traditional
Convulsive	
Tonic-clonic	Grand mal, epilepticus convulsivus
Tonic	—
Clonic	—
Myoclonic	—
Nonconvulsive	
Absence status	Spike and wave stupor, spike and slow wave or 3/s spike and wave status epilepticus, petit mal, epileptic fugue, epilepsia minora continua, epileptic twilight state, minor status epilepticus
Partial status epilepticus	
Elementary	Focal motor status, focal sensory, epilepsia partilis continuans, adversive status epilepticus
Somatomotor	—
Dysphasic	—
Other types	
Complex partial	Epileptic fugue state, prolonged epileptic stupor, prolonged epileptic confusional state, temporal lobe status epilepticus, psychomotor status epilepticus, continuous epileptic twilight state
Unilateral status epilepticus	Hemiclonic status epilepticus, hemiconvulsion-hemiplegia-epilepsy, hemi-grand mal status epilepticus, grand mal
Erratic status epilepticus	Neonatal status epilepticus
(Unclassified)	—

CLASSIFICATION

Because any type of seizure may become prolonged, it may develop into SE. The classification of SE can thus be done in the same manner as individual seizures using the International Classification of the Epileptic Seizures proposed in 1981 and presented by Gastaut in 1982 (Table 14.1).[10, 11] The fundamental distinction is between seizures that are generalized from onset and those that are partial in onset; the latter may or may not be secondarily generalized. Thus, partial onset seizures are thought to originate from a single cortical focus and spread to a greater or lesser extent from that area, whereas seizures that are generalized from onset seem to involve the entire cortex simultaneously. SE characterized by seizures generalized from onset occurs most frequently in children. Partial onset SE—most commonly expressed as secondarily generalized convulsive status—may occur at any age and probably accounts for the overwhelming majority of adult cases.

The classification of patients in whom SE is characterized by only partial or subtle signs of convulsive activity is controversial, even though the seizures are associated with a marked impairment of consciousness and bilateral ictal discharges on the electroencephalographic (EEG) recording. Treiman[9, 12, 13] uses the term *subtle generalized convulsive SE* to describe this condition. Patients with this presentation of generalized convulsive SE have severe encephalopathies associated with underlying systemic illness, primary brain lesions, such as massive cerebral infarctions or infections, or following prolonged uncontrolled convulsive SE. Subtle generalized convulsive SE is clinically characterized by the occurrence of mild motor movements, such as nystagmus, or by clonic twitches, which may be unilateral and are intermittent, brief, and without a true sequential pattern. These subtle movements, however, are associated with marked impairment of consciousness and usually with continuous bilateral ictal patterns on the EEG recording. Our group and others have used the term *nonconvulsive SE* to describe continuing electrographic seizures that do not demonstrate a clinical manifestation. Severely ill adults and neonates[14, 15] show this "electro-clinical dissociation." Treiman,[12, 13] in 1990, described a sequential progression of EEG changes that can be associated with this subtle status, characterized initially by discrete electrographic seizures that coincide temporally with overt clinical convulsions. These discrete seizures merge together to produce a waxing and waning ictal pattern on the EEG recording. This waxing and waning pattern becomes progressively uniform to produce a pattern of continuous ictal discharges and then becomes interrupted by periods of relative flattening; these periods lengthen as the ictal discharges become shorter until the ultimate record is one of periodic epileptiform discharges on a relatively flattened background. Treiman[12] recommends that a patient in status whose EEG recording exhibits only periodic epileptiform discharges should be treated aggressively to prevent progressively severe epileptic brain damage in excess of that caused by the underlying encephalopathy.

Nonconvulsive SE may include complex partial and simple partial seizures along with absences. In complex partial SE, a series of discrete complex partial seizures occurs, and the patient is considered to be in status when complete recovery between seizures is blunted. Complex partial SE may be characterized by an epileptic twilight state in which there is a cyclical variation between periods of (a) partial responsiveness and (b) episodes of seemingly motionless staring and complete unresponsiveness accompanied, at times, by automatic behavior.[9, 15, 16] Simple partial SE is characterized by focal seizures that may persist or be repetitive for at least 30 minutes without impairment of consciousness. A wide variety of simple partial seizures may present as status, including epileptic aphasia. The EEG pattern during simple partial SE may exhibit rhythmic ictal discharges that remain focal and unilateral or abnormalities may not appear on the scalp EEG recording because the area of cortical seizure activity is so small. In complex partial SE, although the spread of ictal activity from the cortical focus involves, to some extent, both cerebral hemispheres, the EEG pattern on scalp recording has some localized features.

Absence, or petit mal, status has also been referred to as spike-wave stupor. This type of nonconvulsive SE may be very difficult to differentiate from complex partial status without EEG evaluation. In absence status, there is a continuous alteration of consciousness without the cyclical variations seen with complex partial SE. The EEG recording exhibits prolonged, sometimes continuous, generalized synchronous 3-hertz (Hz) spike and wave complexes rather than focal ictal discharges.[9, 17]

Myoclonic, generalized clonic, and generalized tonic SE are seen primarily in children; frequently, these children will have encephalopathic epilepsies.[3, 9, 18] Myoclonic status is extremely rare, but recurrent myoclonic seizures are often observed; in the latter, consciousness is preserved throughout the attack and the

Table 14.2   Frequency of status epilepticus (SE) in Richmond, Virginia, and projection for United States

	Actual	*Estimated**
Richmond		
Incidence of SE/100,000	41	61
Episodes of SE/100,000	50	78
Mortality/100,000	9	17
United States		
Cases of SE/year	102,000	152,000
SE events/year	126,000	195,000
Deaths/year	22,200	42,000

*Estimated values were calculated using validation corrections for the Medical College of Virginia and community hospitals.

Source: Reprinted with permission from RJ DeLorenzo, WA Hauser, AR Towne, et al. A prospective, population-based study of status epilepticus in Richmond, Virginia. Neurology 1996;46:1029.

EEG pattern is bilaterally symmetric, revealing polyspike discharges that coincide with the myoclonic jerks. The term *myoclonic SE* should not be used when a patient with severe encephalopathy exhibits repetitive myoclonic jerks not accompanied by ictal discharges on the EEG recording. Rather, these patients have subtle, generalized, convulsive SE as defined by Treiman.[9] About one-half of the cases of generalized clonic SE occur in normal children and are associated with febrile episodes, while the other one-half is equally distributed among those with acute and chronic encephalopathies.[6] The repetitive clonic jerks are of relatively low amplitude and appear bilaterally but are often arrhythmic, asymmetric, or asynchronous. Generalized tonic SE is also relatively common but appears almost exclusively in children, particularly those with Lennox-Gastaut syndrome. Prolonged generalized tonic convulsions have been precipitated by benzodiazepine (BZD) administration. These episodes may last from days to weeks; some episodes are very subtle and require EEG confirmation.

EPIDEMIOLOGY

Hauser[19] reported that SE occurs in 50,000–60,000 individuals in the United States every year, with the highest incidence in children and those older than 60. The prospective population-based study of SE in the city of Richmond, Virginia, revealed the incidence of SE to be 41 patients per year per 100,000 population having 50 episodes per year per 100,000. It is projected that 102,000–152,000 events occur in the U.S., which is an incidence 2.0–2.5 times greater than previously estimated by Hauser's studies (Table 14.2).[8, 20] Approximately one-third of the cases present as the initial seizure of developing epilepsy, one-third occur in patients with a previously established diagnosis of epilepsy, and one-third occur at the time of an acute isolated brain insult. Among those previously diagnosed as having epilepsy, estimates of SE occurrence range from 0.5% to 6.6%. Hauser[19] report-

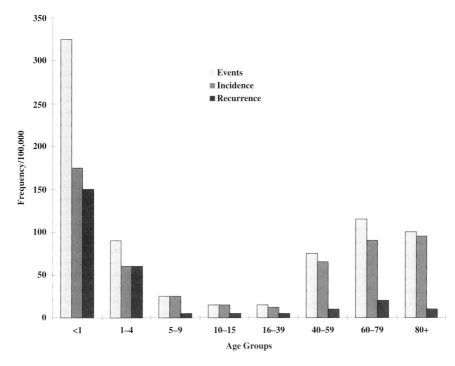

Figure 14.1 Age-specific distribution of the frequency of status epilepticus (SE) events, the incidence of SE, and the frequency of SE recurrence per year per 100,000 in Richmond, Virginia. The population in each group was determined from the National Census Bureau data on the demographics of Richmond, 1990. SE events included all episodes of SE per 100,000 per year. The incidence of SE represents the number of patients that developed SE per 100,000 in Richmond and did not include recurrent episodes of SE. (Reprinted with permission from RJ DeLorenzo, WA Hauser, AR Towne, et al. A prospective, population-based study of status epilepticus in Richmond, Virginia. Neurology 1996;46:1029.)

ed that up to 70% of children who have epilepsy that begins before the age of 1 year will experience an episode of SE. Also, within 5 years of the initial diagnosis of epilepsy, 20% of all patients will experience an episode of SE. Adults with SE as their first unprovoked seizure are likely to develop subsequent epilepsy;[20] however, in a recent prospective study of childhood SE, Maytal et al.[21] reported only a 0.3 probability that children initially presenting with SE will later develop epilepsy. In children, SE is most common in younger children; more than 50% of the cases occurred under the age of 3 years.[22] In the Richmond study, total SE events and incidence per 100,000 individuals per year showed a bimodal distribution with the highest values during the first year of life and during the decades above 60 years of age.[6, 7, 8] As shown in Figure 14.1, infants younger than 1 year of age represent a subgroup of the pediatric population with the highest incidence of SE. As a group, however, the elderly have the highest incidence and total SE events of the four age categories (pediatric, young adult, adult, and elderly), with an incidence of more than 90 per 100,000 per year. The recurrence rate of SE in the Richmond study was 10.8%.[8] Thirty-eight percent of patients younger than 4 years old had repeat episodes. Overall recurrences of SE were more common in the very young and also in the elderly.

Extrapolating these figures world-wide, more than 1 million cases of SE occur throughout the world annually. Because SE is a neurologic emergency that requires immediate, effective treatment to prevent residual neurologic complications or death, SE poses a substantial health risk to a large number of patients.

Mortality rates as high as 50% have been reported, but more recent studies of acute mortality associated with SE have yielded estimates of 8–32%.[4, 19] Overall mortality of SE in the Richmond population was 22%.[20, 21] Mortalities for pediatric and adult patients were 3.4% and 26%, respectively. The highest mortality was seen in elderly patients, with as many as 55 deaths per 100,000 individuals per year in the group aged 80 years and older. Multiple studies confirm the lowered mortality rate in children following adequate emergency treatment.[21–25] Age, etiology, and duration of the episode of SE are also correlated with mortality.[4, 8]

ETIOLOGY

SE is usually (a) a manifestation of an acute precipitating event, primarily or secondarily affecting the central nervous system (CNS) or (b) a manifestation of symptomatic epilepsy, with or without pre-existing neurologic dysfunction. Our recent studies indicate that fewer than 10% of cases of SE in adults and children are truly idiopathic wherein no precipitating or associated cause can be identified.[7, 8] Acute symptomatic causes are most commonly associated with prolonged SE lasting more than 1 hour.[8] A full evaluation for etiology must be undertaken in every case of SE.[2, 3] Even in those patients with pre-existing epilepsy, a precipitating or associated factor may be clearly identified; such identification may help treat this episode of SE and perhaps prevent additional consequences.

Results of retrospective and prospective studies indicate that there is a difference in the etiologies between adults and children[2, 3] (Table 14.3). In the Richmond prospective and retrospective databases, the major cause of SE in the pediatric population was systemic non-CNS infections with fever.[4, 8] Inadequate antiepileptic drug (AED) levels and remote causes, including congenital malformations, also accounted for a significant number of cases in children. It is important to emphasize that many patients with subtherapeutic levels of AEDs had closely followed the instructions of their physicians and recently had drug dosages altered. The distribution of causes in children is highly age dependent.[22] More than 80% of children under age 2 years had SE of a febrile or acute symptomatic cause, whereas cryptogenic or remote symptomatic causes were most common in older children. Thus, even among children, there was a strong effect of age on the frequency and cause of SE as well as on the type of child with SE. In adults, a more even distribution among major causes is seen in the prospective Richmond study.[8] Three major causes emerge: subtherapeutic levels of AEDs, 34%; remote causes, 23%; and cerebrovascular accidents (strokes), 22%. Other relatively common causes in adults include hypoxia, metabolic abnormalities, and ethanol intoxication and withdrawal. In adult patients, the remote group was primarily composed of SE cases that occurred in relationship to stroke. Thus,

Table 14.3   Cause and mortality for pediatric and adult status epilepticus (SE) cases

	Pediatric		Adult	
Etiology	Percentage of SE cases	Mortality	Percentage of SE cases	Mortality
Anoxia	0	0	5	71
Hypoxia	5	0	13	53
CVA	10	0	22	33
Hemorrhage	0	0	1	0
Tumor	0	0	7	30
Infection	52	5	7	10
CNS infection	2	0	3	0
Metabolic	7	0	15	30
LAED	21	0	34	4
Drug OD	2	0	3	25
Etoh	0	0	13	20
Trauma	0	0	3	25
Remote	38	0	25	14
Idiopathic	5	0	3	25

CVA = cerebrovascular accident; CNS = central nervous system; Etoh = alcohol related; LAED = low antiepileptic drug level; OD = overdose.

stroke in adults, as an acute episode or as a remote symptomatic cause, is responsible for a large portion of the cases of SE. Figure 14.2 lists the percentage of causes for SE in children versus adults in retrospective and prospective studies from Richmond.

Recurrence rates for SE are age-specific, as shown in Figure 14.1. Repetition is much more common in those younger than 1 year old. In the Richmond population, 22 patients had repeat episodes of SE; the maximum number of repeat episodes during this 2-year prospective period of study for any individual patient was five. Thirteen percent of patients had a repeat episode of SE. Pediatric, adult, and elderly recurrence rates were 35%, 7%, and 10%, respectively. Recurring SE is more frequent in children with remote symptomatic encephalopathy or progressive degenerative disease.[7, 8]

MANAGEMENT AND THERAPY

The neurologic emergency of SE requires maintenance of respiration, general medical support, and specific treatment of seizures while cause is sought to provide the best outcome.[1, 3, 9, 23, 26] The diagnosis of SE should be made rapidly on clinical grounds, as continuous or repetitive seizures occur within a set period. For study purposes, a 30-minute time span has been selected as a definition of SE. In clinical practice, a 10- to 15-minute duration of seizures may be a more reasonable period to define the need for emergent treatment.[3, 9, 26] It is more difficult to diagnose SE when a patient has had a single, generalized convulsion and then persists with a long period of impaired consciousness. An

274

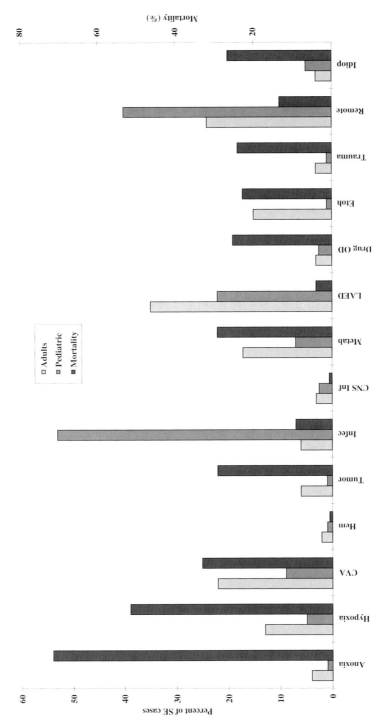

Figure 14.2 Causes of status epilepticus (SE) for adult and pediatric patients and mortality for adult causes. Some patients had more than one cause. (Reprinted with permission from RJ DeLorenzo, WA Hauser, AR Towne, et al. A prospective, population-based study of status epilepticus in Richmond, Virginia. Neurology 1996;46:1029.) (CVA = cerebrovascular accident; Hem = hemorrhage; Infec = systemic infection with fever; CNS Inf = infection of the central nervous system; Metab = metabolic; LAED = low antiepileptic drug level; OD = overdose; Etoh = alcohol related; Idiop = idiopathic.)

Table 14.4   Goals of emergency management for status epilepticus

Ensure adequate brain oxygenation and cardiorespiratory function.
Terminate clinical and electrical seizure activity as rapidly as possible.
Prevent seizure recurrence.
Identify precipitating factors, such as hypoglycemia, electrolyte imbalance, lowered drug
    levels, infection, and fever.
Correct metabolic imbalance.
Prevent systemic complications.
Further evaluate and treat cause of status epilepticus.

electroencephalogram should be obtained urgently whenever possible and, if ictal discharges are noted, the patient should be considered to be in electrographic SE.[9] The goals of SE emergency management are listed in Table 14.4. The principle is to terminate the clinical and electrographic seizure activity as rapidly as possible while ensuring that optimal oxygenation and metabolic balance are preserved. Clinical and electrical seizure activity should be terminated as soon as possible.[12] Numerous studies indicate that the longer an episode of SE continues, the more likely it is to result in permanent neurologic damage.[27] Furthermore, clinical experience suggests that the longer an episode of SE lasts, the more refractory it is to treatment.[4, 8, 12, 19, 26–28]

The most typical and frequent error committed in the treatment of SE is the initial administration of inadequate doses of single AEDs; the physician then waits for more seizures to occur before administering the necessary total dose.[3, 8] The management of SE is best carried out with the use of a predetermined protocol in most settings.[3, 12, 26] For the most part, drugs should be administered intravenously to ensure the most rapid delivery of the highest doses to the brain. The ideal AED for the treatment of SE should optimally have the following properties: rapid onset of action, wide spectrum of activity, intravenous preparation, easy administration, minimal redistribution from the CNS, short elimination half-life, and wide therapeutic safety margin.[1] Because of these desired properties, and in particular because of its being longer acting, lorazepam has become popular in many centers as the initial agent, replacing diazepam.[3, 26] If, however, SE continues after the initial dose of BZD and persists after a primary AED (phenytoin [PHT] or phenobarbital [PB]) is given, a second dose of PHT or PB should be administered before considering a change to an alternative AED. Protocols presently used by our group at the Medical College of Virginia for the management of SE in adults and children are given in Tables 14.5 and 14.6.[23, 26]

Patients in SE must have cardiorespiratory function assessed immediately by vital sign determination, auscultation, airway inspection, determination of arterial gas concentrations, and suction when necessary. Although they may be breathing spontaneously on arrival at the emergency department, patients may already be hypoxic, with respiratory metabolic acidosis, apnea, aspiration, or central respiratory depression. The need for ventilatory support depends not only on respiratory status at the time of presentation, but also on the conditions before arrival and the ability to maintain adequate oxygenation throughout ongoing seizures and during the intravenous administration of AEDs, all of

Table 14.5   Medical College of Virginia status epilepticus treatment protocol for children

Step	Time from beginning of intervention	Procedure
1	0–5 min	Determination of status epilepticus. As soon as the diagnosis is made, institute monitoring of temperature, blood pressure, pulse, respirations, ECG, and EEG. Insert oral airway and administer O_2 if necessary. Insert an IV catheter and draw venous blood for levels of anticonvulsants, glucose (check Dextrostix) electrolytes, calcium, BUN, CBC. Draw arterial antipyretics (acetaminophen). Perform frequent suction.
2	6–9 min	Place an IV line with normal saline. Administer a bolus of 2 ml/kg 50% glucose.
3	10–30 min	Initial treatment consists of an infusion of IV lorazepam given at a rate of 1–2 mg/min (0.1 mg/kg) to a maximum dose of 8 mg. This is followed by IV phenytoin (fosphenytoin; PHT [FPHT]), 18–20 mg/kg, infused at a rate not to exceed 1 mg/kg/min or 50 mg/min. Monitor ECG and blood pressure. May repeat PHT (FPHT), 10 mg/kg before proceeding to next step.
4	31–59 min	If seizures persist, administer a bolus infusion of phenobarbital at a rate not to exceed 50 mg/min until seizures stop or to a loading dose of 20 mg/kg.
5	60 min	If control is still not achieved, other options include: (1) Diazepam (50 mg) is diluted in a solution of 250 ml 0.9% NaCl or D5W and run as a continuous infusion at 1 ml/kg/h (2 mg/kg/h) to achieve blood levels of 0.2–8.0 mg/ml. The IV solution is changed every 6 hours as advised by certain authors, and short-length IV tubing is used. (2) Pentobarbital with an initial IV loading dose of 5 mg/kg with additional amounts given to produce a "burst suppression" pattern on EEG. Maintenance of pentobarbital anesthesia is continued for approximately 4 hours by an infusion of 1–3 mg/kg/hr. The patient is then checked for the reappearance of seizure activity by decreasing the infusion rate. If clinical seizures and/or generalized discharges persist on EEG, the procedure is repeated; if not, the pentobarbital is tapered over 12–24 hours.
6	61–80 min	If seizures are still not controlled, call the anesthesia department to begin general anesthesia with halothane and neuromuscular blockade.

Notes: Continuous monitoring of EEG is recommended in an obtunded patient to ensure that status epilepticus has not recurred. In the management of intractable status, a neurologist who has expertise in status epilepticus should be consulted and advice from a regional epilepsy center should be sought.

Lumbar puncture should be performed as soon as possible, especially in a febrile child or infant below 1 year old.

For infants with a history of neonatal seizures, infantile spasms, or early onset seizures, pyridoxine, 100 mg IV, should be administered while EEG monitoring is being performed to diagnose and treat the rare patient with seizures with a vitamin B_6 deficiency.

ECG = electrocardiogram; EEG = electroencephalogram; IV = intravenous; BUN = blood urea nitrogen; CBC = complete blood count; D5W = 5% dextrose in water.

Table 14.6 Medical College of Virginia status epilepticus treatment protocol for adults

Step	Time from beginning of intervention	Procedure
1	0–5 min	Determination of status epilepticus. As soon as the diagnosis is made, institute monitoring of blood pressure, temperature, pulse, respirations, ECG, and EEG. Insert oral airway and administer O_2 if necessary. Insert an IV catheter and draw venous blood for levels of anticonvulsant, glucose, electrolytes, Ca, Mg, BUN, and CBC. Draw arterial blood for ABG analysis. Obtain urine for urinalysis and toxic screen if indicated. If necessary, nasotracheal suction is performed.
2	6–9 min	Place an IV line with normal saline containing vitamin B complex. Administer a bolus of 50 ml of 50% glucose.
3	10–30 min	Infuse IV lorazepam given at a rate of 2 mg/min (0.1 mg/kg) to a maximum dose of 8 mg or alternatively administer IV diazepam given at a rate not to exceed 2 mg/min until seizures stop or to a total of 20 mg. This is followed by IV phenytoin (fosphenytoin; PHT [FPHT]), 20 mg/kg, at a rate nofaster than 50 mg/min. If seizures are not controlled, a repeat bolus of PHT (FPHT) of 10 mg/kg can be given before proceeding to step 4. Monitor ECG and blood pressure.
4	31–59 min	If seizures persist, perform elective endotracheal intubation before starting a bolus infusion of phenobarbital at a rate not to exceed 100 mg/min until seizures stop or to a loading dose of 20 mg/kg.
5	60 min	If control is still not achieved, other options include: (1) Pentobarbital with an initial IV loading dose of 5–10 mg/kg with additional amounts given to produce a "burst suppression" pattern on EEG. Maintenance of pentobarbital anesthesia is continued for approximately 4 hours by an infusion of 1–3 mg/kg/hr. The patient is then checked for the reappearance of seizure activity by decreasing the infusion rate. If clinical seizures and/or generalized discharges persist on EEG, the procedure is repeated; if not, the pentobarbital is tapered over 12–24 hours. (2) Paraldehyde is given intravenously or rectally at a dose of 0.1–0.15 ml/kg after being diluted in normal saline every 2–4 hours if necessary. (3) Diazepam (50–100 mg) is diluted in a solution of 500 ml 0.9% NaCl or D5W and run as a continuous infusion to achieve blood levels of 0.2–0.8 mg/ml. The IV solution is changed every 6 hours as advised by certain authors and short-length IV tubing is used.
6	61–80 min	If seizures are still not controlled, call the anesthesia department to begin general anesthesia with halothane and neuromuscular blockade.

Note: Continuous EEG monitoring is recommended in an obtunded patient to ensure that status epilepticus has not recurred. In the management of intractable status, a neurologist who has expertise in status epilepticus should be consulted and advice from a regional epilepsy center should be sought.

ECG = electrocardiogram; EEG = electroencephalogram; IV = intravenous; BUN = blood urea nitrogen; CBC = complete blood count; ABG = arterial blood gas; D5W = 5% dextrose in water.

which cause some respiratory depression. In a neurologically depressed patient, elective intubation and respiratory support are urged. In most patients, the placement of an oral airway or nasal oxygen cannula will prove to be insufficient because respiratory drive is depressed.[3] Respiratory arrest and depression are the principle factors contributing to morbidity and mortality.[8] Rapid assessment of vital signs and general neurologic examination findings give clues to the cause of SE. Drawing blood for the determination of blood gases, levels of glucose, calcium, electrolytes, a complete blood count, AED levels, cultures (bacterial and viral), and toxicologic studies helps with the overall determination of etiology. Similarly, urine, drug, and metabolic screening should be performed.

Treatment should be initiated by the establishment of an intravenous (IV) line. Fluid restriction is rarely necessary. In children, immediately following placement of an IV line, 25% glucose (2–4 ml/kg) should be given by bolus.[1, 3] In adults, the IV line is typically kept open with normal saline and the patient should then be given 100 mg of thiamine followed by 50 ml of 50% glucose by slow IV push if hypoglycemia is possible.[9, 26] Whenever the IV route cannot be established, the intraosseous route, which has been shown to be efficient for fluid and medication administration, may be substituted.[29]

Because of the substantial incidence of febrile SE resulting from CNS infections in infants and young children, a lumbar puncture should be done early in the course of management, although not necessarily in the initial phase of stabilization. In children, only rarely should one wait for imaging studies to be obtained before performing the lumbar puncture. In adults, the process of obtaining cerebrospinal fluid samples is dependent on the overall patient presentation. Hyperpyrexia may become significant during the course of SE, even in the absence of prior febrile illness. Rectal temperature should be monitored and fever should be aggressively treated because significant temperature elevation may contribute to brain damage.[2]

Electrocardiographic (ECG) and EEG monitoring optimizes the management of SE and when available should be continued expectantly. As noted earlier, EEG monitoring is extremely useful in initial and subsequent management of SE.[1, 9, 23, 30] Classification of the patient's SE and clues to cause and prognosis may be suggested from the EEG recording. This may be especially useful in managing patients with hysterical attacks or those with overdoses of drugs or focal pathologic entities. EEG findings may clearly define seizures as being mainly partial versus primarily or secondarily generalized, and, in nonconvulsive cases, the EEG recording should establish the diagnosis of complex partial versus absence. Use of EEG monitoring is mandatory when muscular blockade is contemplated or whenever the recurrence of seizures cannot be documented by clinical observation. A seeming electroclinical dissociation may exist after large doses of AEDs have been given so that the clinical manifestations are absent while electrographic seizures continue. EEG patterns, such as paroxysmal lateralized epileptiform discharges (PLEDs), periodic discharges, and evidence of continued post-SE ictal discharges without clinical correlation while the patient remains in coma, may be helpful in establishing the etiologic diagnosis and prognosis. ECG changes seen in adults during and after SE range from evidence of ischemia to tachyarrhythmias.[31, 32] These must be recognized promptly and appropriately treated.

DRUG THERAPY OF STATUS EPILEPTICUS

The choice of the optimal pharmacologic agent for each patient with SE may not be identical. Although BZDs and PHT as initial therapy are preferred by our group at the Medical College of Virginia, others may wish to continue alternative agents if the patient is known to be on maintenance therapy or has already received smaller doses of PHT or PB. A brief review of each of the major medications follows. Discussion concerning the optimal or first-choice drug therapy of SE examines the morbidity, mortality, and practical issues of drug administration and adverse effects. As recently reviewed, no one drug of choice may be acceptable to all clinicians and investigators.[33] Certainly lorazepam, diazepam, PHT, and PB are all accepted agents for initial and continued therapy of SE. The large SE treatment study sponsored by the U.S. Veterans Administration suggests that when comparing four IV drug regimens (1) diazepam, 0.15 mg/kg, and PHT, 18 mg/kg; (2) lorazepam, 0.1 mg/kg; and (3) PB, 15 mg/kg, were found superior to PHT, 18 mg/kg, alone for initial management of generalized convulsive SE.[28] Thus, the choice of an initial agent may depend on individual patient characteristics, prior AED therapy, and physician preference. In the near future, medications with neuronal protective properties may be added to the classic AEDs for treatment of SE, and fosphenytoin (FHPT) administration will most likely replace PHT (see below).

Benzodiazepines

As a group, the BZDs are the most potent and efficacious in the treatment of SE.[12, 28] Lasting control of SE is achieved in approximately 80% of patients treated with lorazepam, diazepam, or clonazepam. All three, however, cause a transient depression of consciousness after IV injection. Lorazepam is the most likely to cause transient amnesia.[9]

Lorazepam

Lorazepam is a potent BZD with rapid onset of action and a more prolonged duration of anticonvulsant action compared with diazepam. Although the half-life of approximately 10–15 hours in adults and children is less than that of diazepam, lorazepam enters the brain nearly as rapidly as diazepam and continues to have effective brain level concentrations and clinical efficacy for at least 8 hours in most patients. A more favorable smaller volume of distribution of unbound drug and distribution coefficient allows lorazepam to remain in the brain longer than diazepam, which redistributes more rapidly. The recommended IV bolus dose is 0.1 mg/kg up to a total dose of 8 mg. Tachyphylaxis may develop, making repeated doses less effective.[3, 34]

Adverse effects of lorazepam include ataxia, vomiting, amnesia, lethargy, respiratory depression, and hypotension. These side effects are exacerbated when other depressant drugs, such as barbiturates, are administered before lorazepam. Following its rectal administration, lorazepam has a more prolonged onset of action than diazepam.[35] Sedation that follows IV administration of lorazepam is longer than that following diazepam,[34] but it has been used successfully through this route for prehospital treatment of prolonged seizures.[36]

Diazepam

Diazepam enters the brain within seconds after IV administration and successfully stops convulsive and nonconvulsive seizures in the majority of adults and children.[12] Its primary advantages are similar to those of lorazepam. The disadvantage is that seizures frequently recur after 15–20 minutes because of its rapid redistribution from the brain, requiring that a repeat diazepam dose or an alternative, longer-acting AED be given. Respiratory support should be available when this drug is used to treat SE because of adverse effects similar to those with lorazepam, including respiratory depression, especially when diazepam is administered rapidly or in conjunction with other sedating compounds. Recommended dosage estimates are given in Table 14.5; doses range from 0.4 mg/kg per dose in children to a total initial adult dose of 20 mg or greater. In children, an initial estimate of the dose may be made according to the patient's age, giving 1 mg/year plus 1 mg. In addition to respiratory depression, laryngeal spasm may develop during the administration of diazepam.[37]

Although lorazepam and diazepam are usually suggested as the initial drugs of choice, they are sometimes useful as a second or third agent when seizures continue. Respiratory support should be provided because of probable apnea or respiratory arrest, and hypotension should be expected. Diazepam may also be given by intraosseous[29] or rectal routes[35] or by continuous IV infusion.[9, 12] Rectal administration of diazepam may be used as home therapy for those with recurrent SE, prolonged seizures, or acute repetitive seizures.[38]

Midazolam

Midazolam is a new and effective BZD that may be used to treat SE in children and adults.[39] Some suggest it is superior to other BZDs because of its very rapid onset of anticonvulsant action and seeming success when more conventional therapies fail,[40] but no controlled comparative studies are available. Midazolam may be given by IV bolus (0.15 mg/kg) followed by continuous infusion using 1.0 mg/kg per hour with dose escalation every 15 minutes until clinical seizures are controlled.[41] In one series of 24 patients, all had SE controlled using this schedule within the average of 0.78 hours (range 0.25–4.5 hours), using a mean infusion rate of 2.3 mg/kg per minute (range 1–18 mg/kg per minute). Adverse effects are similar to those of other BZDs. Tachyphylaxis is quite remarkable, requiring an escalation of midazolam dosage when continuous infusions are continued.

Phenobarbital

PB remains the drug of choice in some institutions for treatment of childhood SE.[18] Its onset of action is longer than that of the BZDs and PHT with peak brain levels being obtained in 20–60 minutes. Slow IV bolus infusion of 20–25 mg/kg is suggested, repeat doses of 10–20 mg/kg should be administered as necessary. The principal side effects of intravenous PB are hypotension and respiratory and sensorial depression. PB should be administered by IV push no faster than 100 mg per minute. In a randomized trial comparing diazepam and PHT versus PB and optional PHT in adults, the PB regimen was thought to have practical advantages.[42]

Phenytoin

PHT is administered intravenously following lorazepam in the protocol used at our institution. It is an excellent agent for the treatment of convulsive SE, partial and generalized, but it is not indicated in the treatment of absence SE.[3] The drug rapidly enters the brain because of its lipid solubility, reaching peak brain levels in 15 minutes.[43, 44] A marked advantage of PHT is that it is not as depressant as other IV AEDs. Loading doses of approximately 20 mg/kg provide initial serum PHT levels greater than 20 µg/ml, and this dosage is effective in maintaining serum levels of at least 10 µg/ml or greater for up to 24 hours.[45] Because of reported hypotension and cardiac conduction disturbances, primarily noted in adults or children with pre-existing cardiac disease, blood pressure and ECG monitoring should be performed during IV administration of PHT. The rate of infusion should be less than 50 mg per minute in adults or 1–3 mg/kg per minute in children. IV injection should be directly into the vein or IV line close to venous access because precipitation is likely to occur in most IV solutions. Intramuscular administration of PHT is discouraged because of crystallization, muscle destruction, and unpredictable absorption.[46] Extravasation from the vein may cause tissue injury because of the caustic alkaline solution in which PHT is delivered (pH 12).

FPHT is a water-soluble prodrug of PHT delivered in a neutral pH solution.[47] Many think that fosphenytoin will replace the present injectable PHT preparation.[48] Dosing is safe at 150 mg per minute (3 mg/kg per minute), a rate three times more rapid than the administration rate of PHT. Fosphenytoin is administered in "PHT equivalents" to obtain similar PHT levels, so that 20 mg/kg of fosphenytoin is administered to equal the derived amount of PHT equal to a dose of 20 mg/kg of PHT. This compound may be given intramuscularly or by the IV route because there is no local irritation or tissue destruction noted. Fosphenytoin is rapidly converted to PHT by systemic phosphatases, and higher unbound PHT peak levels are more rapidly available after the IV infusion of fosphenytoin than with the classic PHT preparation.[48]

Pentobarbital

Pentobarbital is used at many institutions for refractory SE. It should be used only in intensive care settings. After an IV loading dose of 5–20 mg/kg, 1–2 mg/kg per hour is given to keep the serum level between 20 and 40 µg/ml in order to produce electrographic suppression of burst suppression patterns.[26, 49] The half-life of pentobarbital is approximately 20 hours. Although the length of coma varies, most authorities stop pentobarbital-induced coma at 24–48 hours to observe if the clinical and electrographic SE has subsided.[49] At pentobarbital levels above 40 μg/ml, cardiac output and blood pressure are compromised. Treatment requiring coma with pentobarbital or other anesthetic agents to produce EEG suppression is associated with a higher rate or morbidity and mortality.[50]

Other Agents

When SE is resistant to BZDs, barbiturates, and PHT, additional agents have been given; the results have been unpredictable. Although the IV solution of paraldehyde is no longer commercially available in the United States, rectal solution is sometimes still used. Lidocaine may alternatively be used for the treatment of SE, but toxic levels produce an increased number of seizures.[51] An initial bolus of 2–3 mg/kg followed by a slow infusion of 4–10 mg/kg per hour is given. The principal side effect is cardiovascular dysfunction. A number of anesthetic agents, including propofol, have also been used for the control of SE; these agents are used to produce EEG suppression.[52]

Valproate (VPA) is useful in the management of generalized epilepsy, including absence SE.[23] After the administration of a BZD, VPA administration by the oral, nasogastric, or rectal route is often successful. An IV VPA preparation has been developed, but its role in the treatment of SE is not yet defined.[53] In one study of patients with recurrent episodes of absence SE as a manifestation of their primary generalized epilepsy, chronic therapy with VPA markedly reduced seizure recurrence.[54]

MEDICAL COMPLICATIONS OF STATUS EPILEPTICUS

The treatment of SE requires close monitoring of physiologic variables and excellent nursing to prevent secondary complications.[3, 9, 23] Besides underlying diseases that trigger or are associated with SE, other medical complications are quite common. Pulmonary care, proper positioning, and careful observation of seizures noting possible changes in seizure pattern are a must. Constant maintenance of IV fluids with adequate glucose and electrolytes is mandatory. Optimal oxygenation and expectant observation for treatment of hyperthermia and other medical complications directly lead to a lessening of morbidity and mortality. Cardiovascular, respiratory, and renal effects may be severe. Medical complications of SE are listed in Table 14.7. When hyperthermia is resistant to rectally administered antipyretics and cooling blankets, muscular blockade may be necessary. In this case, EEG monitoring is a necessity. A rise in blood pressure may physiologically accompany seizures but rarely requires antihypertensive medications unless the patient is at risk for malignant hypertension. Treatment, however, may result in hypotension and reduce cerebral perfusion pressure. Only infrequently does cerebral edema or increased intracranial pressure become problematic. Thus, osmotic diuretics and steroids are rarely indicated for the treatment of SE.

Table 14.7 Medical complications of status epilepticus

Tachycardia	Apnea
Bradycardia	Anoxia
Cardiac arrhythmia	Hypoxia
Cardia arrest	CO_2 narcosis
Conduction disturbance	Intravascular coagulation
Congestive heart failure	Metabolic and respiratory acidosis
Hypertension	Cerebral edema
Hypotension	Excessive perspiration
Altered respiratory pattern	Dehydration
Pulmonary edema	Endocrine failure
Pneumonia	Altered pituitary function
Oliguria	Elevated prolactin
Uremia	Elevated vasopressin
Renal tubular necrosis	Hyperglycemia
Lower nephron nephrosis	Hypoglycemia
Rhabdomyolysis	Increased plasma cortisol
Increased creatine phosphokinase	Autonomic dysfunction
Myoglobinuria	Fever

Source: Reprinted with permission from JM Pellock. Status Epilepticus. In JM Pellock, EC Meyer (eds), Neurologic Emergencies in Infancy and Childhood (2nd ed). New York: Demos, 1993.

OUTCOME

SE is recognized as a medical emergency because of the associated significant morbidity and mortality. Common sequelae of SE include intellectual dysfunction, permanent neurologic deficits, and continuing recurrent seizures. Neuropathologic studies in animals have demonstrated that prolonged electrical activity in the CNS can result in irreversible neuronal damage.[55] These experimental studies suggest that seizures lasting for less than 1 hour may produce neuronal injuries that are reversible. Seizures lasting longer than 1 hour produce neuronal death.[55, 56] The biochemical basis and pathophysiologic features underlying the means by which chronic seizures evolve to SE remain unclear. There seems to be a loss of inhibitory mechanisms, and the neuronal metabolism is unable to keep up with the demand of continuing ictal activity. During prolonged seizures, inadequate blood flow and decreased glucose use and oxygen consumption lead to impairment of oxygen use by mitochondria at the epileptic focus.[57, 58] The classic pathologic findings of laminar necrosis and neuronal damage after prolonged seizures are similar to those seen after cerebral hypoxia. Meldrum[55] clearly demonstrated that brain pathologic features were marked by damage in the middle layers of the neocortex, cerebellum, and hippocampus. Damage in the cerebellum correlated with the degree of hyperthermia. Excitatory amino acid neurotransmitters released during SE most probably also account for neuronal destruction in some adult animals.[59] Whereas some suggest that young animals may be less likely to develop brain damage after SE,[60] studies using alternative models demonstrate hippocampal cellular injury in immature rodents.[61] Nevertheless, the length of convulsions and the subject's age correlate well with the extent of neuropathologic changes in experimental SE and also predict clinical outcome in humans.[4]

Retrospective and prospective studies done at the Medical College of Virginia/Virginia Commonwealth University have carefully explored the relationship among seizure duration, seizure type, etiology, age, race, and sex with mortality and morbidity in patients with SE.[4, 7, 8] In the prospective population-based epidemiologic study, incidence of SE was 41 patients per year per 100,000 population and incidence of total SE episodes was 50 per year per 100,000. The mortality rate for the population was 22% overall, with 3% in children and 26% in adults. Based on the incidence of SE actually determined in Richmond, it was projected that there are 126,000–195,000 SE events with 22,000–42,000 deaths per year in the United States. The majority of SE patients had no previous history of epilepsy. The highest mortality rate was seen in the elderly, with as many as 55 deaths per 100,000 individuals per year in the "over 80 year old group." Although the overall mortality is extremely low in children, children 1–4 years old have the highest mortality among the pediatric age group. Recurrences of SE following a single episode were more common in the very young and also the elderly. These patients in general have chronic neurologic disability and rarely died. In those patients who died, death was rarely during the acute episode of SE. Rather, most deaths occurred within 15–30 days after the beginning of SE. Some remained in a coma, but many did not. Certain causes have a higher mortality in adults as shown in Table 14.2. Those with chronic epilepsy and low AED levels have the lowest mortality rate.

Concurrent disease states are certainly more common in adults versus children who develop SE. Recent studies at our institution suggest that cardiovascular changes occurring during the stress of SE may play an important role in the overall mortality of adults, particularly the elderly.[31, 32]

Morbidity of SE in children was examined in retrospective and prospective groups in the Medical College of Virginia Status Epilepticus database. Before their SE event, 81% of children with no prior seizure were neurologically normal in contrast to only 31% of children with a seizure history. Of the neurologically normal children with no prior seizures, more than 25% deteriorated after their first SE event, in comparison with less than 15% of neurologically normal children with a seizure history. Children who were neurologically abnormal without prior seizures deteriorated further in 6.7% compared with 11.3% of the abnormal children with a seizure history. Morbidity was determined at the time of hospital discharge, and in some children the abnormalities noted would certainly improve, as minor degrees of ataxia, incoordination, or motor deficits can be attributed to the acute therapies or clinical changes after a prolonged seizure that may not persist. It is more difficult to determine whether language deficits and difficulty performing school work was a transient or more permanent effect of SE. Interestingly, our previous retrospective study yielded a higher rate of morbidity of nearly 30%, suggesting a sampling bias.[62] In the prospective study, 11–15% had a significant morbidity after an episode of SE. Our recent findings suggest a neurologic morbidity substantially lower than the "greater than 50%" rate previously reported in children.[63]

CONCLUSION

SE is a neurologic emergency that must be treated aggressively. Significant morbidity and mortality are associated with SE in children and adults. In addition to treating the seizure in the most optimal way, the clinician must investigate the cause of the SE and design specific treatments depending on the underlying cause. An emergency SE treatment and evaluation plan should be established and followed to ensure expedited care. Anticonvulsant agents, although successful in treating the majority of SE cases, are not completely successful, and new agents must be developed. In addition, future therapies may well include agents for systemic and neuroprotection to improve the morbidity and mortality of SE. Rapid recognition and treatment offer the best opportunity to improve the outcome of those afflicted with this world-wide neurologic emergency.

REFERENCES

1. Pellock JM. Status Epilepticus. In JM Pellock, EC Myer (eds), Neurologic Emergencies in Infancy and Childhood (2nd ed). New York: Demos, 1993;167.
2. Dodson WE, DeLorenzo RJ, Pedley TA, et al. For The Epilepsy Foundation of America's Working Group on Status Epilepticus. Treatment of convulsive status epilepticus. JAMA 1993;270:854.
3. Pellock JM. Status epilepticus in children: update and review. J Child Neurol 1994;9(Suppl 2):S27.
4. Towne AR, Pellock JM, Ko D, DeLorenzo RJ. Determinants of mortality in status epilepticus. Epilepsia 1994;35:27.
5. Wilson JVK, Reynolds EH. Translation and analysis of a cuneiform text forming part of a Babylonian treatise on epilepsy. Med Hist 1990;34:185.
6. DeLorenzo RJ, Towne AR, Pellock JM, Ko D. Status epilepticus in children, adults, and the elderly. Epilepsia 1992;33(Suppl 4):S15.
7. DeLorenzo RJ, Pellock JM, Towne AR, Boggs JG. Pathophysiology of status epilepticus. J Clin Neurol 1995;12:316.
8. DeLorenzo RJ, Hauser WA, Towne AR, et al. A prospective, population-based study of status epilepticus in Richmond, Virginia. Neurology 1996;46:1029.
9. Treiman DM. Status Epilepticus. In J Laidlaw, A Richens, D Chadwick (eds), A Textbook of Epilepsy. Edinburgh: Churchill Livingstone, 1993;205.
10. Commission on Classification and Terminology of the International League Against Epilepsy. Proposal for revised clinical and electroencephalographic classification of epileptic seizures. Epilepsia 1981;22:489.
11. Gastaut H. Classification of Status Epilepticus. In AV Delgado-Escueta, RJ Porter, CG Wasterlain (eds), Status Epilepticus: Mechanisms of Brain Damage and Treatment. New York: Raven, 1982;15.
12. Treiman DM. The role of benzodiazepines in the management of status epilepticus. Neurology 1990;40(Suppl 2):32.
13. Treiman DM, Walton NY, Kendrick C. A progressive sequence of electroencephalogenic changes during generalized convulsive status epilepticus. Epilepsy Res 1990;5:49.
14. Mizrahi EM, Kellaway P. Characterization and classification of neonatal seizures. Neurology 1987;37:1837.
15. Scher MS, Aso K, Beggarly ME, et al. Electrographic seizures in preterm and full-term neonates: clinical correlates, associated brain lesions, and risk for neurological sequelae. Pediatrics 1993;91:128.
16. Delgado-Escueta AV, Treiman DM. Focal Status Epilepticus: Modern Concepts. In H Lüders, RP Lesser (eds), Epilepsy: Electroclinical Syndromes. London: Springer, 1987;347.
17. Porter RJ, Peury JK. Petit Mal Status. In AV Delgado-Escueta, CG Wasterlain, et al. (eds), Status Epilepticus. New York: Raven, 1983;61.
18. Lockman LA. Treatment of status epilepticus in children. Neurology 1990;40(Suppl 2):43.
19. Hauser WA. Status epilepticus: epidemiologic considerations. Neurology 1990;40(Suppl 2):9.

20. Hauser WA, Rich SS, Annegers JF, Anderson VE. Seizure recurrence after a first unprovoked seizure: an extended follow-up. Neurology 1990;40:1163.
21. Maytal J, Shinnar S, Moshé SL, Alverez LA. Low morbidity and mortality of status epilepticus in children. Pediatrics 1989;83:323.
22. Shinnar S, Pellock JM, Berg AT, et al. An inception cohort of children with febrile status epilepticus: cohort characteristics and early outcomes [abstract]. Epilepsia 1995;36(Suppl 4):31.
23. Pellock JM. Status Epilepticus. In WE Dodson, JM Pellock (eds), Pediatric Epilepsy, Diagnosis and Therapy. New York: Demos, 1993;197.
24. Dunn W. Status epilepticus in children: etiology, clinical features, and outcome. J Child Neurol 1988;3:167.
25. Phillips SA, Shanahan RJ. Etiology and mortality of status epilepticus in children. Arch Neurol 1989;46:74.
26. DeLorenzo RJ. Status Epilepticus. In RJ Johnson (ed), Current Therapy in Neurologic Disease 3. Philadelphia: BC Decker, 1990;47.
27. Treiman DM, Meyers PD, Walton NY, et al. Duration of generalized convulsive status epilepticus: relationship to clinical symptomatology and response to treatment [abstract]. Epilepsia 1992;33(Suppl 3):66.
28. Treiman DM, Meyers PD, Walton NY, et al. Treatment of generalized convulsive status epilepticus: a multicenter comparison of four drug regimens [abstract]. Neurology 1996;46(Suppl):A219.
29. Orlowski JP, Porembha DT, Gallagher BB, et al. Comparison study of intraosseous, central intravenous and peripheral intravenous infusions of emergency drugs. Am J Dis Child 1990;144:112.
30. Jaitly R, Sgro JA, Towne AR, DeLorenzo RJ. A prospective study of prolonged (24 hour) EEG monitoring in a large population of status epilepticus patients [abstract]. Neurology 1994; 44(Suppl):A172.
31. Boggs JG, Painter JA, DeLorenzo RJ. Analysis of electrocardiographic changes in status epilepticus. Epilepsy Res 1993;14:87.
32. Boggs JG, Painter JA, Wood MA, et al. Signal-averaged electrocardiograms in patients with status epilepticus [abstract]. Neurology 1994;44(Suppl):A205.
33. Holmes GL. Drug of choice for status epilepticus. J Epilepsy 1990;3:1.
34. Homan RW, Treiman DM. Lorazepam. In RH Levy, RH Mattson, BS Meldrum, et al. (eds), Antiepileptic Drugs (4th ed). New York: Raven, 1995;779.
35. Graves NM, Kriel RL. Rectal administration of antiepileptic drugs in children. Pediatr Neurol 1987;3:321.
36. Lowenstein DH, Allridge B, Gel A, et al. Prehospital treatment of status epilepticus. Neurology 1995;45(Suppl 4):A390.
37. Schmidt D. Diazepam. In RH Levy, RH Mattson, BS Meldrin, et al. (eds), Antiepileptic Drugs (4th ed). New York: Raven, 1995;705.
38. Driefus FE, Kuzniecky RI, Pellock JM, et al. A double-blind, placebo-controlled trial of Diastat diazepam viscous solution administered rectally to children and adults for acute repetitive seizures. 1997 (submitted).
39. Crisp CB, Gannon R, Kauft F. Continuous infusion of midazolam hydrochloride to control status epilepticus. Clin Pharmacol 1933;7:322.
40. Chaing CWJ, Bleck TP. Status epilepticus. Neurol Clin 1995;13:529.
41. Rivera R, Segnini M, Baltodano A, Perez V. Midazolam in the treatment of status epilepticus in children. Crit Care Med 1993;21:991.
42. Shaner DM, McCurdy SA, Herring MO, Gabor AJ. Treatment of status epilepticus: a prospective comparison of diazepam and phenytoin versus phenobarbital and optional phenytoin. Neurology 1988;38:202.
43. Wilder BJ, Ramsay RE, Willmore LJ, et al. Efficacy of intravenous phenytoin in the treatment of status epilepticus: kinetics of central nervous system penetration. Ann Neurol 1977;1:51.
44. Ramsay RE, Hammond EJ, Perchalski RJ, et al. Brain uptake of phenytoin, phenobarbital, and clonazepam. Arch Neurol 1979;36:535.
45. Cranford RE, Leppik IE, Patrick B, et al. Intravenous phenytoin: clinical and pharmacokinetic aspects. Neurology 1979;29:1474.
46. Wilensky AJ, Lowden JA. Inadequate serum levels after intramuscular administration of diphenylhydantoin. Neurology 1973;23:318.
47. Leppik IE, Boucher BA, Wilder BJ, et al. Pharmacokinetics and safety of a phenytoin products given IV or IM in patients. Neurology 1987;37:500.
48. Pellock JM (ed). Formulary report: issues in the management of acute seizures. Pharmacol Ther 1996;(Suppl 5):1S.

49. Raskin MC, Younger C, Penovich P. Pentobarbital treatment of refractory status epilepticus. Neurology 1987;37:500.
50. VanNess PC. Pentobarbital and EEG burst suppression in treatment of status epilepticus refractory to benzodiazepines and phenytoin. Epilepsia 1990;31:61.
51. Lemmen LJ, Klasen M, Duiser B. Intravenous lidocaine in the treatment of convulsions. JAMA 1978;239:2025.
52. Mäkelä JP, Iivanainen M, Pieninkeroinen IP, et al. Seizures associated with propofol anesthesia. Epilepsia 1993;34:832.
53. Devinsky O, Leppik I, Wilmore LJ, et al. Safety of intravenous valproate. Ann Neurol 1995;38:670.
54. Berkovic SF, Andermann F, Griberman A, et al. Valproate prevents the recurrence of absence status. Neurology 1989;39:1294.
55. Meldrum BS. Metabolic Factors During Two Prolonged Seizures and Their Relationship to Nerve Cell Death. In AV Delgado-Escueta, CG Wasterlain, DM Treiman, RJ Porter (eds), Status Epilepticus: Mechanisms of Brain Damage and Treatment. New York: Raven, 1983;261.
56. Simon RP. Physiologic consequences of status epilepticus. Epilepsia 1985;26(Suppl 1):S58.
57. Wasterlain CG. Glucose and Energy Metabolism of the Immature Brain During Status Epilepticus. In AV Delgado-Escueta, CG Wasterlain, DM Treiman, RJ Porter (eds), Status Epilepticus: Mechanisms of Brain Damage and Treatment. New York: Raven, 1983;241.
58. Dwyer BE, Wasterlain CG, Fajikawa DG, et al. Brain Protein Metabolism in Epilepsy. In AV Delgado-Escueta, AA Ward, DM Woodburg, et al. (eds), Basic Mechanisms of the Epilepsies: Molecular and Cellular Approaches. New York: Raven, 1986;903.
59. Lothman E. The biochemical basis and pathophysiology of status epilepticus. Neurology 1990;40(Suppl 2):13.
60. Moshé SL. Epileptogenesis and the immature brain. Epilepsia 1987;28(Suppl 1):S3.
61. Thompson K, Wasterlain CG. A model of status epilepticus that produces neuronal necrosis in the immature brain [abstract]. Neurology 1994;44:A273.
62. Fortner C, Pellock JM, Driscoll SM, DeLorenzo RJ. Morbidity in children after a first episode of status epilepticus [abstract]. Epilepsia 1993;34(Suppl 6):55.
63. Aicardi JF, Chevrie JJ. Convulsive status epilepticus in infants and children: a study of 239 cases. Epilepsia 1987;11:187.

15
Febrile Convulsions: A Pragmatic Approach

Christopher M. Verity

> *Pragmatic:* "dealing with matters according to their practical significance or immediate importance."
>
> *—The Concise Oxford Dictionary*

It is certainly of practical significance to discuss the management of febrile convulsions because they present the single most common problem in pediatric neurology.[1] How serious are they for the child? Opinions have changed with time. In 1950, Ekholm and Niemineva[2] reported that after convulsions in early childhood, "only a fraction of the patients later developed quite normally." In 1949, Lennox[3] wrote, "febrile convulsions may cause brain pathology as evidenced by transient or permanent neurological deficit." In contrast, Robinson, in 1991,[4] referred to children with febrile convulsions as having a "generally excellent prognosis."

Why has there been this change in opinion? One reason is that earlier reports of the relatively poor prognosis for children with more severe problems attending specialized clinics or hospitals have been balanced by the more optimistic findings of population-based studies of unselected groups of children.[5–17] Another reason is that the results of studies depend on the way that febrile convulsions are defined—some researchers have included children with underlying meningitis or encephalitis in their studies of febrile convulsions. The issues have been discussed in recent reviews.[18–21]

DEFINITIONS

In this chapter, the term *febrile convulsion* is used synonymously with the term *febrile seizure.*

Febrile convulsions are a heterogeneous group, and it is important to know the type of febrile convulsion and the clinical context in which it occurs. There has been debate whether febrile convulsions are genetically separate from epilepsy.[21–24]

289

Febrile Convulsions

It has become generally accepted that seizures that are known to be symptomatic of an underlying central nervous system (CNS) infection should *not* be called febrile convulsions.[25, 26] In 1993, the Commission on Epidemiology and Prognosis of the International League Against Epilepsy[27] defined a febrile seizure (convulsion) as:

> "an epileptic seizure … occurring in childhood after age 1 month, associated with a febrile illness not caused by an infection of the CNS, without previous neonatal seizures or a previous unprovoked seizure, and not meeting criteria for other acute symptomatic seizures."

Convulsions with Fever

Some authors have used a definition of febrile convulsions that includes those that occur when children are febrile because of an underlying meningitis or encephalitis[21, 28]—these would not meet the definition of febrile convulsions given above. The joint working group that met in the Royal College of Physicians in London in 1991[26] considered that it was important to define a broader group of "convulsions with fever" as "any convulsion in a child of any age with fever of any cause."

Simple Versus Complex Febrile Convulsions

Febrile convulsions can be subclassified.[3, 29, 30] In the National Collaborative Perinatal Project (NCPP), the large American prospective population study,[12] *complex febrile seizures (convulsions)* were defined as those that had one or more of the following: (1) duration of more than 15 minutes; (2) recurrence within 24 hours; and (3) focal features. The British Child Health and Education Study (CHES) adopted a very similar definition,[15–17] and so did Forsgren in his Swedish study.[8–10] *Simple febrile convulsions* are those that do not have complex features.

Are these definitions robust when used by investigators? Berg et al.[31] asked three pediatric neurologists to classify febrile convulsions and found that there was excellent agreement whether the convulsions were multiple or prolonged and fair to good agreement on the occurrence of focal features.

"Febrile Status Epilepticus" Versus "Status Epilepticus Associated with Fever"

There are studies that have dealt specifically with febrile convulsions that are prolonged enough to be regarded as status epilepticus.[32–35] Maytal and Shinnar[33] used the term "febrile status epilepticus" for febrile convulsions that lasted longer than 30 minutes. However, not all children who are febrile during an episode of status epilepticus are having seizures that would meet the definition of febrile convulsions given above. The following definitions are therefore proposed:

Status epilepticus associated with fever. Status epilepticus preceded by hyperthermia or (if the temperature was not taken before the convulsion) when fever is present at the initial medical examination. In childhood, some cases of status epilepticus associated with fever are *lengthy febrile convulsions* and some are *acute symptomatic febrile status epilepticus.*

Lengthy febrile convulsions. Febrile convulsions that last longer than 30 minutes. (Nelson and Ellenberg[13] were perhaps the first to use the term in this way.)

Acute symptomatic febrile status epilepticus. An episode of status epilepticus that is preceded and accompanied by fever and that is concurrent with and considered to be the consequence of an acute disorder of the CNS (usually an intracranial infection).

INCIDENCE, PREVALENCE, AND RECURRENCE

Overall Rates

Between 2% and 4% of all children have one or more febrile convulsions by 5 years of age.[8, 13–16, 36, 37] Some studies have found higher rates in boys than in girls,[8, 13, 38] but others have not.[14, 15, 37] The NCPP[13] reported racial differences, the prevalence rates being 3.5% in white children and 4.2% in black children (*p* <0.001). There are geographical differences—a prevalence of 8.3% by 3 years of age in Tokyo, for instance.[38]

Age

Febrile convulsions most commonly start in the second year of life. Children are at greatest risk between 6 months and 3 years of age.[21] The age of onset has been reported to vary between 2 months of age and 7 years 9 months.[17]

Type of Febrile Convulsion

In Wallace's study,[30] 62% of 131 children admitted to the hospital because of febrile convulsions had "complicated" (complex) convulsions. Chevrie and Aicardi[39] also found a high incidence of convulsions with partial features in their hospital study. Population-based studies that include children who are not admitted to the hospital have found that a smaller proportion of first febrile convulsions are complex—18% in the United States,[12] 22% in Britain,[17] and 8.6% in Sweden.[8] The fact that a higher proportion of complex cases are found in the hospital-based series suggests that the more severe cases are admitted to the hospital. Alternatively, it could be that in population-based studies, lateralizing or focal features are not recognized and are therefore underreported.[21]

Febrile Recurrences

"Recurrence" in this context means more than one episode of febrile convulsions, as opposed to "multiple," which means more than one convulsion during an episode of fever (see definition of complex febrile convulsions above).

Berg et al.[40] performed a meta-analysis of 14 studies that reported on the risk of recurrent febrile convulsions. The overall risk of a recurrence was 34.3%. Young age at onset (1 year or less) and a family history of febrile seizures each predicted increased risk. Focal, prolonged, and multiple convulsions were only associated with a small increase. Other studies have found similar results.[7, 8, 41–44] Most recurrences occur within 3 years of the first.[21]

ETIOLOGY

Genetic Factors

Berg et al.[45] performed a case control study and found that a family history of febrile convulsions in a first-degree relative was a significant risk factor for first febrile convulsions in patients seen at hospital emergency departments. Population-based studies also suggest that family history is important and that febrile convulsions and epilepsy each provide an independent contribution to the familial risk of febrile convulsions.[46–48] Forsgren et al.[9] concluded that multifactorial inheritance was most likely. Tsuboi and Endo[49] agreed and calculated that the heritability (the estimated genetic contribution to the expression of febrile convulsions) was 75%—very similar to the 76% calculated by Fukuyama et al.[50] Concordance rates for febrile convulsions in monozygotic twins are higher than in dizygotic twins.[49, 51, 52]

Prenatal Factors

Maternal ill health, parental subfertility,[21] prenatal maternal cigarette smoking, and alcohol intake[53] have been associated with the occurrence of febrile convulsions in offspring. Nelson and Ellenberg[46] found that maternal smoking during the pregnancy was associated with increased risk of febrile convulsions in the child. However, in general, population-based cohort studies do not find much evidence that social and maternal factors are of practical significance.[10, 16, 46]

Perinatal Factors

A hospital-based series suggested that an abnormal pregnancy or birth history predisposes an individual to febrile convulsions in general and complicated initial febrile convulsions in particular.[30, 54] In contrast, the American NCPP[46] concluded that pregnancy and birth factors contribute little to the risk of febrile convulsions. In Sweden,[10] a community-based, case-control study found that in pregnancy, proteinuria and preeclampsia/eclampsia occurred more often in mothers of children with febrile convulsions. A similar association of maternal preeclampsia with febrile convulsions in the child has been found in the 10-year data obtained by the British CHES cohort.[55] In China,[56] a case-control study did not identify important prenatal or perinatal risk factors for febrile convulsions. In Canada, a case control study[48] found that discharge from the hospital of neonates at 28 days or later (a marker of difficulties in the neonatal period) was associated with increased risk of first febrile convulsions (odds ratio [OR], 5.6).

Postnatal Factors

Bethune et al.[48] identified children presenting with their first febrile seizure to a hospital emergency department and performed a case-control study to investigate risk factors. They found that parental report of slow development (OR, 4.9) and day-care attendance (OR, 3.1) were both associated with a significant increase in risk of a first febrile seizure. Forsgren et al.[10] did not find evidence that developmental delay was a significant risk factor, but living in an apartment and attending day care was significant (possibly because of increased exposure to infections). Berg et al.[45] did not find that day care was a risk factor for first febrile convulsions.

Precipitating Factors

The height or duration of the fever may be important,[18, 21] but there are problems in evaluating the temperature recordings because febrile convulsions usually occur randomly at home. Viral infections commonly cause the fever that is associated with febrile convulsions.[57, 58] Synthesis of immunoglobulin in the cerebrospinal fluid (CSF) of children with febrile convulsions has been demonstrated, suggesting that encephalitis may sometimes occur but is not recognized.[21] There is evidence that human herpesvirus-6 (HHV-6) is linked with exanthem subitum, a condition that is frequently complicated by febrile convulsions.[59] More recent work suggests that acute HHV-6 infection is a cause of febrile convulsions in young children who do not have the signs of exanthem subitum.[60] Bacterial infections may be associated with febrile convulsions—urinary tract infections, *Shigella* and pneumococcal bacteremia, for instance. Children with bacterial meningitis sometimes have convulsions, and it is important to remember this when deciding whether to perform a lumbar puncture. Immunization can lead to an elevated temperature, which can trigger a febrile convulsion.[61]

OUTCOME AFTER FEBRILE CONVULSIONS

In 1971, Taylor and Ounsted[62] wrote, "We think that convulsive hypoxia sustained during prolonged febrile convulsions causes the death of vulnerable neurones in the cerebellum, the thalamus, and in mesial temporal structures." However, more recent experimental data do not support the poor prognosis perceived a few years ago,[63] and population-based studies also give a more optimistic view.

Evidence that Febrile Convulsions May Damage the Brain

Human Pathology: Postmortem Studies

There are reports of neuronal necrosis in the brains of children who died after prolonged "febrile convulsions."[64] The neuronal necrosis is described as particularly involving the cerebral cortex, the hippocampus, and the cerebellum.[65] These authors were describing extreme cases that were far from typical of the majority of febrile convulsions.

Retrospective Study of Patients with Temporal Lobe Epilepsy

In 1964, Falconer et al.[66] reported on pathologic findings in the resected temporal lobes of 100 adults with refractory temporal lobe epilepsy. About one-half had "mesial temporal sclerosis" (MTS), which varied from loss of nerve cells in the Sommer (H1) sector of the hippocampus to wider involvement of the temporal lobe. In 40% of the patients with MTS there was a history of "infantile convulsions," suggesting a causal relationship. Similarly, Taylor[67] and Taylor and Ounsted[62] concluded that hypoxia during convulsions in childhood caused MTS, some of the evidence coming from the retrospective study of temporal lobectomy patients. Harbord and Manson,[68] in a retrospective study of patients with temporal lobe epilepsy, found that previous complicated febrile convulsions were the most common predisposing factor. In their 1995 series, Kodama et al.[69] found that five children who had "early" onset of temporal lobe epilepsy at 10 years or less and who had magnetic resonance imaging (MRI) findings of MTS all had a history of complex febrile convulsions. Kuks et al.[70] studied 107 patients with drug-resistant epilepsy using high-resolution, volumetric MRI scanning. Forty-five of the patients had focal or diffuse hippocampal volume loss, and there was a strong association between hippocampal sclerosis and a history of childhood febrile convulsions. The authors pointed out that this association does not prove a causal relationship and that 64% of their patients with hippocampal volume loss gave no history of febrile convulsions, so if childhood febrile convulsions cause some cases of hippocampal sclerosis, this cannot be the only mechanism. Possibly in some children preexisting minor cerebral abnormalities, such as focal cortical microdysgenesis,[71] predispose the children to complex febrile convulsions and to later epilepsy.[4]

Studies Performed on Cerebrospinal Fluid of Patients with Febrile Convulsions

Simpson et al.[72, 73] found elevated CSF lactate levels or lactate/pyruvate ratios in some children with febrile convulsions, suggesting cerebral hypoxia. Other workers have not found evidence of metabolic disturbances in the CSF of children with febrile convulsions.[74–76]

Imaging Studies

Radiologic studies (pneumoencephalograms and computed tomographic scans) have shown brain swelling and then atrophy in children (some of whom were febrile) after episodes of status epilepticus.[77] Dierckx et al.[78] used single photon emission computed tomography (SPECT) to study 19 children with febrile convulsions. Two patients with complex febrile convulsions showed focal lesions on SPECT scans contralateral to the neurologic deficit. In 9 of 17 children with simple febrile convulsions, focally disturbed perfusion was shown, suggesting that brain tissue is regionally more vulnerable to fever, even in convulsions that are clinically generalized.

Studies of Outcome After Febrile Convulsions

Deaths

A mortality rate of 11% was reported by Ekholm and Niemineva in 1950.[2] This was in a group of hospitalized children with "infection convulsions." In contrast, two large population-based studies found no deaths that were directly attributable to febrile convulsions.[13, 17] The rate partly depends on how febrile convulsions are defined—some studies have included seizures complicating known meningitis or encephalitis.

Subsequent Afebrile Seizures

Incidence   In hospital-based series, rates of subsequent afebrile seizures or epilepsy (defined as "recurrent" afebrile seizures) have varied from 7% to 40%.[21] In the population-based American NCPP, the rate of epilepsy after febrile convulsions was 2% by 7 years of age,[12] and in the British CHES it was 2.5% by 10 years of age.[17] Annegers et al.[6] found that the risk of "unprovoked seizures" after febrile convulsions steadily increased with age—2% at 5 years, 4.5% at 10 years, 5.5% at 15 years, and 7% by age 25. There is evidence that up to 85% of afebrile seizures occur within 4 years of febrile convulsions,[21] but it seems that determination of the true incidence of afebrile seizures requires long follow-up.

Predisposing Factors for Later Afebrile Seizures
    1.   *Family history of epilepsy.* The information from population-based studies is conflicting. The NCPP[13] found that a history of seizures without fever in a parent or prior-born sibling was associated with a threefold increase in the rate of subsequent epilepsy after febrile convulsions. However, Annegers et al.[6] found only a weak association.

2. *Age of onset of febrile convulsions.* There is evidence that early onset of febrile convulsions[21] and "late" onset (after 6 years of age)[79] are associated with increased risk of later afebrile seizures. In the population-based NCPP,[12] there was an increased rate of epilepsy by 7 years of age in children whose febrile convulsions began in the first year and especially in the first 6 months (57 per 1,000 in the first 6 months versus 15 per 1,000 after the first year; chi-square 7.6, $p = 0.006$). However, there was a tendency for abnormal children to have convulsions early, which might explain the increased risk of epilepsy in this group. Annegers et al.[6] found that most of the increased rates associated with age were the result of confounding by complex features of the febrile convulsions.

3. *Abnormal neurologic or developmental status.* In the American NCPP,[12] children who had neurologic or developmental abnormalities before the first febrile convulsion were three times more likely to be epileptic by age 7 years than those who were previously normal.

4. *Characteristics of the febrile convulsions.* Afebrile seizures occur with increased frequency after convulsions that are *complicated* or *complex*. In the American NCPP,[12] the rate of spontaneous epilepsy, not preceded by febrile convulsions, was 5 per 1,000; after febrile convulsions that were not complex, epilepsy developed in 15 per 1,000, while after complex febrile convulsions, epilepsy developed in 41 per 1,000. The outcome also varied according to the type of complex febrile convulsion—when the first convulsion had prolonged, multiple, or focal features, epilepsy developed in 31, 42, and 71 per 1,000, respectively. The British CHES[17] found very similar results and so did Annegers et al.[6]—they found that the risk of what they called "unprovoked seizures" ranged from 2.4% among those who had simple febrile convulsions to 6–8% for those with a single complex feature, 17–22% for those with two complex features, and 49% for those with all three complex features.

5. *Recurrent episodes of febrile convulsions.* There are reports that an increase in the number of febrile recurrences is associated with an increased risk of later epilepsy.[21] However, neither the NCPP[12] nor the Rochester study[6] found much evidence for this. It has been suggested that each convulsion predisposes the patient to further convulsions. However, the sequence of brief first febrile convulsion followed by prolonged febrile recurrence followed by epilepsy was not seen once among 1,706 children with febrile convulsions.[80] In the CHES study,[17] only 4 of 382 children with febrile convulsions had a first simple febrile convulsion followed by a complex febrile recurrence and then by an afebrile seizure; also, the proportion of first febrile convulsions that were complex was 20%, whereas the proportion of recurrent febrile convulsions that were complex was lower—17%. Thus, there was little evidence in the American or the British study that there was progressive "damage" leading to more severe attacks.

Type of Afebrile Seizure After Febrile Convulsions   Some studies suggest that febrile convulsions can cause temporal lobe damage and lead to afebrile complex partial seizures (see above). In a hospital-based study, Wallace[81] reported that there was a correlation between the occurrence of a prolonged (>30 minutes) initial febrile convulsion with unilateral features and later development of temporal lobe epilepsy. However, cohort studies have shown that distribution of generalized and complex partial seizures in those who have had febrile convulsions was similar to that in the general population that was studied (i.e., there was no excess of complex partial seizures in the febrile convulsion group).[5, 17, 82] This suggests that febrile convulsions do not contribute appreciably to the occurrence of complex partial seizures in the general population.[83]

Annegers et al.[6] did find that children with febrile convulsions had a higher risk of later partial, rather than generalized, afebrile ("unprovoked") seizures. The prognostic factors for partial and generalized seizures were different. Febrile convulsions that were focal, repeated, or prolonged were strongly associated with *partial* afebrile seizures, whereas only the number of febrile convulsions was significantly associated with *generalized-onset* seizures. Verity and Golding[17] also reported an association between the occurrence of focal febrile convulsions and later afebrile complex partial seizures.

Neurologic Impairment

Hospital-based studies show that outcome is poor for some children with febrile convulsions. Wallace[84] studied children with febrile convulsions who were admitted to the hospital and concluded that perhaps 5% of the children acquired new abnormalities. However, Wallace included convulsions complicating a known infection of the CNS. Aicardi and Chevrie[85] excluded such children, but nevertheless outcome was poor for many in their series—of 402 children with febrile convulsions who were hospitalized or seen as outpatients, 37 had neurologic sequelae, including 24 with hemiplegia.

Population-based studies report a much better outcome. The NCPP[12] found that febrile convulsions often occur in children who are abnormal or suspected of being abnormal—22% of the 1,621 whose prior status was known. However, no child in the NCPP developed persisting hemiplegia or other motor deficits during or immediately after a febrile convulsion.[13] In the CHES cohort, 398 children had febrile convulsions. Nineteen (4.8%) had lengthy febrile convulsions (>30 minutes); in this group there was no evidence of neurologic sequelae in those who had been normal before the lengthy attacks except for one atypical case—a child who became very hyperpyrexial after he was put into a hot bath while having a convulsion.[34]

Maytal and Shinnar[33] in their study of "febrile status epilepticus" (febrile convulsions lasting longer than 30 minutes) reported that no child died or developed new neurologic deficits after the episodes of status. Subtle signs of neurologic dysfunction can be missed—Schiottz-Christensen[86] studied 14 pairs of monozygotic twins discordant for febrile convulsions. There was an increased incidence of "soft signs" and behavior disturbances in the twins who had experienced a febrile convulsion—these may have preceded the convulsions.

Intellectual Outcome

After hospital admission or attendance with febrile convulsions, mental retardation was found at follow-up in 22% by Lennox,[3] in 13.4% by Aicardi and Chevrie,[85] and in 8% by Wallace and Cull.[87] Aldridge-Smith and Wallace[88] reported that continuing febrile convulsions were more likely to be detrimental to overall intellectual development than continuous prophylactic treatment with phenobarbitone or sodium valproate. Schiottz-Christensen and Bruhn[89] studied 14 monozygotic twin pairs and found significant intellectual impairments in those with febrile convulsions, although the deficits were small.

In contrast, Ellenberg and Nelson[11] tested 431 sibling pairs who were discordant for febrile convulsions in the NCPP and found that at 7 years of age children who were normal before any febrile convulsion did not differ in intelligence quotient (IQ) from their normal, seizure-free siblings. Children who were abnormal or suspected of being abnormal before the first febrile convulsion scored significantly lower IQs than their siblings. Neither recurrent convulsions nor those lasting longer than 30 minutes were associated with IQ deficit. Population-based studies in Britain[16, 36] also found little difference in intellectual outcome between children who had febrile convulsions and their peers if the children with febrile convulsions had no other known neurologic abnormality.

Behavior

Immediate and short-term effects on behavior have been reported in up to 35% of children after febrile convulsions.[90] Schiottz-Christensen and Bruhn[89] studied twin-pairs who were discordant for febrile convulsions. Febrile convulsions did not seem to have influenced later behavior, as intra-pair differences were only found in a few cases. In the CHES cohort, an extensive questionnaire found that at 5 years of age the behavior of children with febrile convulsions differed very little from that of their peers.[16]

Outcome After Febrile Convulsions—Conclusions

Authors who have reported a poor outcome tend to have studied selected groups of children attending specialized hospitals or clinics. Sometimes they have included children who have suffered with convulsions that complicate meningitis or encephalitis. Some have included children who were known to be developmentally or neurologically abnormal before they had their first febrile convulsion. In contrast, population-based studies that have studied a less-selected group of children give a much more positive view. Such studies show that most children who have febrile convulsions are normal individuals who have *simple febrile convulsions,* the majority of which do not recur. In such children, there is little evidence of long-term effects on behavior or intelligence, and the increased risk of later epilepsy is slight. The minority of children have *complex febrile convulsions,* and for most of them the outlook is good. However, within this group there are a few children who are at particular risk of later having epilepsy, the risk being greatest for those who have febrile convulsions with focal features, which tend to be prolonged and to occur at a younger age.

CLINICAL CHARACTERISTICS

Aicardi[18] stated that febrile convulsions are all tonic-clonic or possibly hypotonic in type and are never myoclonic seizures, spasms, or nonconvulsive attacks.

Most are brief and bilateral, but long-lasting and partial (unilateral) febrile convulsions do occur. Most long-lasting febrile convulsions (70–75%) are the initial seizure experienced by the child.

Simple febrile convulsions are the most common type of febrile convulsion. They are brief (<15 minutes), generalized seizures that do not occur more than once during a single febrile episode. Some just consist of staring, perhaps accompanied by stiffening of the limbs, and they may not cause the parents great concern. Often they are much more dramatic, and many parents think that their child is dying when having a first febrile convulsion.[91] In the CHES birth cohort,[17] there were 382 children who were neurologically normal before their first febrile convulsion. Of these children, 287 (75%) had only simple febrile convulsions and 58% of them were admitted to the hospital—in other words, about 40% were not considered sufficiently severe to necessitate admission. About two-thirds of the children suffered with only one febrile convulsion ever.

Complex febrile convulsions may be more severe than simple febrile convulsions. In the CHES cohort, 95 children (25% of the children with febrile convulsions) had complex convulsions and 78% of them were admitted to the hospital—a higher proportion than was found in those with simple convulsions.[17] In these 95 children, the complex features were as follows: 55 (58%) multiple, 32 (34%) prolonged, and 17 (18%) focal (some had more than one complex feature). It is important to emphasize that the most severe attacks made up a very small proportion of all febrile convulsions.

MANAGEMENT

The management of children with febrile convulsions remains controversial (see reviews by Aicardi,[1, 18] Camfield and Camfield,[92] Hirtz,[93] Hirtz and Nelson,[61] Millichap and Colliver,[94] Nealis,[95] O'Donohoe,[19] Rosman,[96] Verity,[20] and Wallace[21]). Two groups of experts have published guidelines—the Consensus Development Panel that met at the National Institutes of Health in America,[25] and the Joint Working Group of the Research Unit of the Royal College of Physicians (RCP) and the British Paediatric Association (BPA).[26]

Initial Assessment

First, the convulsion should be stopped if it is continuing. Then the temperature should be measured to confirm that the child is febrile (the rectal temperature is more reliable than oral or axillary). It is important to determine whether the fever preceded the convulsion. The parents/caregivers may report a febrile illness, and they may have measured the child's temperature before the seizure started. The history and the general physical examination findings may provide clues: There may be an exanthematous rash or evidence of an upper respiratory tract infection. If the child is in a convulsion, the situation should be reassessed when it has stopped. Even when there is evidence of an infection outside the nervous system, it may be important to exclude an intracranial infection by performing a lumbar puncture.

Admission to the Hospital

Febrile convulsions that last for more than a few minutes should be stopped; if the convulsion cannot be stopped, the child should be admitted to the hospital. If the convulsion has stopped, it must then be decided whether to admit the child. According to the RCP/BPA Joint Working Group,[26] the following factors would favor admission after a first convulsion: (a) complex convulsion, (b) child aged less than 18 months, (c) early review by a doctor at home not possible, (d) home circumstances inadequate or unusual parental anxiety, or parents' inability to cope. Hirtz[93] suggested similar guidelines but thought that most children are better off at home if awake and alert after the seizure.

Investigations

According to the Joint Working Group of the RCP/BPA, "No investigations are routinely necessary in all children after a febrile convulsion."[26] This statement seems to be representative of the views of most commentators. It may be appropriate to check the blood glucose concentration or the electrolytes in some children with continuing convulsions.

Lumbar Puncture

Lumbar puncture is still a controversial subject. Rosman[96] recommended a very active approach—lumbar puncture for all children younger than 2 years old with febrile convulsions and all those older than 3 years old after a first febrile convulsion. He suggested the need for a second lumbar puncture in some children suspected of having meningitis, quoting evidence from Lorber and Sunderland,[97] who reported that sometimes the CSF is normal early in the course of meningitis, although their general advice was that "lumbar puncture should not be carried out as a routine procedure." Rutter and Smales[98] also reported that two children in their series developed meningitis within 1 or 2 days of negative results on lumbar puncture, so false reassurance can be derived from a lumbar puncture. Clinical vigilance seems to be all-important, together with the awareness that clinical signs of meningism are much less likely to be found in younger children.

The RCP/BPA Joint Working Group[26] recommended that a lumbar puncture should be performed (a) if there are clinical signs of meningism; (b) after a complex convulsion; (c) if the child is unduly drowsy or irritable or systemically ill; and (d) if the child is younger than 18 months (probably) and almost certainly if the child is aged younger than 12 months. The group considered that ideally a decision should be made by an experienced physician. If the decision is made not to perform a lumbar puncture, it should be reviewed within a few hours. The risk of coning in a comatose child should be borne in mind.

Camfield and Camfield[92] recommended a lumbar puncture for the majority of children under 1 year of age with a first febrile seizure because in a child younger than 1 year of age, meningitis may be accompanied by very little nuchal rigidity or other findings of meningeal irritation. Stenklyft and Carmona[99] stressed the importance of clinical judgment and made the point that lumbar puncture is indicated when there is the possibility of a partially treated meningitis in a child who has already been given antibiotics.

It may be decided that lumbar puncture is contraindicated in a febrile child who does not return to normal consciousness after a prolonged convulsion—there is a risk of cerebral herniation if the intracranial pressure is elevated. The RCP/BPA group did not give specific guidelines about this. It is my practice in this situation to take a sample of blood for bacterial culture (as well as throat and urine cultures if possible), to treat the patient with adequate doses of broad-spectrum antibiotics, and *not* to perform a lumbar puncture immediately. Brain imaging is then performed to look for cerebral edema or a collection of pus (possibly an intracerebral abscess or infected subdural fluid). Depending on the scan findings, a neurosurgeon may be asked about the need for a surgical drainage operation. Even if the scan findings are reassuring, the lumbar puncture is postponed until the clinical situation is improving—scans are not a reliable means of ensuring that intracranial pressure is normal in children. In a retrospective review of the progress of 445 children admitted to the hospital with bacterial meningitis, Rennick et al.[100] concluded that lumbar puncture may cause cerebral herniation in some cases, and normal results on computed tomography (CT) do not mean that it is safe to perform a lumbar puncture in a child with bacterial meningitis.

Electroencephalography

As Camfield and Camfield noted, "There appears to be no benefit from routine electroencephalography (EEG) in children with febrile seizures."[92] Reviewers have concluded that EEG studies are not helpful in assessing the prognosis of children who have febrile convulsions.[18, 21, 101, 102] Studies have shown that a proportion of children who have had febrile convulsions show spike and wave discharges as they fall asleep,[103] but this pattern has no long-term significance.[104] An EEG recording is therefore not recommended as part of the assessment of a child with febrile convulsions.

Although experts have concluded that EEG studies are not usually helpful,[26] a recent review of the management of febrile seizures by pediatric neurologists in North America revealed that 45.2% of respondents still used EEG recordings to determine the need for long-term prophylactic phenobarbital therapy.[94]

Brain Imaging

A child with a preceding or underlying neurologic problem may first come to medical attention because of a febrile convulsion. Underlying pathologic entities may therefore be suspected on the basis of the history or examination findings, and it may then be appropriate to perform a scan to investigate. This situation will exist in only a small minority of children with febrile convulsions.

It could be argued that a scan should be performed after prolonged or focal febrile convulsions because of the concern that these may be associated with MTS (see above). In order to investigate this, an MRI scan with special views of the temporal lobes would have to be obtained. It does not seem justified to recommend this. There is no clear evidence that it would change management.[20, 92]

Acute Therapy

Management of Fever

Fever should be treated for the comfort of the child. Kinmonth et al.[105] found that advising the parents to give the child paracetamol (acetaminophen) was more effective than sponging or unwrapping in controlling temperature in children at home and was more acceptable to parents. The RCP/BPA Joint Working Group did not recommend physical methods, such as fanning, cold bathing, and tepid sponging.

Rectal Diazepam to Abort Febrile Convulsions

The home use of rectal diazepam to abort seizures in children with convulsive disorders has been shown to be effective.[42, 106, 107] Some members of the RCP/BPA Joint Working Group[26] advised parents to give the drug as soon as possible; others advised that the parents wait for 5 minutes, by which time most convulsions will have stopped and the drug will be unnecessary.

Intermittent Prophylaxis

One approach to preventing recurrent febrile convulsions is to intervene at the onset of febrile illnesses in the child at risk. Active steps to lower the body temperature have been advocated and so has the prophylactic use of diazepam.

Antipyretic Measures   Camfield et al.[108] studied antipyretic instruction plus phenobarbitone or a placebo to prevent recurrence after the first febrile seizure. Despite verbal and written instructions about temperature control and demonstration of the use of the thermometer, there was little evidence that antipyretic counseling decreased seizure recurrence among patients receiving the placebo. The RCP/BPA Joint Working Group met in 1990, and at that time the members knew of no evidence that antipyretic treatment influenced the recurrence of febrile seizures.[26] More recently, Uhari et al.[109] showed that low doses of acetaminophen were ineffective for preventing febrile seizures. Camfield et al.[110] concluded that there was no evidence that the usual methods of fever control have any effect on recurrences of febrile seizures. In their opinion, the continuing recommendation that parents document fever and use antipyretic agents was likely to increase parental anxiety and "fever phobia."

Intermittent Prophylactic Anticonvulsants   Intermittent prophylactic rectal diazepam reduces the number of febrile recurrences[41, 42, 111, 112] and so does oral diazepam.[113] The guidelines published by the British Joint Working

Group[26] acknowledged that rectal diazepam could be effective in preventing convulsions when given at the onset of fever and a large oral dose of phenobarbitone may produce an effective drug concentration in the blood in 90 minutes, but the group did not recommend the use of either drug in this way because both cause drowsiness.

Rosman et al. performed a randomized placebo-controlled trial and concluded that oral diazepam, given only when fever is present, is safe and reduces the risk of recurrent febrile seizures.[114] On the basis of the results, the authors recommended starting oral diazepam at the first sign of illness. Treatment with diazepam should then continue if the child becomes febrile, and should stop after a day or two if no fever develops. In the paper, the authors stated that diazepam has no serious side effects, but 38.6% of the 153 children who received at least one dose of diazepam had what the authors termed moderate side effects. These included ataxia (30.0%), lethargy (28.8%), and irritability (24.2%). In the subsequent correspondence, Rosman et al.[115] emphasized that the 153 children had 661 fevers with moderate side effects in "only" 16.8% of these fever episodes.

In an editorial review, Camfield et al.[110] commented that the use of phenobarbitone at the time of illness appears ineffective, probably because of the delay in achieving appropriate serum levels; the only placebo-controlled trials of intermittent administration have been with orally administered diazepam. A meticulous study by Uhari et al.[109] has shown that intermittent diazepam was of no benefit in preventing recurrence, even when the oral diazepam was combined with acetaminophen. Autret et al.[116] also found no benefit from diazepam—the authors concluded that the failure was the result of the difficulties of early identification of the fever and the logistics of administering medication intermittently to children with multiple caregivers, rather than to the ineffectiveness of the drug. In this respect, the findings of Berg et al.[117] are of interest. They performed a prospective study of recurrent febrile seizures and found that the shorter the duration of the fever before the first febrile convulsion and the lower the child's temperature, the greater was the risk of a febrile recurrence. This information might be used to identify the children who are at particular risk of recurrence, but in this context it may not be of practical value, as the work of Autret et al.[116] suggests that intervention is unlikely to happen in time to prevent recurrence.

Continuous Prophylactic Anticonvulsants

The RCP/BPA Joint Working Group[26] suggested, "The vogue for long-term anticonvulsant prophylaxis against febrile convulsions seen in the 1970s and early 1980s has passed." Camfield et al.[110] offered, "Our efforts should focus on strategies to reduce parental anxiety about this benign disorder, rather than offering children ineffective medication." Despite these statements, Millichap and Colliver[94] found that long-term phenobarbital was still prescribed by 89% of North American child neurologists for the prevention of recurrence after complex febrile convulsions and by 43% after simple febrile seizures. What is the basis for making the decision about giving medication to prevent recurrences? Aicardi[18] and Wallace[21] have reviewed the research into the continuous oral use of drugs to prevent recurrence of febrile convulsions. This can be summarized as follows:

- *Phenobarbitone* at a dose of 4–5 mg/kg per day reduces the number of febrile recurrences;[112,118–120] phenobarbitone has a number of behavioral side effects, with intolerable behavior being reported in from 9% to 21% of children taking the drug.[21]
- *Sodium valproate* has been shown to prevent febrile recurrences.[119, 121, 122]
- *Other continuous anticonvulsants:* experience is limited and unsatisfactory.[18]

Despite the evidence that drugs can reduce recurrences, there are good arguments that prophylactic medication is rarely indicated. Some of these are:

1.   In the American NCPP cohort,[80] there were 1,706 children with febrile convulsions who were assessed at 7 years of age. Not one child had a brief initial febrile convulsion that was followed by a prolonged recurrence and then by epilepsy. This undermines the argument that prevention of febrile recurrences will prevent "brain damage" and thus reduce the risk of developing epilepsy.

2.   In the NCPP,[80] 90% of children who were epileptic after febrile convulsions by 7 years had never had a febrile convulsion that lasted as long as 30 minutes. The minority who became epileptic after having had a lengthy seizure had it as the first seizure of their lives.

3.   Similar conclusions have been reached as a result of the population-based CHES.[17] In that study, only a small proportion of the children were prescribed anticonvulsants for more than 1 month, so it seemed unlikely that these drugs had much effect on outcome. Only 4 of the 287 children who had simple febrile convulsions later had afebrile seizures—this provides little support for prescribing anticonvulsants after simple febrile convulsions. Only 9 of the 95 children with complex febrile convulsions developed afebrile seizures, and in five of the nine children the first febrile convulsion was complex, so in these five any damage that might have been caused by a complex convulsion would probably have occurred before prophylactic medication could be considered.

4.   There is particular concern that prolonged febrile convulsions cause MTS. In the CHES cohort,[17] there were just three children who had prolonged (>15 minutes) febrile convulsions and then had afebrile complex partial seizures by 10 years of age. In two of them, the prolonged febrile convulsions occurred in the first year of life and also had focal features. In both these cases, they were the first and most severe febrile convulsions suffered by that child. There are three points to be made from this: (1) if prolonged febrile convulsions actually cause temporal lobe damage (rather than being the first overt evidence of such damage), it happens relatively rarely (3 children out of 392 with febrile convulsions in the cohort); (2) if damage does occur, it is likely to have happened by the time the child first gets to a physician; and (3) recommendations that have been made about the use of prophylactic anticonvulsants in children with febrile convulsions have been unduly and inappropriately influenced by the anxiety about this very small group of children.

5.   A number of authors published recommendations that only selected high-risk children should receive prophylactic anticonvulsants. In 1981, Ellenberg and Nelson[123] showed that most of these "selective" recommendations would result in one-third to two-thirds of children with febrile convulsions receiving chronic therapy, even though most of the children selected for chronic treatment would never have an afebrile seizure without treatment.

6.   Recent studies have cast doubt on the effectiveness of anticonvulsants in preventing febrile recurrences. A British study of the use of sodium valproate and phenobarbitone in preventing recurrence of febrile convulsions was analyzed on an intention-to-treat basis. The overall risk of recurrence was 30%, and prophylactic treatment did not lessen this risk.[124] Newton[125] pooled the results from six British trials of phenobarbitone and four of valproate and analyzed them on an intention-to-treat basis. They showed little overall value in treating children who have febrile convulsions with anticonvulsants.

7.   Farwell et al.[126] studied the use of phenobarbitone in children who had had at least one febrile convulsion and were at heightened risk of further convulsions. The results showed that phenobarbitone depressed cognitive performance in children treated for febrile convulsions and that this could outlast the administration of the drug by several months. There was no reduction in the rate of recurrence of febrile convulsions in the phenobarbitone group compared with the group receiving a placebo.

Immunization

The RCP/BPA Joint Working Group[26] recommended that, when assessing suitability for immunization, babies having convulsions with fever before the age of 4 months should be assessed by a pediatrician. Children who have febrile convulsions before their immunizations have been given should still be immunized after their parents have been instructed about the management of fever and the use of rectal diazepam.

Information for Parents

Freeman[127] noted, "I believe it is finally time to stop prescribing medication and to begin providing families with solid information and reassurance about the consequences and outcomes of febrile seizures." Camfield and Camfield[92] stated, "The treatment for most children with a febrile seizure is reassurance." After seeing their child in a febrile convulsion, many parents think that the child has died,[91] and there is often panic.[128, 129] Subsequently, parents are concerned that there will be further febrile convulsions, epilepsy, and mental retardation.[128] Camfield et al.[130] aimed to reassure parents and produced an audiotape-slide show to supplement the interview with the doctor. The RCP/BPA Joint Working Group[26] agreed that advice to parents should be given verbally and that a supplementary leaflet would be helpful; a suitable leaflet has now been prepared by the BPA.

THE PRAGMATIC APPROACH

General Outcome

Febrile convulsions are common. The majority are simple febrile convulsions—brief, generalized seizures that occur just once in the lifetime of normal children.

Most children who have febrile convulsions of any type (simple or complex) are subsequently normal in intellect, neurologic function, and behavior.

Subsequent Epilepsy

For most children with febrile convulsions, the risk of later developing epilepsy is little different from that in the general population. A small minority of children who have febrile convulsions are at increased risk of developing epilepsy—those who are neurologically or developmentally abnormal before the convulsions and some of those who have febrile convulsions with complex features, particularly if focal.

Initial Management

Most febrile convulsions stop spontaneously, and not all children need to be admitted to the hospital. It is reassuring if the child seems neurologically normal after the convulsion. However, prolonged seizures should be stopped by appropriate acute treatment, and if there is any other concern about the child's neurologic state, hospital assessment is appropriate. A lumbar puncture may be necessary to exclude meningitis in the minority of cases, particularly in children younger than 18 months of age. Ideally, this decision should be made by an experienced physician. Investigations are not routinely indicated after febrile convulsions—EEG is not helpful and brain scans are rarely indicated.

Subsequent Medication

If febrile convulsions are frequent or prolonged, it may be appropriate to teach parents to administer rectal diazepam at home. There is no convincing evidence that antipyretic measures reduce the frequency of febrile recurrences or that the administration of intermittent or continuous prophylactic anticonvulsant medication reduces the risk of later developing epilepsy. Prophylactic medication is not generally advised for children with febrile convulsions.

Information for the Caregivers

Many parents or caregivers are very distressed when they witness febrile convulsions in their children, and it should be a priority to inform them about the essentially benign nature of most febrile convulsions. When assessing the prognosis, it is relevant to consider the type of febrile convulsion and the clinical context in which it occurs, but parents can be reassured that for the majority of children with febrile convulsions the outcome is good and that medication is rarely indicated. Ideally, written information should supplement the interview, and there are now excellent videotapes that provide advice and support for parents.

REFERENCES

1. Aicardi J. Diseases of the Nervous System in Children. London: MacKeith, 1992;958.
2. Ekholm E, Niemineva K. On convulsions in early childhood and their prognosis. Acta Paediatr 1950;39:481.
3. Lennox MA. Febrile convulsions in childhood: their relationship to adult epilepsy. J Pediatr 1949;35:427.
4. Robinson RJ. Febrile convulsions. Further reassuring news about prognosis. Leader. BMJ 1991;303:1345.
5. Annegers JF, Hauser WA, Elveback LR, et al. The risk of epilepsy following febrile convulsions. Neurology 1979;29:297.
6. Annegers JF, Hauser WA, Shirts SB, et al. Factors prognostic of unprovoked seizures after febrile convulsions. N Engl J Med 1987;316:493.
7. Annegers JF, Blakley SA, Hauser WA, et al. Recurrence of febrile convulsions in a population-based cohort. Epilepsy Res 1990;5:209.
8. Forsgren L, Sidenvall R, Blomquist HK, et al. A prospective incidence study of febrile convulsions. Acta Paediatr Scand 1990;79:550.
9. Forsgren L, Sidenvall R, Blomquist HK, et al. An incident case-referent study of febrile convulsions in children: genetical and social aspects. Neuropediatrics 1990;21:153.
10. Forsgren L, Sidenvall R, Blomquist HK, et al. Pre- and perinatal factors in febrile convulsions. Acta Paediatr Scand 1991;80:218.
11. Ellenberg JH, Nelson KB. Febrile seizures and later intellectual performance. Arch Neurol 1978;35:17.
12. Nelson KB, Ellenberg JH. Predictors of epilepsy in children who have experienced febrile seizures. N Engl J Med 1976;295:1029.
13. Nelson KB, Ellenberg JH. Prognosis in children with febrile seizures. Pediatrics 1978;61:720.
14. Offringa M, Hazebroek-Kampschreur AAJM, Derksen-Lubsen G. Prevalence of febrile seizures in Dutch schoolchildren. Paediatr Perinat Epidemiol 1991;5:181.
15. Verity CM, Butler NR, Golding J. Febrile convulsions in a national cohort followed up from birth. I. Prevalence and recurrence in the first five years of life. BMJ 1985;290:1307.
16. Verity CM, Butler NR, Golding J. Febrile convulsions in a national cohort followed up from birth. II. Medical history and intellectual ability at 5 years of age. BMJ 1985;290:1311.
17. Verity CM, Golding J. Risk of epilepsy after febrile convulsions: a national cohort study. BMJ 1991;303:1373.
18. Aicardi J. Epilepsy in Children (2nd ed). International Review of Child Neurology Series. New York: Raven, 1994;212.
19. O'Donohoe NV. Febrile Convulsions. In J Roger, M Bureau, C Dravet, et al. (eds), Epileptic Syndromes in Infancy, Childhood and Adolescence. London: John Libbey, 1992;45.
20. Verity CM. Febrile Convulsions. In A Hopkins, S Shorvon, G Cascino (eds), Epilepsy (2nd ed). London: Chapman & Hall, 1995;353.
21. Wallace SJ. The Child with Febrile Seizures. London: John Wright, 1988.
22. Berg AT. Febrile seizures and epilepsy: the contributions of epidemiology. Paediatr Perinat Epidemiol 1992;6:145.
23. Degen R, Degen HE, Hans K. A contribution to the genetics of febrile seizures: waking and sleep EEG in siblings. Epilepsia 1991;32:515.
24. Ounsted C. Genetic and social aspects of the epilepsies of childhood. Eugenics Rev 1955;47:33.
25. National Institutes of Health. Consensus Statement. Febrile seizures: long-term management of children with fever-associated seizures. BMJ 1980;281:277.
26. Joint Working Group of the Research Unit of the Royal College of Physicians and the British Paediatric Association. Guidelines for the management of convulsions with fever. BMJ 1991;303:634.
27. Commission on Epidemiology and Prognosis of the International League Against Epilepsy. Guidelines for epidemiologic studies on epilepsy. Epilepsia 1993;34:592.
28. Stephenson JBP. Fits and Faints. Clinics in Developmental Medicine No. 109. London: MacKeith, 1990;169.
29. Livingston S. Convulsive disorders in infants and children. Adv Pediatr 1958;10:113.
30. Wallace SJ. Factors predisposing to a complicated initial febrile convulsion. Arch Dis Child 1975;50:943.

31. Berg AT, Steinschneider M, Kang H, et al. Classification of complex features of febrile seizures: interrator agreement. Epilepsia 1992;33:661.
32. Maytal J, Shinnar S, Moshe SL, et al. Low morbidity and mortality of status epilepticus in children. Pediatrics 1989;83:323.
33. Maytal J, Shinnar S. Febrile status epilepticus. Pediatrics 1990;86:611.
34. Verity CM, Ross EM, Golding J. Outcome of childhood status epilepticus and lengthy febrile convulsions: findings of national cohort study. BMJ 1993;307:225.
35. Viani F, Beghi E, Romeo A, et al. Infantile febrile status epilepticus: risk factors and outcome. Dev Med Child Neurol 1987;29:495.
36. Ross EM, Peckham CS, West P, Butler NR. Epilepsy in childhood: findings from the National Child Development Study. BMJ 1980;280:207.
37. van den Berg BJ, Yerushalmy J. Studies on convulsive disorders in young children. Pediatr Res 1969;3:298.
38. Tsuboi T. Epidemiology of febrile and afebrile convulsions in children in Japan. Neurology 1984;34:175.
39. Chevrie JJ, Aicardi J. Duration and lateralization of febrile convulsions. Etiological factors. Epilepsia 1975;16:781.
40. Berg AT, Shinnar S, Hauser WA, et al. Predictors of recurrent febrile seizures: a meta-analytic review. J Pediatr 1990;116:329.
41. Knudsen FU. Recurrence risk after first febrile seizure and effect of short term diazepam prophylaxis. Arch Dis Child 1985;60:1045.
42. Knudsen FU. Intermittent diazepam prophylaxis in febrile convulsions. Pros and cons. Acta Neurol Scand 1991;83(Suppl.135):1.
43. Offringa M, Derksen-Lubsen G, Bossuyt PM, Lubsen J. Seizure recurrence after a first febrile seizure: a multivariate approach. Dev Med Child Neurol 1992;34:15.
44. Wallace SJ. Recurrence of febrile convulsions. Arch Dis Child 1974;49:763.
45. Berg AT, Shinnar S, Shapiro ED, et al. Risk factors for a first febrile seizure. A matched case-control study. Epilepsia 1995;36:334.
46. Nelson KB, Ellenberg JH. Prenatal and perinatal antecedents of febrile seizures. Ann Neurol 1990;27:127.
47. Hauser WA. The Natural History of Febrile Seizures. In KB Nelson, JH Ellenberg (eds), Febrile Seizures. New York: Raven, 1981;5.
48. Bethune P, Gordon K, Dooley J, et al. Which child will have a febrile seizure? Am J Dis Child 1993;147:35.
49. Tsuboi T, Endo S. Genetic Studies of Febrile Convulsions: Analysis of Twin and Family Data. In VE Anderson, WA Hauser, IE Leppik, et al. (eds), Genetic Strategies in Epilepsy Research (Epilepsy Research Supplement 4). Amsterdam: Elsevier, 1991;119.
50. Fukuyama Y, Kagawa K, Tanaka T. A genetic study of febrile convulsions. Eur Neurol 1979;18:166.
51. Corey LA, Berg K, Pellock JM, et al. The occurrence of epilepsy and febrile seizures in Virginian and Norwegian twins. Neurology 1991;41:1433.
52. Tsuboi T. Genetic analysis of febrile convulsions: twin and family studies. Hum Genet 1987;75:7.
53. Cassano PA, Koepsell TD, Farwell JR, et al. Risk of febrile seizures in childhood in relation to prenatal maternal cigarette smoking and alcohol intake. Am J Epidemiol 1990;132:462.
54. Wallace SJ. Etiological aspects of febrile convulsions. Arch Dis Child 1972;47:171.
55. Greenwood R, Golding J, Ross E, et al. Prenatal and perinatal antecedents of febrile convulsions and afebrile seizures: data from a national cohort study. 1996, Submitted for publication.
56. Zhao F, Emoto SE, Lavine L, et al. Risk factors for febrile seizures in the People's Republic of China: a case control study. Epilepsia 1991;32:510.
57. Stokes MJ, Downham MAPS, Webb JKG, et al. Viruses and febrile convulsions. Arch Dis Child 1977;52:129.
58. Lewis HM, Parry JV, Parry RP, et al. Role of viruses in febrile convulsions. Arch Dis Child 1979;54:869.
59. Kondo K, Nagafuji H, Hata A, et al. Association of human herpesvirus 6 infection of the central nervous system with recurrence of febrile convulsions. J Infect Dis 1993;167:1197.
60. Barone SR, Kaplan MH, Krilov LR. Human herpesvirus-6 infection in children with first febrile seizures. J Pediatr 1995;127:95.
61. Hirtz DG, Nelson KB. The natural history of febrile seizures. Annu Rev Med 1983;34:453.
62. Taylor DC, Ounsted C. Biological mechanisms influencing the outcome of seizures in response to fever. Epilepsia 1971;12:33.
63. Moshe SL. Epileptogenesis and the immature brain. Epilepsia 1987;28(Suppl 1):S3.

64. Fowler M. Brain damage after febrile convulsions. Arch Dis Child 1957;32:67.
65. Meldrum BS. Secondary Pathology of Febrile and Experimental Convulsions. In MAB Brazier, F Coceani (eds), Brain Dysfunction in Infantile Febrile Convulsions. New York: Raven, 1976;213.
66. Falconer MA, Serafetinides EA, Corsellis JAN. Etiology and pathogenesis of temporal lobe epilepsy. Arch Neurol 1964;10:233.
67. Taylor DC. Differential rates of cerebral maturation between sexes and between hemispheres. Lancet 1969;2:140.
68. Harbord MG, Manson JL. Temporal lobe epilepsy in childhood: reappraisal of etiology and outcome. Pediatr Neurol 1987;3:263.
69. Kodama K, Murakami A, Yamanouchi N, et al. MR in temporal lobe epilepsy: early childhood onset versus later onset. AJNR Am J Neuroradiol 1995;16:523.
70. Kuks JB, Cook MJ, Fish DR, et al. Hippocampal sclerosis in epilepsy and childhood febrile seizures. Lancet 1993;342:1391.
71. Hardiman O, Burke T, Phillips J, et al. Microdysgenesis in resected temporal neocortex: incidence and clinical significance in focal epilepsy. Neurology 1988;38:1041.
72. Simpson H, Habel AH, George EL. Cerebrospinal fluid acid-base status and lactate and pyruvate concentrations after short (<30 minutes) first febrile convulsions. Arch Dis Child 1977;52:836.
73. Simpson H, Habel AH, George EL. Cerebrospinal fluid acid-base status and lactate and pyruvate concentrations after convulsions of varied durations and etiology in children. Arch Dis Child 1977;52:844.
74. Livingston JH, Brown JK, Harkness RA, et al. Cerebrospinal fluid nucleotide metabolites following short febrile convulsions. Dev Med Child Neurol 1989;31:161.
75. Rodriguez-Nunez A, Camina F, Lojo S, et al. Purine metabolites and pyrimidine bases in cerebrospinal fluid of children with simple febrile seizures. Dev Med Child Neurol 1991;33:908.
76. Castro-Gago M, Cid E, Trabazo S, et al. Cerebrospinal fluid purine metabolites and pyrimidine bases after brief febrile convulsions. Epilepsia 1995;36:471.
77. Aicardi J, Chevrie JJ. Consequences of Status Epilepticus in Infants and Children. In AV Delgado-Escueta, CG Wasterlain, DM Treimann, RJ Porter (eds), Advances in Neurology. Volume 34: Status Epilepticus. New York: Raven, 1983;115.
78. Dierckx RA, Melis K, Dom L, et al. Technetium-99m hexamethylpropylene amine oxime single photon emission tomography in febrile convulsions. Eur J Nucl Med 1992;19:278.
79. Pavone L, Cavazutti GB, Incorpora G, et al. Late febrile convulsions: a clinical follow up. Brain Dev 1989;11:183.
80. Nelson KB, Ellenberg JH. The Role of Recurrences in Determining Outcome in Children with Febrile Seizures. In KB Nelson, JH Ellenberg (eds), Febrile Seizures. New York: Raven, 1981;19.
81. Wallace SJ. Spontaneous fits after convulsions with fever. Arch Dis Child 1977;52:192.
82. Lee K, Diaz M, Melchior JC. Temporal lobe epilepsy—not a consequence of childhood febrile convulsions in Denmark. Acta Neurol Scand 1981;63:231.
83. Leviton A, Cowan LD. Do Febrile Seizures Increase the Risk of Complex Partial Seizures? An Epidemiologic Assessment. In KB Nelson, JH Ellenberg (eds), Febrile Seizures. New York: Raven, 1981;65.
84. Wallace SJ. Neurological and Intellectual Deficits: Convulsions with Fever Viewed as Acute Indications of Life-Long Developmental Defects. In MAB Brazier, F Coceani (eds), Brain Dysfunction in Infantile Febrile Convulsions. New York: Raven, 1976;259.
85. Aicardi J, Chevrie JJ. Febrile Convulsions: Neurological Sequelae and Mental Retardation. In MAB Brazier, F Coceani (eds), Brain Dysfunction in Infantile Febrile Convulsions. New York: Raven, 1976;247.
86. Schiottz-Christensen E. Neurological findings in twins discordant for febrile convulsions. Acta Neurol Scand 1973;49:368.
87. Wallace SJ, Cull AM. Long-term psychological outlook for children whose first fit occurs with fever. Dev Med Child Neurol 1979;21:28.
88. Aldridge Smith J, Wallace SJ. Febrile convulsions: intellectual progress in relation to anticonvulsant therapy and to recurrence of fits. Arch Dis Child 1982;57:104.
89. Schiottz-Christensen E, Bruhn P. Intelligence, behaviour and scholastic achievement subsequent to febrile convulsions: an analysis of discordant twin-pairs. Dev Med Child Neurol 1973;15:565.
90. Millichap JG. Febrile Convulsions. New York: Macmillan, 1968.
91. Baumer JH, David TJ, Valentine SJ, et al. Many parents think their child is dying when having a first febrile convulsion. Dev Med Child Neurol 1981;23:462.
92. Camfield PR, Camfield CS. Febrile Seizures. In EM Ross, RC Woody (eds), Baillière's Clinical Paediatrics (Vol 2/No 3), Epilepsy. London: Baillière Tindall, 1994;547.

93. Hirtz DG. Generalized tonic-clonic and febrile seizures. Pediatr Clin North Am 1989;36:365.
94. Millichap JG, Colliver JA. Management of febrile seizures: survey of current practice and phenobarbital usage. Pediatr Neurol 1991;7:243.
95. Nealis JGT. Management of Febrile Seizures by Pediatricians in the United States. In KB Nelson, JH Ellenberg (eds), Febrile Seizures. New York: Raven, 1981;81.
96. Rosman NP. Febrile seizures. Emerg Med Clin North Am 1987;5:719.
97. Lorber J, Sunderland R. Lumbar puncture in children with convulsions associated with fever. Lancet 1980;1:785.
98. Rutter N, Smales ORC. Role of routine investigations in children presenting with their first febrile convulsion. Arch Dis Child 1977;52:188.
99. Stenklyft PH, Carmona M. Febrile seizures. Emerg Med Clin North Am 1994;12:989.
100. Rennick G, Shann F, de Campo J. Cerebral herniation during bacterial meningitis in children. BMJ 1993;306:953.
101. Binnie CD. Neurophysiological Investigation of Epilepsy in Children. In EM Ross, RC Woody (eds), Baillière's Clinical Paediatrics, International Practice and Research (Vol 2/No 3), Epilepsy. London: Baillière Tindall, 1994;585.
102. Stores G. When does an EEG contribute to the management of a febrile seizure? Arch Dis Child 1991;66:554.
103. Doose H, Ritter K, Volzke E. EEG longitudinal studies in febrile convulsions, genetic aspects. Neuropediatrics 1983;14:81.
104. Frantzen E, Lennox-Buchthal M, Nygaard A, et al. Longitudinal EEG and clinical study of children with febrile convulsions. Electroencephalogr Clin Neurophysiol 1968;24:197
105. Kinmonth A-L, Fulton Y, Campbell MJ. Management of feverish children at home. BMJ 1992;305:1134.
106. Hoppu K, Santavuori P. Diazepam rectal solution for home treatment of acute seizures in children. Acta Paediatr Scand 1981;70:369.
107. Camfield S, Camfield PR, Smythe E, et al. Home use of rectal diazepam to prevent status epilepticus in children with convulsive disorders. J Child Neurol 1989;4:125.
108. Camfield PR, Camfield CS, Shapiro SH, et al. The first febrile seizure—antipyretic instruction plus either phenobarbital or placebo to prevent recurrence. J Pediatr 1980;97:16.
109. Uhari M, Rantala H, Vainionpaa L, et al. Effect of acetaminophen and of low intermittent doses of diazepam on prevention of recurrences of febrile seizures. J Pediatr 1995;126:991.
110. Camfield PR, Camfield CS, Gordon K, et al. Prevention of recurrent febrile seizures. J Pediatr 1995;126:929.
111. Knudsen FU, Vestermark S. Prophylactic diazepam or phenobarbitone in febrile convulsions: a prospective, controlled study. Arch Dis Child 1978;53:660.
112. Thorn I. Prevention of Recurrent Febrile Seizures: Intermittent Prophylaxis with Diazepam Compared with Continuous Treatment with Phenobarbital. In KB Nelson, JH Ellenberg (eds), Febrile Seizures. New York: Raven, 1981;119.
113. Dianese G. Prophylaxis of febrile convulsions: searching for the best [letter]. Arch Dis Child 1986;61:621.
114. Rosman NP, Colton T, Labazzo J, et al. A controlled trial of diazepam administered during febrile illnesses to prevent recurrence of febrile seizures. N Engl J Med 1993;329:79.
115. Rosman NP, Colton T, Labazzo J. Diazepam to prevent febrile seizures [correspondence]. N Engl J Med 1993;329:2033.
116. Autret E, Billard C, Bertrand P, et al. Double-blind randomized trial of diazepam versus placebo for prevention of recurrence of febrile seizures. J Pediatr 1990;117:490.
117. Berg AT, Shinnar S, Hauser WA, et al. A prospective study of recurrent febrile seizures. N Engl J Med 1992;327:1122.
118. Bacon CJ, Mucklow JC, Rawlins M, et al. Placebo-controlled study of phenobarbitone and phenytoin in the prophylaxis of febrile convulsions. Lancet 1981;2:600.
119. Wallace SJ, Aldridge Smith JA. Successful prophylaxis against febrile convulsions with valproic acid or phenobarbital. BMJ 1980;280:353.
120. Wolf SM, Carr A, Davis DC, et al. The value of phenobarbital in the child who has had a single febrile seizure: a controlled prospective study. Pediatrics 1977;59:378.
121. Cavazutti GB. Prevention of febrile convulsions with dipropylacetate (Depakine). Epilepsia 1975;16:647.
122. Ngwane E, Bower B. Continuous sodium valproate or phenobarbitone in the prevention of 'simple' febrile convulsions. Arch Dis Child 1980;55:171.

123. Ellenberg JH, Nelson KB. The Efficiency of Published Recommendations for the Treatment of Febrile Seizures. In KB Nelson, JH Ellenberg (eds), Febrile Seizures. New York: Raven, 1981;97.

124. McKinlay I, Newton RW. Intention to treat febrile convulsions with rectal diazepam, valproate or phenobarbitone. Dev Med Child Neurol 1989;31:617.

125. Newton RW. Randomized controlled trials of phenobarbitone and valproate in febrile convulsions. Arch Dis Child 1988;63:1189.

126. Farwell JR, Lee YJ, Hirtz DG, et al. Phenobarbital for febrile seizures—effects on intelligence and on seizure recurrence. N Engl J Med 1990;322:364.

127. Freeman JM. The best medicine for febrile seizures [editorial]. N Engl J Med 1992;327;1161.

128. Clare M, Aldridge Smith J, Wallace SJ. A child's first febrile convulsion. Practitioner 1978;221:775.

129. Rutter N, Metcalf DH. Febrile convulsions—what do parents do? BMJ 1978;277:1345.

130. Camfield PR, Camfield CS, Buchholz K, et al. Information on Febrile Seizures for Parents and Caretakers. In KB Nelson, JH Ellenberg (eds), Febrile Seizures. New York: Raven, 1981;245.

16
Pregnancy and Epilepsy

Martha J. Morrell

Clinical management of the pregnant woman with epilepsy can be challenging. Severity and frequency of seizures may increase as a result of changes in sex steroid hormones, in antiepileptic drug (AED) pharmacokinetics, and in compliance. Fetal exposure to AEDs increases the risk for major malformations, minor anomalies, and, possibly, neurodevelopmental disability.[1] Yet most women with seizure disorders must continue to take AEDs in order to control seizures. Knowledge of the mechanisms of AED-mediated teratogenesis permits treatment modifications that will optimize pregnancy and fetal outcome.

SEIZURE CONTROL AND ANTIEPILEPTIC DRUGS IN THE MOTHER

During pregnancies, seizure frequency may increase in as many as one-third of women with epilepsy.[2, 3] Women with localization-related epilepsy (LRE) may be more likely to experience a seizure exacerbation than women with primary generalized epilepsy (PGE).[4] Seizures may become more frequent or severe in response to (a) increases in neuroactive hormones, such as the sex steroid hormones, (b) physiologic stress associated with sleep deprivation, or (c) reduction in AED concentrations as a result of changes in pharmacokinetics and compliance.

Neuroactive steroids modulate cortical excitability and alter the probability that a seizure will occur. Ovarian steroid hormones have potent neuromodulatory effects. Estrogenic compounds increase neuronal excitability, and progestogenic compounds decrease neuronal excitability.[5] A pregnant woman experiences a substantial increase in the serum concentration of these sex steroid hormones as well as a change in the particular type of hormone within each class. The principal estrogenic hormone in pregnancy is estriol, whereas estradiol predominates during the nonpregnant state. For certain women with hormonally sensitive seizures, these changes may alter the seizure threshold to a clinically significant degree.

313

ANTIEPILEPTIC DRUG PHARMACOKINETICS IN PREGNANCY

AED levels decline throughout pregnancy,[6] increasing again in the first few weeks after birth.[7, 8] Total AED serum concentrations fall because of significant increases in volume of distribution, metabolism, and clearance during pregnancy. Intravascular and extravascular volume of distribution and the renal glomerular filtration rate increase by up to 50%. Resting cardiac output rises from a mean of 6 liters per minute to 7.5 liters per minute. Drugs metabolized by the hepatic cytochrome P450 enzyme system (cyP450) are more rapidly cleared. This enzyme system is induced by high serum levels of progesterone[9] and because the hepatic smooth endoplasmic reticulum proliferates during pregnancy.[10] Hepatic clearance is most likely to be increased in women taking AED polytherapy.[11] Metabolic pathways for AEDs are also altered during pregnancy. For example, production of carbamazepine (CBZ) epoxide increases, as does the mean percentage excreted as unmetabolized CBZ.[11] Finally, drug-taking behavior may change. Hyperemesis gravidarum may cause AED levels to fall. AED serum concentrations may also fall because of reduced compliance—usually prompted by fears that AEDs will harm the developing fetus.[2]

Although total serum concentrations for most AEDs fall during pregnancy, the rate and extent of decline differ for the protein-bound and nonprotein-bound fraction. Total phenytoin (PHT) and phenobarbital (PB) concentrations decrease steadily over all three trimesters, with less reduction in the free concentration.[4, 7, 12–14] Total CBZ concentrations drop in the second and third trimesters, while free CBZ concentrations remain stable.[4, 12] Steady-state serum concentrations of valproate (VPA) decrease significantly from the first to the third trimester, but free VPA levels may actually increase.[8]

This dissociation between the total and free AED concentrations occurs because plasma protein binding falls throughout pregnancy.[13] AEDs bind to albumin and other circulating plasma proteins, such as sex hormone-binding globulin (sHBG). Serum albumin concentrations decrease during pregnancy and competition with sex steroid hormones for binding sites increases. Therefore, less AED is bound, and more of the total concentration represents the unbound, biologically active fraction. For AEDs that are highly protein-bound, such as PHT and VPA, measurement of the free AED fraction is required to accurately portray the level in the central nervous system (CNS).

EFFECT OF SEIZURES AND MATERNAL EPILEPSY ON FETUS AND NEONATE

Infants of mothers with epilepsy may be at higher risk for adverse pregnancy outcome, although studies evaluating pregnancy outcome in women with epilepsy are confounded by the lower socioeconomic status of women with epilepsy compared with the nonepileptic population. Nevertheless, women with epilepsy appear to be more likely to experience fetal wastage,[15] to deliver preterm, and to have children with low birth weight.[16, 17] A study based in the Netherlands found that abortion and ectopic pregnancies were twice as likely to occur in the pregnancies of epileptic women than in those of controls.[18] Neonatal and perinatal

Table 16.1 Commonly used drugs recognized as known human teratogens

Alcohol
Angiotensin converting enzyme inhibitors
Antibiotics
    Aminoglycoside (streptomycin)
    Tetracycline
Anticancer drugs
    Alkylating agents
    Antimetabolites
        Propylthiouracil, methimazole
Antiepileptic drugs
    Benzodiazepines
    Carbamazepine
    Phenobarbital
    Phenytoin
    Primidone
    Trimethadione
    Valproate
Antithyroid drugs
    Propylthiouracil, methimazole
Cocaine
Coumarin anticoagulants
Disulfiram
Hormones
    Androgens
    Diethylstilbestrol
    Progestins
Lithium
Penicillamine
Retinoids
Thalidomide

Source: Adapted from TH Shepard (ed). Catalog of Teratogenic Agents. Baltimore: Johns Hopkins University Press, 1995; and JL Shardein. Drugs Affecting the Central Nervous System: Anticonvulsants. In FJ DiCarlo, FW Oehme (eds), Chemically-Induced Birth Defects. New York: Marcel Dekker, 1985;142.

and colleagues, who reported that more than 50% of fetuses exposed to trimethadione displayed dysmorphic features, poor speech development, and mental retardation.[26, 27] Fetal hydantoin syndrome was next identified in a small series of infants exposed in utero to PHT alone or in combination with PB.[28] These children had facial clefts, facial and digital anomalies, microcephaly, and growth retardation. Fetal PB, fetal primidone, fetal VPA, and fetal CBZ syndromes have been subsequently described.[29] These syndromes have been striking in the similarities of dysmorphisms, which include lip and palatal malformations, cardiac malformations, and facial and digital anomalies.

Four to 6% of infants born to epileptic mothers are born with a major malformation, compared with 2–4% of infants born to nonepileptic mothers. Although the maternal trait of epilepsy increases the likelihood of a malformation, much of the risk is attributed to exposure to AEDs. The rate of facial clefts, including cleft lip, cleft palate, or both, is increased sixfold in infants of epileptic mothers over the background rate. Facial clefts appear to be primarily related to AED exposure, with genetic factors of minor importance.[30, 31] Children of fathers with epilepsy and siblings of epileptic children had no more facial clefts than expected.[31] Congenital heart defects show a threefold to fourfold increase over the background population rate and include atrial septal defect, tetralogy of Fallot, ventricular septal defect, coarctation of the aorta, patent ductus arteriosus, and pulmonary stenosis.[32]

The only class of major malformation specific to an AED is the association of VPA and CBZ with neural tube defects (NTD). VPA (valproic acid and divalproex sodium) is associated with a 1–2% incidence of spina bifida, anencephaly, or both.[33–35] Spina bifida may arise in 0.5–1.0% of infants exposed to CBZ.[36]

As is illustrated in Figure 16.1, NTDs and the other major malformations associated with AED exposure occur very early in gestation. The posterior neuropore is closed by day 26, meaning that NTDs are established in the first month of gestation, before many women are aware that they are pregnant.

Congenital anomalies represent relatively minor cosmetic deviations from normal morphology and are more frequent than malformations. Depending on the study—and how closely the children are examined—anomalies can be detected in 5–30% of infants of epileptic mothers.[18, 29, 37] Minor anomalies in infants of epileptic mothers involve eyes, nose, ears, and fingers.[38] Ocular abnormalities include ocular hypertelorism and epicanthal folds. Nasal growth deficiency manifests as anteverted nares, small nose, and a low nasal bridge. Ears may be low-set, show abnormal cartilaginous folding, or have posteriorly angulated auricles. The hairline may be abnormally low. Digit anomalies include distal phalangeal hypoplasia, nail hypoplasia, and low arched fingertip dermatoglyphic patterns. These dysmorphisms may recede with growth. In infants of epileptic mothers followed over the first several years of life, craniofacial hypoplasia and nail and phalangeal hypoplasia tend to resolve with age.[1]

COGNITIVE DEVELOPMENT OF INFANTS OF EPILEPTIC MOTHERS EXPOSED TO ANTIEPILEPTIC DRUGS

In vitro, animal, and human studies raise the possibility that fetal AED exposure leads to long-term cognitive disability. However, limitations in experimental design and a lack of well controlled clinical studies do not permit a conclusive answer. Animal and in vitro studies suggest that at certain concentrations, and during critical periods of exposure, AEDs may adversely affect the developing CNS. Neuronal loss, changes in neuronal morphology, a reduction of transmitter-related enzymatic activity, and long-term behavioral changes occur after AED exposure in these experimental systems.[39] Yet animal and in vitro studies may not be applicable to humans because of differences in CNS structure and function or in AED pharmacokinetics and because AED exposures in animal models are often significantly higher than would be expected in a human receiving usual therapeutic dosages.

Studies of AED effects on neurocognitive development do not provide consistent findings. Most studies have used intelligence quotient (IQ) and head circumference as objective measures of human brain development. IQ at 4 years of

319

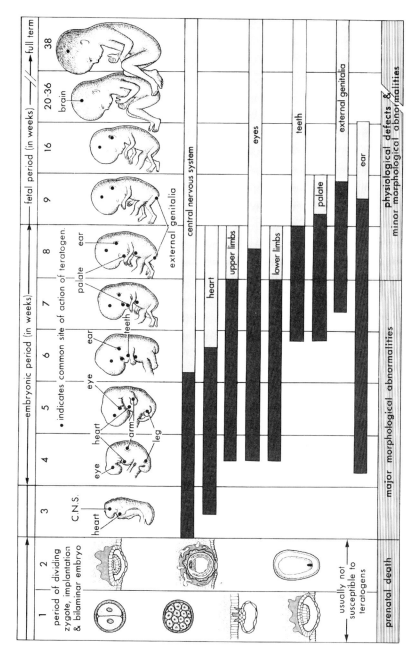

Figure 16.1 Human development and organogenesis by gestational age. (Reprinted with permission from KL Moore. The Developing Human: Clinically Oriented Embryology [5th ed]. Philadelphia: Saunders, 1993.)

age varies with head circumference at 1 year, suggesting that small head circumference may be linked to mental retardation.[40] Maternal epilepsy and use of AEDs may be associated with microcephaly, but these observations are somewhat controversial.[41, 42] Uncontrolled studies have reported reduced head circumference in infants exposed to PHT with or without other AEDs[28] and to CBZ alone or in combination with a barbiturate.[43]

Hiilesmaa and colleagues[41] assessed fetal head growth at birth and at 18 months in infants of epileptic mothers who had been exposed to AEDs and in a control group of infants of nonepileptic mothers. There was no significant difference between epileptic mothers and controls in maternal stature, head circumference, weight, weight gain during pregnancy, pregnancy complications, smoking, alcohol or drug use, cesarean section, or duration of labor. Although the mean head circumference in the majority of AED-exposed infants was normal, CBZ or CBZ combined with PB was associated with smaller mean head circumference, which persisted at 18 months. In a follow-up study, Gaily and colleagues[42] evaluated head circumference at birth and at age 5 in children of epileptic mothers exposed to PHT or CBZ, with or without PB; in a group of infants of epileptic mothers not exposed to AEDs; and in a control group. Maternal and paternal head circumference was also determined. Microcephaly was no more likely to occur in the infants of epileptic mothers as in the general population when controlled for paternal head circumference.

Using IQ scores as an indicator of neurodevelopment, many population-based studies find no association between AED exposure and low intelligence.[25, 38, 44] Gaily and colleagues[38] evaluated IQ in 148 infants of epileptic mothers, 131 of whom were exposed to AEDs. The prevalence of mental deficiency (IQ less than 71) was the same as the general population. Although the mean IQ was lower in infants of epileptic mothers at age 5.5 years, this was associated with a high number of minor anomalies but was not related to exposure to AEDs or to brief maternal convulsions. These findings led the authors to suggest that low IQ was not associated with AED exposure but was instead related to maternal epilepsy.

Nelson and Ellenberg assessed head circumference and IQ in infants of epileptic mothers and in controls evaluated as part of the Collaborative Perinatal Project.[44] Infants of epileptic mothers were below the mean for birth weight and gestational age and were twice as likely to have microcephaly at 1 year of age and to have low IQ. This was independent of drug exposure, suggesting that fetal head size and IQ are related, at least in part, to the maternal trait of epilepsy.

Studies assessing the intelligence of children born to epileptic mothers describe variable results, perhaps because of inconsistent methodologies. Studies have not always controlled for fetal exposure to AEDs (monotherapy versus polytherapy), have typically not determined drug levels or evaluated compliance, have not classified the maternal epilepsy syndrome or determined maternal seizure frequency or severity, and have not controlled for maternal and paternal IQ and for socioeconomic status. These studies are also limited by lack of long-term follow-up.

Mechanisms of Teratogenesis

Mechanisms by which AEDs mediate teratogenicity have not been entirely elucidated. AEDs may cause malformations through the action of cytotoxic metabolites, such as free radicals, by inducing folate deficiency, or by interfering with folate-mediated biologic processes. In addition, a genetic susceptibility may predispose a fetus to AED-related teratogenicity.

Genetic predisposition to epilepsy may confer increased susceptibility to development of malformations. Genetics may determine the specific malformation elicited by a particular environmental factor. In addition, liability genes may place specific organ systems at risk for abnormal morphogenesis given exposure to a teratogen. Genetics also determines AED pharmacokinetics within an individual, such as propensity to produce oxide metabolites.

Clinical observation suggests that infants with fetal anticonvulsant syndrome have a genetic predisposition to develop malformations. There is a higher prevalence of malformations in relatives of affected children than unaffected children,[30] and malformation rates are higher in infants of untreated epileptic mothers than in controls,[1, 25] particularly for cardiovascular malformations.[30] Spina bifida occulta, a form of NTD, arises significantly more often in patients with genetic epilepsies than in those with symptomatic epilepsy syndromes.[45] Twenty-five percent of infants born with spina bifida who have been exposed to AEDs also have a family history of NTDs.[46]

Variability in patterns of malformations after exposure to AEDs may reflect individual genetic susceptibility. Three genetic mouse strains given constant environmental conditions and standard PHT exposures developed varied patterns of malformations and anomalies,[47] suggesting that genes determine sensitivity to teratogens and patterns of teratogenesis.

Another mechanism of AED teratogenesis may involve formation of oxidative intermediates.[48] AEDs are metabolized to chemically reactive oxidative metabolites that covalently bind embryonic macromolecules, such as nucleic acids, and disrupt normal developmental processes. Lymphocytes of children with PHT-induced major malformations are more sensitive to toxic PHT metabolites in vitro, suggesting that these children were deficient in enzymes required to detoxify metabolites.[49] In three inbred mouse strains, combination therapy with PHT and a potent inhibitor of the cyP450 enzyme system (stiripentol) lowered the incidence of soft-tissue and skeletal malformations, supporting the hypothesis that PHT teratogenic effects arise at least partly through metabolism to toxic intermediates.[50]

Oxide metabolites are normally eliminated by the enzyme epoxide hydrolase, and deficiencies in this enzyme may place fetuses at risk for AED-mediated teratogenicity. Epoxide hydrolase activity can be assayed in cultured fibroblasts and amniocytes. A single gene for this enzyme has two allelic forms. The enzyme displays a trimodal distribution with individuals showing a high, intermediate, or low level of activity. Epoxide hydrolase activity in a fetal liver is lower than in an adult;[51] furthermore, fetuses that are homozygous for the recessive allele have even lower enzyme activity and appear to be at greatest risk to develop malformations associated with fetal anticonvulsant syndrome.[47, 49, 52] A complementary deoxyribonucleic acid (cDNA) probe may soon allow determination of this enzyme activity from lymphocytes and will permit prenatal identification of individuals at risk.[53]

Serum folate is reduced in up to 90% of patients receiving PHT, CBZ, or barbiturates.[54] VPA does not reduce folate levels but does interfere with folate metabolism by inhibiting glutamate formyl transferase, an enzyme mediating the pathway that produces folinic acid.[55] Lamotrigine (LTG), an AED that has weak folate properties in vitro, had no effects on serum or red blood cell folate in 14 patients on short-term treatment and in an additional 14 patients who had been treated up to 5 years.[56]

Folate deficiency induced experimentally in animals by folate antagonists or by a folate-deficient diet produces intrauterine growth retardation and congenital malformations, even with a period of deficiency as short as 2 days early in gestation.[57] Low serum and red blood cell folate levels are associated with an increased incidence of spontaneous abortions and malformations in women with epilepsy.[54, 58, 59]

Occurrence[60–62] and recurrence studies[63, 64] have conclusively shown that folate supplementation significantly reduces the risk of NTDs in nonepileptic women. The risk of occurrent NTDs is reduced by 60% with doses as low as 0.4 mg per day,[62] and risk of recurrent NTDs reduced by 72% with a 4-mg per day supplement.[64] Occurrence of other major malformations (except cleft lip and cleft palate) are also reduced by periconceptional folate supplementation.[65]

A dose-response effect of plasma folate levels on the risk of an NTD has been demonstrated in a large case control study of NTDs in women giving birth in Ireland.[66] Serum and red blood cell (RBC) folate concentrations were determined at a median of 15 weeks gestation. The RBC folate level was included in order to determine folate turnover during the previous 120 days. As shown in Figure 16.2, although risk was highest in women with RBC folate levels of less than 340 nmol/L (150 ng/mL), there was a continuous gradation of risk, suggesting that folate supplementation may have wide-reaching benefit. According to these data, folate supplementation in women with RBC folate levels of less than 340 nmol/L will reduce the risk of an NTD by more than 85%.

Folate may protect against birth defects by overcoming an abnormality in homocysteine metabolism (Figure 16.3). In one study, women with fetuses with NTDs had lower vitamin B_{12} as well as folate levels.[67] A second study found that mothers of children with NTDs had significantly elevated homocysteine levels.[68] The defect may be related to abnormalities in the activity of the enzyme methionine synthetase. Methionine synthetase is critical for methylation in a number of biologic processes, including production of myelin basic protein and DNA biosynthesis. Folate and vitamin B_{12} are required as cofactors for methionine synthetase. Further work will elucidate whether the most effective periconceptional prophylaxis to prevent NTDs also requires vitamin B_{12} as well as folic acid.

VARIABLES INFLUENCING RISK OF TERATOGENESIS

The risk of teratogenicity in infants of epileptic mothers increases with exposure to AEDs. Infants of epileptic mothers are at higher risk for birth defects if their mothers are treated with AEDs than if they are not treated.[32] Risk is increased if fetuses are exposed to higher AED doses or to AED polytherapy.

AED-mediated teratogenesis appears to be related to peak rather than cumulative exposure. Mice exposed to constant infusions of valproic acid were compared with mice receiving repeated high injections. Incidence of NTDs was related to the peak level of valproic acid, not the total daily dosage.[69] Also, infants born with NTDs are more likely to have been exposed to significantly higher daily doses of VPA than unaffected infants.[33, 70]

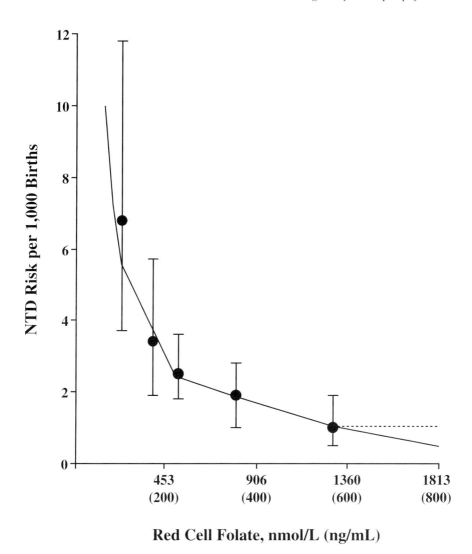

Figure 16.2   Risk of neural tube defects (NTDs) varies inversely with red blood cell folate. (Reprinted with permission from LE Daily, PN Kirke, A Molloy, et al. Folate levels and neural tube defects: implications for treatment. JAMA 1995;274:1698.)

Polytherapy confers a substantially increased risk of teratogenicity.[1, 70, 71] In one study in Japan, the risk of a malformation was 2% in mothers receiving one AED but increased to 25% with exposure to four or more AEDs.[72] Polytherapy leads to metabolic interactions, such as induction of the cytochrome P450 enzyme system and inhibition of the breakdown of oxidative metabolites by epoxide hydrolase (Figure 16.4).

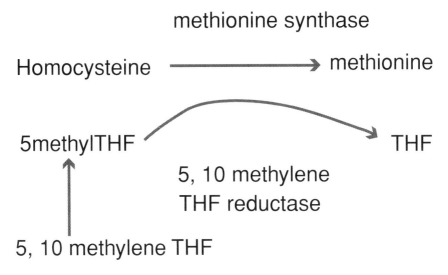

Figure 16.3   Metabolic pathways for synthesis of methionine from homocysteine require vitamin B_{12} and folate as cofactors. (THF = tetrahydrofolate.) (Adapted from JL Mills, JM McPartlin, PN Kirke, et al. Homocysteine metabolism in pregnancies complicated by neural tube defects. Lancet 1995;345:149.)

Mechanisms of Teratogenesis: Toxic Metabolites

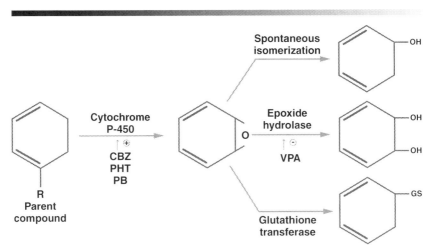

Figure 16.4   Antiepileptic drugs (AEDs) form reactive arene oxide intermediates, which are further metabolized to nonreactive metabolites by a variety of pathways. AEDs that induce cytochrome P450, such as carbamazepine (CBZ), phenytoin (PHT), and phenobarbital (PB), induce formation of these unstable intermediates. Valproate (VPA) inhibits activity of the enzyme epoxide hydrolase, reducing the rate of formation of a nonreactive dihydrodiol.

For example, the most significant metabolic pathway for CBZ is through formation of the 10,11-epoxide via the hepatic microsomal (P450) enzyme system. The epoxide is converted to trans-10,11-dihydroxy-10,11-dihydro-CBZ, which is excreted in the urine. Polytherapy with PHT or PB induces the P450 system and enhances epoxide formation.[73] Polytherapy may also compound folate deficiency.

NEONATAL PROBLEMS RELATED TO EXPOSURE TO ANTIEPILEPTIC DRUGS: HEMORRHAGIC DISEASE OF THE NEWBORN

Infants of epileptic mothers are at higher risk of developing hemorrhagic disease of the newborn. Fetal hemorrhage within the first 24 hours of life is associated with maternal use of liver enzyme–inducing AEDs.[74] An AED-mediated deficiency of vitamin K leads to a reduction in factors II, VII, IX, and X.[75] The mechanism of AED-mediated coagulopathy is presumed to be related to competitive inhibition of vitamin K transport across the placenta or because of induction of fetal cyP450 liver enzymes, leading to increased oxidative degradation of vitamin K in the fetus. The mother rarely experiences vitamin K deficiency because of abundant hepatic stores of vitamin K_2 (menaquinones).[76] Although almost always asymptomatic in the mother, the protime may be prolonged in the fetus. Vitamin K deficiency can be detected prenatally by assays for PIVKA proteins (protein induced by vitamin K absence), which represent decarboxylated forms of vitamin K–dependent coagulation factors.[76] When PIVKA proteins are present, vitamin K is deficient. In one study, 54% of neonates exposed to AEDs had detectable PIVKA proteins in cord blood samples.[75]

Fetal coagulopathy can be overcome by maternal oral supplementation of vitamin K_1 (10–20 mg per day) during the last month of gestation.[77] Maternal supplementation with vitamin K_1 at 10 mg per day raises maternal levels of vitamin K_1 by 60-fold and cord blood levels by 15-fold. The infant should receive 1 mg of vitamin K_1 parenterally immediately after delivery, and cord blood specimens should be assayed for clotting factors. If deficient, the neonate should receive fresh frozen plasma at a dose of 20 mg/kg over 1–2 hours.[76]

CHOICE OF ANTIEPILEPTIC DRUGS

AEDs are teratogens, but seizures pose a risk to the mother and to the fetus. Therein lies the clinical dilemma. Will the new AEDs prove a desirable alternative for a woman with uncontrolled seizures who is contemplating pregnancy? There have been few human pregnancy exposures to the new AEDs. Nevertheless, favorable animal toxicology data and pharmacokinetic characteristics of the new AEDs suggests that these drugs will have an important role in the treatment of epilepsy in women of child-bearing potential.

Animal models of teratogenicity are not necessarily predictive of the human response in terms of dysmorphology and, especially, neurocognitive development. Nevertheless, the new drugs do not appear to be teratogenic in animals.

Table 16.2   U.S. Food and Drug Administration pregnancy risk categories for antiepileptic drugs

---

Category C
Risk cannot be ruled out. Human studies are lacking, and animal studies are positive for
   fetal risk or lacking as well. However, potential benefits may justify the potential risk.
      Carbamazepine
      Felbamate
      Gabapentin
      Lamotrigine
      Phenobarbital
Category D
Positive evidence of risk. Investigational or postmarketing data show risk to the fetus.
   Nevertheless, potential benefits may outweigh the potential risk.
      Valproate
      Phenytoin
Not categorized
      Ethosuximide
      Clonazepam (Klonopin)
      Diazepam (Valium)

Felbamate (FBM), gabapentin (GBP), and LTG are associated with delayed ossification in the skull and hind limbs and with reduced fetal weight at maternal toxic doses (package inserts).

The U.S. Food and Drug Administration (FDA) provides pregnancy risk categories for all AEDs. Most AEDs fall into pregnancy risk category C. VPA and PHT receive a higher risk category. All the marketed new AEDs have received a class C category from the FDA, meaning that they should be used by pregnant women only if the benefits outweigh the risks (Table 16.2).

Experience with human pregnancies is very limited for the new AEDs. Reported pregnancy exposures to FBM and GBP are limited to unintentional pregnancies occurring during the preclinical testing period. Some were therapeutically terminated and only a few carried to term. Sixty-nine first trimester pregnancy exposures have been reported with LTG. Of the pregnancies carried to term (34), several had birth defects—each exposed to AED polytherapy and showing birth defects consistent with exposure to the concomitant AED (information on file, Glaxo-Wellcome). Seventy-two human pregnancies had been reported after exposure to vigabatrin as of spring, 1995. Fifty-two had normal outcomes, seven terminated in a spontaneous abortion, and five in an induced abortion—two of these pregnancies were terminated because of birth defects. Seven infants were born with malformations or anomalies. There has been no consistent pattern of maldevelopment, and all of these infants had been exposed to polytherapy (information on file, Hoescht Marion Roussel, Inc.).

Information regarding the teratogenic effects of newly released AEDs relies almost entirely on postmarketing experience. However, it is estimated that no more than 10% of serious adverse effects to pharmacologic compounds are ever reported to the FDA. The lack of well-organized, accessible postmarketing epidemiologic safety monitoring may account for the 15-year and greater delay from release of the older AEDs to recognition of their teratogenicity. Since pregnant women are systematically excluded from investigational drug trials, the only data on human teratogenicity available at the time a drug is released comes from the very few unintentional pregnancies that occur during the investigational trials, which is always an insufficient number to understand true teratogenic potential. Data from animal reproductive toxicology may not accurately represent human risks. Therefore, it is essential that data be acquired on every human pregnancy exposure to a new pharmacologic compound. Only with establishment of postmarketing pregnancy registries that are easily accessible to health care providers can adverse outcomes, such as fetal teratogenesis, be identified in an appropriately short period. Information should be obtained regarding time and duration of exposure, maximal dose, exposure to polytherapy, and determination of other variables affecting fetal outcome, including adequacy of prenatal care. Glaxo-Wellcome initiated an international pregnancy registry to identify pregnancy exposures to LTG and follow outcome. Other pharmaceutical companies are following suit.

MANAGEMENT OF PREGNANT WOMEN WITH EPILEPSY

Comprehensive care of a pregnant woman with epilepsy begins well before conception. Prenatal counseling addresses contraception choice, AED selection and dosage, and AED-related teratogenicity. The patient is informed about prenatal diagnostic testing to detect fetal malformation.

Several principles govern selection of an AED for a woman of child-bearing potential. The goal must be effective control of maternal seizures while conferring the least risk to the fetus. Since every established AED is teratogenic, the medication that is most effective for that woman's epilepsy and seizure type is selected and used as monotherapy at the lowest possible dose.[78] Because human teratogenicity has not been established, the newer AEDs (GBP, LTG, and VGB) should probably be reserved for women who have not experienced acceptable seizure control or tolerability on the established AEDs.

Preconception is the ideal time to re-evaluate the need for any AED. AED withdrawal should be considered in any woman planning pregnancy who has been seizure-free for at least 2 years. Women who are at high risk for relapse, in whom withdrawal should not be attempted, can be identified. This includes women with epilepsy syndromes that are unlikely to remit, such as juvenile myoclonic epilepsy.[79] Other variables that predict a high likelihood of relapse include abnormality on neurologic examination, structural brain abnormality on magnetic resonance imaging (MRI) studies, and a history of prolonged convulsive seizures and status epilepticus. If AED treatment is no longer indicated, withdrawal should be accomplished before conception, if possible. There is a 12% risk of seizure relapse in the first 6 months of drug withdrawal and a 32% risk during the first year.[80] Withdrawal can be attempted over 1–3 months, depending on the AED. Barbiturates and benzodiazepines typically require a longer period of withdrawal.

If an AED is needed, the most effective drug for the seizure type is used in monotherapy and at the lowest possible dose. If a woman requiring AED treatment is seen after conception and is taking a single drug that is effective for her seizure type, a medication change should not be attempted. Since major malformations arise from early exposure, there is no benefit from medication change after conception. Risk may be added by exposure to a second agent and there also might be a risk of breakthrough seizures during the change. If a woman is seen after conception who is on AED polytherapy and is seizure-free, then serious consideration should be given to the possibility that monotherapy can be achieved. Any AED reduction and discontinuation should be accomplished with appropriate regard for changes in the total and unbound levels of the remaining AED.

If there is a family history of NTDs, and there are acceptable treatment alternatives, VPA and CBZ should be avoided. VPA particularly should be used at the lowest effective dose because teratogenicity may be related to peak dose rather than cumulative exposure.[70] If a high daily dose is needed, then this should be administered as frequent smaller individual doses.

Folate supplementation should be provided at a dose of 0.4–4.0 mg per day. Folate must be present within the first 25 days after conception in order to protect against malformations of the neural tube. A missed menstrual cycle is usually not noticed until the 15th day after conception. Up to 40% of pregnancies are unplanned, and 50% of women with planned pregnancies do not consult a health care provider before conception.[81] In the United Kingdom, 67% of those attending an antenatal clinic for the first time were unaware of recommendations regarding folate supplementation and only 37% of those who were aware received that information before conception.[82]

Given these realities, it seems prudent that folate supplementation be given routinely to women of child-bearing potential. The Canadian College of Medical Geneticists recommends that 0.8–5.0 mg per day of folic acid be given to women who are at increased risk of having offspring with NTDs and who are planning a pregnancy. The United States Public Health Service recommends that all women of child-bearing age in the United States who are capable of becoming pregnant consume 0.4 mg per day of folic acid for the purpose of reducing their risk of having a child affected with a NTD.[83] Women who have already had a child with a NTD are encouraged to consult their physician regarding appropriate folate dosage and to refer to the 1991 Centers for Disease Control guideline suggesting a dosage of 0.4 mg per day based on the Medical Research Council recurrent risk study. Whether women with epilepsy require a dosage higher than 0.4 mg per day is not known.

Prenatal testing will detect major malformations in the first trimester. In most high-risk perinatal centers, high resolution ultrasound and testing of maternal serum for alpha-fetoprotein are sufficient to detect more than 95% of cases of NTDs. A level II ultrasound study will also detect most oral clefts and heart anomalies. In some cases, amniocentesis will also be required.

Vitamin K_1, 10–20 mg per day, is supplemented in the last month of gestation. The infant is given vitamin K_1, 1 mg intramuscularly, at birth.

Women with epilepsy in most cases may be encouraged to breast feed. Breastfeeding does not usually pose a hazard to the neonate because of the relatively low concentration of most AEDs in breast milk. AEDs cross into breast milk in inverse relation to their degree of maternal serum protein binding (Table 16.3). However, because of the longer elimination half-life and reduced protein binding in neonates, concentrations in the neonate may equal or exceed those in

Table 16.3 Concentration of antiepileptic drugs in breast milk expressed as a percentage of maternal plasma concentration

Antiepileptic drug	Concentration in breast milk
Phenytoin	24–45[a]
Carbamazepine	40[b]
Carbamazepine epoxide	100[b]
Ethosuximide	>90[b]
Phenobarbital	40–60[b]
Valproate	<20[a]

[a]Data from H Nau, W Kuhnz, HJ Egger, et al. Anticonvulsants during pregnancy and lactation. Clin Pharmokinet 1982;7:508.

[b]Data from S Kaneko, K Suzuki, T Sato, et al. The Problems of Anticonvulsant Medication at the Neonatal Period: Is Breast Feeding Advisable? In D Janz, M Dam, A Richens, et al. (eds), Epilepsy, Pregnancy and the Child. New York: Raven, 1981;343.

the mother. Neonates, particularly those exposed to PB, must be carefully observed for poor feeding and irritability.

CONCLUSION

Family planning for women with epilepsy is accomplished most successfully when undertaken well before conception. The woman and her physician must consider the optimal medical treatment for that woman's seizure type and frequency. Some women can be successfully withdrawn from AEDs, others may be satisfactorily controlled with monotherapy, and many are able to reduce medication dosage. Folate supplementation should be routinely provided to every woman of childbearing potential. Prenatal diagnostic testing can detect most morphologic abnormalities, and prenatal testing of AED pharmacokinetics in mother and fetus may ultimately provide a means by which physicians can select the AED expected to have the fewest teratogenic effects. It is the responsibility of every physician caring for women of reproductive age with epilepsy to report adverse fetal outcomes after exposure to AEDs. Complete ascertainment of AED-related birth defects is required in order to define the role of newer AEDs in treating epilepsy in women.

REFERENCES

1. Koch S, Loesche G, Jager-Roman E, et al. Major and minor malformations and antiepileptic drugs. Neurology 1992;42(S5):83.
2. Schmidt D, Canger R, Cornaggia C, et al. Seizure Frequency During Pregnancy and the Puerperium. The Role of Noncompliance and Sleep Deprivation. In R Porter, AA Ward, RH Mattson, et al. (eds), Advances in Epileptology: XVth Epilepsy International Symposium. New York: Raven, 1984.

3. Schmidt D, Beck-Mannagetta G, Janz D, Koch S. The Effect of Pregnancy on the Course of Epilepsy: A Prospective Study. In D Janz, M Dam, A Richens, et al. (eds), Epilepsy, Pregnancy and the Child. New York: Raven, 1982;39.

4. Tomson T, Lindbom U, Ekquist B, Sundquist A. Disposition of carbamazepine and phenytoin in pregnancy. Epilepsia 1994;35:131.

5. Morrell MJ. Hormones and epilepsy through the lifetime. Epilepsia 1992;33:S38.

6. Yerby MS, Friel PN, McCormick K. Antiepileptic drug disposition during pregnancy. Neurology 1992;42(S5):12.

7. Battino D, Binelli S, Bossi L, et al. Monitoring of Antiepileptic Drugs and Hormones in Pregnant Epileptic Women. In RJ Porter, AA Ward, RH Mattson, et al. (eds), Advances in Epileptology: XVth Epilepsy International Symposium. New York: Raven, 1984;227.

8. Nau H, Schmidt-Gollwitzer M, Kuhnz W, et al. Antiepileptic Drug Disposition, Protein Binding, and Estradiol/Progesterone Serum Concentration Ratios During Pregnancy. In RJ Porter, AA Ward, RH Mattson, et al. (eds), Advances in Epileptology: XVth Epilepsy International Symposium. New York: Raven, 1984;239.

9. Cooney AH. Pharmacological implications of microsomal enzyme induction. Pharmacol Rev 1967;9:317.

10. Perez B, Gorodisch S, Casavilla F, Maruffo C. Ultrastructure of the human liver at the end of normal pregnancy. Am J Obstet Gynecol 1971;110:428.

11. Bernus I, Hooper WD, Dickinson RG, Eadie MJ. Metabolism of carbamazepine and co-administered anticonvulsants during pregnancy. Epilepsy Res 1995;21:65.

12. Tomson T, Lindbom U, Ekquist B, Sundquist A. Epilepsy and pregnancy: a prospective study of seizure control in relation to free and total plasma concentrations of carbamazepine and phenytoin. Epilepsia 1994;35:122.

13. Yerby MS, Leppik I. Epilepsy and the outcome of pregnancy. J Epilepsy 1990;3:193.

14. Ramsey RE, Perchalski RJ, Resillez M, Cohen H. Changes in Hormone Levels and Anticonvulsant Metabolism During Pregnancy. In RJ Porter, AA Ward, RH Mattson, et al. (eds), Advances in Epileptology: XVth Epilepsy International Symposium. New York: Raven, 1984;233.

15. Yerby MS, Koepsell T, Daling J. Pregnancy complications and outcomes in a cohort of women with epilepsy. Epilepsia 1985;26:631.

16. Battino D, Granata T, Binelli S, et al. Intrauterine growth in the offspring of epileptic mothers. Acta Neurol Scand 1992;86:555.

17. Philbert A, Dam M. The epileptic mother and her child. Epilepsia 1982;23:85.

18. Steegers-Theunissen RPM, Renier WO, Borm GF, et al. Factors influencing the risk of abnormal pregnancy outcome in epileptic women: a multi-centre prospective study. Epilepsy Res 1994;18:261.

19. Hiilesmaa VK. Pregnancy and birth in women with epilepsy. Neurology 1992;42(S5):8.

20. Yerby MS, Cawthon ML. Infant mortality of infants of mothers with epilepsy. Ann Neurol 1994;36:330.

21. Minkoff H, Schaffer RM, Delke I, Grunebaum AN. Diagnosis of intracranial hemorrhage in utero after a maternal seizure. Obstet Gynecol 1985;64(Suppl 3):22S.

22. Teramo K, Hiilesmaa V, Brady A, Saarikoski S. Fetal heart rate during a maternal grand mal epileptic seizure. J Perinatal Med 1979;7:3.

23. Nau H, Kuhnz W, Egger HJ, et al. Anticonvulsants during pregnancy and lactation. Clin Pharmacokinet 1982;7:508.

24. Pienimaki P, Hartikainen A, Arvela P, et al. Carbamazepine and its metabolites in human perfused placenta and in maternal and cord blood. Epilepsia 1995;36:241.

25. Shapiro S, Slone D, Hartz SC, et al. Anticonvulsants and parental epilepsy in the development of birth defects. Lancet 1976;1:272.

26. German J, Kowal A, Ellers KH. Trimethadione and human teratogenesis. Teratology 1970;3:349.

27. Zackai EH, Mellman WJ, Neiderer B, Hanson JW. The fetal trimethadione syndrome. J Pediatr 1975;87:280.

28. Hanson JW, Myrianthopoulos NC, Sedgwick Harvey MA, Smith DW. Risks to the offspring of women treated with hydantoin anticonvulsants, with emphasis on the fetal hydantoin syndrome. J Pediatr 1976;89:662.

29. Yerby MS, Leavitt A, Erickson DM, et al. Antiepileptics and the development of congenital anomalies. Neurology 1992;42(S5):132.

30. Dansky LV, Finnell RH. Parental epilepsy, anticonvulsant drugs, and reproductive outcome: epidemiologic and experimental findings spanning three decades; two human studies. Reprod Toxicol 1991;5:301.

31. Friis ML. Facial clefts and congenital heart defects in children of parents with epilepsy: genetic and environmental etiologic factors. Acta Neurol Scand 1989;79:433.

32. Annegers JF, Hauser WA, Elveback LR, et al. Congenital malformations and seizure disorders in the offspring of parents with epilepsy. Int J Epidemiol 1978;7:241.
33. Omtzigt JGC, Los FJ, Grobee DE, et al. The risk of spina bifida aperta after first trimester exposure to valproate in a prenatal cohort. Neurology 1992;42(S5):119.
34. Lindhout D, Schmidt D. In-utero exposure to valproate and neural tube defects. Lancet 1986;1:1392.
35. Robert E, Giubaud P. Maternal valproic acid and congenital neural tube defects. Lancet 1982;2:937.
36. Rosa FW. Spina bifida in infants of women treated with carbamazepine during pregnancy. N Engl J Med 1991;324:674.
37. Kelly TE. Teratogenicity of anticonvulsant drugs III: radiographic hand analysis of children exposed in utero to diphenylhydantoin. Am J Med Genet 1984;19:445.
38. Gaily E, Kantola-Sorsa E, Granstrom ML. Intelligence of children of epileptic mothers. J Pediatr 1988;113:677.
39. Ransom BR, Elmore JG. Effects of Antiepileptic Drugs on the Developing Nervous System. In D Smith, D Treiman, M Trimble (eds), Advances in Neurology. New York: Raven, 1991;225.
40. Nelson KB, Deutschberger J. Head size at one year as a prediction of four year IQ. Neurology 1970;12:487.
41. Hiilesmaa VK, Teramo K, Granstrom ML, Bardy AH. Fetal head growth retardation associated with maternal antiepileptic drugs. Lancet 1981;2:165.
42. Gaily EK, Granstrom ML, Hiilesmaa VK, Bardy AH. Head circumference in children of epileptic mothers: contributions of drug exposure and genetic background. Epilepsy Res 1990;5:217.
43. Jones KL, Lacro RV, Johnson KA, Adams J. Pattern of malformations in the children of women treated with carbamazepine during pregnancy. N Engl J Med 1989;320:1661.
44. Nelson KB, Ellenberg JH. Maternal seizure disorder, outcome of pregnancy, and neurologic abnormalities in the children. Neurology 1982;32:1247.
45. Klepel H, Freitag G. Spina bifida occulta in epilepsy syndromes. Neurology 1992;42(S5):119.
46. Lindhout D, Omizigt JG, Cornel MC. Spectrum of neural-tube defects in 34 infants prenatally exposed to antiepileptic drugs. Neurology 1992;42(S5):111.
47. Finnell RH, Chernoff GF. Variable patterns of malformations in the mouse fetal hydantoin syndrome. Am J Med Genet 1984;19:463.
48. Wong M, Wells PG. Modulation of embryonic glutathione reductase and phenytoin teratogenicity by 1,3-bis-(2-chloroethyl)-1-nitrosourea (BCNU). J Pharmacol Exp Ther 1989;250:336.
49. Strickler SM, Miller MA, Andermann E, et al. Genetic predisposition to phenytoin-induced birth defects. Lancet 1985;2:746.
50. Finnell RH, Kerr BM, Van Waes M, et al. Protection from phenytoin-induced congenital malformations by coadministration of the antiepileptic drug stirpentol in a mouse model. Epilepsia 1994;35:141.
51. Pacifici M, Colizzi C, Giuliani L, Rane A. Cytosolic epoxide hydrolase in fetal and adult human liver. Arch Toxicol 1983;54:331.
52. Buehler BA, Delimont D, Van Waes M, Finnell RH. Prenatal prediction of risk of the fetal hydantoin syndrome N Engl J Med 1990;322:1567.
53. Buehler BA, Rao V, Finnell RH. Biochemical and molecular teratology of fetal hydantoin syndrome. Neurol Clin 1994;12:741.
54. Ogawa Y, Kaneko S, Otani K, Fukushima Y. Serum folic acid levels in epileptic mothers and their relationship to congenital malformations. Epilepsy Res 1991;8:75.
55. Wegner C, Nau H. Alteration of embryonic folate metabolism by valproic acid during organogenesis: implications for mechanism of teratogenesis. Neurology 1992;42(S5):17.
56. Sander JWAS, Patsalos PN. An assessment of serum and red blood cell folate concentrations in patients with epilepsy on lamotrigine therapy. Epilepsy Res 1992;13:89.
57. Jordan RL, Wilson JG, Schumacher HJ. Embryotoxicity of the folate antagonist methotrexate in rats and rabbits. Teratology 1977;15:73.
58. Dansky LV, Andermann E, Rosenblatt D, et al. Anticonvulsants, folate levels, and pregnancy outcome: a prospective study. Ann Neurol 1987;21:176.
59. Reynolds EH. Anticonvulsants, folic acid and epilepsy. Lancet 1973;1:1376.
60. Mulinare J, Corder JF, Erickson JD, et al. Periconceptional use of multivitamins and the occurrence of neural tube defects. JAMA 1988;260:3141.
61. Milunsky A, Jick H, Jick SS. Multivitamin/folic acid supplementation in early pregnancy reduces the prevalence of neural tube defects. JAMA 1989;262:2847.
62. Werler MM, Shapiro S, Mitchell AA. Periconceptional folic acid exposure and risk of occurrent neural tube defects. JAMA 1993;269:1257.
63. Laurence KM, James N, Miller MH, et al. Double-blind, randomized controlled trial of folate treatment before conception to prevent the recurrence of neural-tube defects. BMJ 1981;282:1509.

64. Medical Research Council Vitamin Research Group. Prevention of neural tube defects: results of the Medical Research Council Vitamin Study. Lancet 1991;338:131.
65. Czeizel AE, Dudas I. Prevention of the first occurrence of neural tube defects by periconceptional vitamin supplementation. N Engl J Med 1992;327:1832.
66. Daily LE, Kirke PN, Molloy A, et al. Folate levels and neural tube defects: implications for treatment. JAMA 1995;274:1698.
67. Kirke PN, Molloy AM, Daly LE, et al. Maternal plasma folate and vitamin B_{12} are independent risk factors for neural tube defects. QJM 1993;86:703.
68. Mills JL, McPartlin JM, Kirke PN, et al. Homocysteine metabolism in pregnancies complicated by neural tube defects. Lancet 1995;345:149.
69. Nau H. Teratogenetic valproic acid concentrations: infusion by implanted minipumps versus conventional injection regimes in the mouse. Toxicol Appl Pharmacol 1985;80:243.
70. Oguni M, Dansky L, Andermann E, et al. Improved pregnancy outcome in epileptic women in the last decade: relationship to maternal anticonvulsant therapy. Brain Dev 1992;14:371.
71. Kaneko S, Otani K, Fukushima Y. Teratogenicity of antiepilepsy drugs—analysis of possible risk factors. Epilepsia 1988;29:459.
72. Nakane Y, Okuma T, Takahaski R, et al. Multiinstitutional study on the teratogenicity and fetal toxicity of antiepileptic drugs; a report of a collaborative study group in Japan. Epilepsia 1980;21:663.
73. Liu H, Delgado M. Interactions of phenobarbital and phenytoin with carbamazepine and its metabolites' concentrations, concentration ratios, and level/dose ratios in epileptic children. Epilepsia 1995;36:249.
74. Moslet U, Hansen ES. A review of vitamin K, epilepsy, and pregnancy. Acta Neurol Scand 1992;85:39.
75. Cornelissen M, Steegers-Theunissen R, Kollee L, et al. Increased incidence of neonatal vitamin K deficiency resulting from maternal anticonvulsant therapy. Am J Obstet Gynecol 1993;168:923.
76. Thorp JA, Gaston L, Caspers DR, Pal ML. Current concepts and controversies in the use of vitamin K. Drugs 1995;49:376.
77. Cornelissen M, Steegers-Theunissen R, Kollee L, et al. Supplementation of vitamin K in pregnant women receiving anticonvulsant therapy prevents neonatal vitamin K deficiency. Am J Obstet Gynecol 1993;168:884.
78. Delgado-Escueta AV, Janz D. Consensus guidelines: preconception counseling, management, and care of the pregnant woman with epilepsy. Neurology 1992;42(S5):149.
79. Janz D. Juvenile Myoclonic Epilepsy. In M Dam, L Gram (eds), Comprehensive Epileptology. New York: Raven, 1990;171.
80. Chadwick D. The Discontinuation of AED Therapy. In TA Pedley, BS Meldrum (eds), Recent Advances in Epilepsy (Vol 2). Edinburgh: Churchill Livingstone, 1985;111.
81. Grimes DA. Unplanned pregnancies in the U.S. Obstet Gynecol 1986;67:438.
82. Clark N, Fisk N. Minimal compliance with the Department of Health recommendation for routine prophylaxis to prevent fetal neural tube defects. Br J Obstet Gynaecol 1994;101:709.
83. Centers for Disease Control. Recommendations for the use of folic acid to reduce the number of cases of spina bifida and other neural tube defects. MMWR 1992;41:1.

17
When to Refer Your Patients for Epilepsy Surgery

Michael R. Sperling and Roger J. Porter

In spite of recent advances in antiepileptic drug therapy, a surprisingly large number of patients have uncontrolled seizures or are intolerant of medication. For many of these individuals, surgical intervention offers the only hope for a more normal life—the only chance for total freedom from seizures.

Although epilepsy surgery has been available for more than half a century, only in the past decade has it become widely available in the United States and elsewhere in the industrialized world. Ward,[1] for example, estimated that only about 100 operations were performed yearly in the United States in the early 1980s, although more than 50,000 people might benefit from this therapeutic approach. In contrast, representatives from more than 50 epilepsy surgical centers attended the Palm Desert conference in 1986,[2] and many more centers have since initiated activities. Now, many patients undergo a variety of surgical procedures for medically refractory seizures. Several forces propelled the increase in availability, including the increased safety and efficacy of surgical treatment, the rise in the number of neurologists and neurosurgeons, and the trend toward subspecialization within neurology that fostered the development of specialized procedures. In any case, patients have generally been the winners. Not only has improved accessibility to surgical intervention become a reality, but perhaps the biggest single contribution has been the demythologizing of epilepsy surgery, from the experimental and dangerous to the routine and the safe. In the setting of these accomplishments, this chapter addresses the critical issue of when surgery should be considered for a patient.

The issues for patient and treating physician can be divided into three fundamental areas. These are the medical criteria for surgical intervention, the social and motivational factors, and the choice of the center for the presurgical evaluation and surgery. Important at the outset is the understanding that referral does not automatically lead to surgery, but rather that the surgical center will fully evaluate the suitability of each patient for such an intervention. This chapter concludes with a discussion of important recent advances in epilepsy surgery.

MEDICAL CRITERIA FOR SURGICAL INTERVENTION

Inherent in considering an epileptic patient as a candidate for surgical intervention is the understanding that the patient is inadequately responsive to available medications. Surgery offers no measurable benefit to patients whose seizures are well controlled by medication and who experience no significant side effects from their therapy.

Predictors of Intractability

Certain patients respond less well to antiepileptic drugs than others. Those patients whose seizures are more likely to be intractable to medications often have one or more of the following features: abnormal neurologic examination findings, low intelligence quotient (IQ), psychiatric abnormalities, history of status epilepticus, symptomatic epilepsy (such as that caused by head trauma, meningitis, or a structural lesion), early secondary generalization of seizures, clusters of seizures, or poorly localized electroencephalogram (EEG) abnormalities.[3] Some of these factors may also contribute to the likelihood of a poor surgical outcome.[4] In outlining these factors, one must keep in mind that patients with epilepsy are heterogeneous and that each patient requires an individual assessment.

Diagnostic Re-Evaluation and the Importance of the Medical History

In the case of most patients, the diagnosis is apparent from the description of the seizure and from the prolonged history available because of medical unresponsiveness. Nevertheless, it behooves the physician to re-evaluate the diagnosis in all potential surgical candidates; occasional surprises occur, and it is the obligation of the surgical team to be certain not only that the patient has the kind of epilepsy appropriate for surgical intervention, but that the patient does not instead have some other disorder, such as psychogenic seizures (Table 17.1).

In an era of increasing sophistication and reliance on machines, technicians, and specialists, the power of the appropriate historical information that can be gleaned from the patient is often ignored. Recognizing that such information is subjective and potentially misleading, a considerable storehouse of information awaits the physician who is willing to take the time to probe for the data. The experienced physician should critically and logically ascertain the facts, some of which might only be obtained by a thorough repetitive interrogation.[3] First, a detailed description of the seizures must be obtained. Many patients are not prepared for this line of questioning; others will give a terminology-oriented description, using such terms as "petit mal" or "temporal lobe." The physician must orient the patient to more fundamental, descriptive terms. The doctor may begin by asking the patient, "What is the first thing that happens in a typical seizure?" The entire sequence of symptoms must be gotten through, and patients should be questioned about changes in the character of their auras through the years. Patients with simple partial seizures are often able to describe the entire event by themselves in logical sequence. Patients with complex partial seizures usually

Table 17.1 Common causes of anticonvulsant therapy failures and appropriate management of such failures

Cause	Detection	Management
Noncompliance	History Monitoring of anti- convulsant drug levels	Patient instruction and education
Nonepileptic seizures or combination of epileptic and nonepileptic seizures	History CCTV/EEG Suggestion Seizure markers (prolactin)	Psychological counseling Psychotherapy
Incorrect seizure sub- classification	History	Medication adjustment
Incorrect choice or combination of drugs	CCTV/EEG	Medication adjustment
Inappropriate drug dosage	Monitoring of anticon- vulsant drug levels	Medication adjustment

CCTV = closed circuit television; EEG = electroencephalogram.

Source: Reprinted with permission from P Boon, P Williamson. Presurgical evaluation of patients with partial epilepsy. Indications and evaluation techniques for resective surgery. Clin Neurol Neurosurg 1989;91:3.

need assistance, from persons who have seen the attacks or from a knowledge of what they have been told. The physician may ask, for example, "What do other people see when you have a seizure? What do they observe?" It is most helpful to have a relative or friend who has witnessed seizures present for the interview. Finally, it is important to learn whether the attack ends abruptly or whether it tapers into a postictal state. One good question is, "Do you feel bad or tired after an attack?" A positive response strongly suggests the presence of an abnormal postictal state, which may guide the physician away from absence seizures, for example, and suggest seizure types such as complex partial.[3] It is not usually necessary, except when psychogenic seizures are considered in the differential diagnosis, to obtain a detailed description of generalized tonic-clonic (grand mal) seizures; such seizures tend to be more stereotyped than other attacks and are often secondary to a wide variety of more fundamental seizure types. Also, generalized tonic-clonic seizures are more responsive to medical therapy than many other seizure types.[3]

All of this history gathering will lead the physician to a first impression—often, but not always, a correct one of the nature of the patient's seizures. Obtaining the seizure diagnosis is the first step in learning what is important about the patient's epilepsy. The international classification of epileptic seizures has been developed over many years with great effort; it is pragmatic and provides the physician with an appropriate framework for taking a seizure history and finding the correct category for the attacks. This is, however, only one important step in the process of the diagnostic effort. Each patient with seizures must be evaluated for potential causes of the seizures. The "etiologic" diagnosis may be almost any pathologic process that can injure the brain—from birth injuries to tumors to infections to congenital or hereditary abnormalities. Establishing the "seizure diagnosis" can be a first important step toward finding the etiologic diagnosis. When the cause is uncovered (and we are not always able to do so), action that is quite independent of care for the seizures may be needed to treat the cause. In patients who turn out to be candidates for surgical intervention, the etiologic process may be of special importance in planning the invasive diagnostic procedures and the surgery.

Most important, the process of taking a history permits the physician to think not only about the type of seizures that occur and the likely etiologic process, but to consider the syndromic diagnosis, which involves the entire patient rather than just a fragment. The epilepsy syndrome is most important for determining prognosis, type of treatment, and duration of therapy. Before thinking about offering surgery, it must be clear that the individual neither suffers from a type of epilepsy that spontaneously remits with the passage of time nor has a progressive condition for which surgery would provide little return.

Medical Treatment and Unresponsiveness

One of the most controversial of issues is that of defining intractability in patients, which is a necessary precondition to considering surgery. Clearly, no patient can be or should be tried on all medications. With the arrival of several new drugs in the 1990s, the issue grows even more complex. How many drugs should a patient try? How many combinations should be used? There are several approaches to this issue.

A reasonable initial approach is the mechanism-based strategy, which is grounded on the assumption that the patient's condition is declared intractable after failing to respond to a series of drugs that are different in their known mechanisms of action. This logical approach observes that the causes of epilepsy are diverse, that our ability to predict the basic mechanism of seizure generation in a patient is poor, and that a variety of drugs with different mechanisms of action should be attempted before declaring intractability. Using this logic for patients with partial seizures, clearly at least one drug should be used whose primary action is to block voltage-dependent sodium channels (i.e., phenytoin, carbamazepine, lamotrigine, and topiramate). In addition, drugs that affect gamma-aminobutyric acid (GABA) function, such as the barbiturates, or newer drugs, such as vigabatrin or tiagabine, should be considered. Finally, consideration should be given to drugs whose mechanism is less certain, such as valproate and gabapentin. For patients who have generalized epilepsy, for whom corpus callosotomy is under consideration, the drugs to be tested may differ from those for partial epilepsies; valproate should be used, and felbamate, although risky, might be considered. This mechanism-based approach, however, is flawed in that it assumes that our current understanding of the drug mechanisms consistently bears some meaningful relationship to seizure control, which thus far is an entirely unproved contention.

Once drugs of different types have failed when used as monotherapy, most physicians will next employ combinations of various drugs. Drugs usually considered for this purpose are the older combinations of carbamazepine with phenobarbital, phenytoin, or valproate. Largely unexplored are the myriad possibilities of combinations of new drugs, with each other or with the older, established medications. Such newer combinations are very unlikely to confer sustained seizure control, and indeed the preliminary evidence points in that direction. However, we are only beginning to evaluate these combinations, and controlled trials are warranted.

The usual patient who is a candidate for surgery has been treated with both approaches to ensure that medication cannot control seizures. It takes many months to accomplish this task with this method. The task has proved easier than it would seem, as patients who fail to respond to reasonable doses of one or two appropriate major drugs nearly always fail with subsequent medication efforts.[5] Considering the present state of knowledge of medical therapy and factoring in the risks of uncontrolled seizures, it seems reasonable to conclude that a patient has medically intractable seizures after three appropriate drugs have been given in monotherapy and perhaps one combination has been used. How long should each medication be tried before concluding that it has failed? This conclusion can probably be reached after lack of response to the maximum tolerated dose for 1–2 months. Consequently, medical failure is usually obvious within 1 year once frequent seizures have begun. When the patient has unacceptable side effects at relatively low serum levels, the drug must be considered inadequate; if the levels are extremely low, however, (e.g., a phenytoin level of 2 g/ml), then that drug might be disregarded when counting the number of agents that have failed. It is very important to confirm the diagnosis of epilepsy when medications appear inadequate and to critically question the syndromic diagnosis.

One rarely addressed issue is that of the capability of physicians to deliver medications at adequate but nontoxic levels. Although training in pharmacologic principles is improving, the level of skill required to deliver antiepileptic medications properly is higher than for most other therapeutic areas. The reason is primarily the narrow therapeutic range of these drugs, compounded by their variability in clearance and frequent drug-drug interactions. Some patients are dramatically improved by the appropriate delivery of standard medications. Failure to attain maximal tolerated serum concentrations, for example, is a common treatment deficiency in referred patients.[5] More needs to be done to educate physicians to ensure proper prescribing techniques.

Having noted that a vigorous and thorough medical plan is needed to ensure surgical candidacy, it is also true that intractable epilepsy is a serious and occasionally life-threatening disorder. All major surgical centers have observed that some patients will die while waiting in line for epilepsy surgery; recent data suggest that the mortality rate for patients with uncontrolled seizures exceeds 1 in 100 per year.[6] Uncontrolled seizures can also lead to nonlethal injuries, such as fractures, aspiration pneumonia, cognitive decline, and psychological disturbances. Such complications mandate that intractability be established quickly so that referral to a surgical center is not delayed.

The patient also plays an important role in the medical aspects of determining surgical eligibility. Compliance with medication instructions is critical. The physician is aided greatly in assessing compliance by frequent determinations of plasma levels of antiepileptic drugs during the intensive period of medical re-evaluation (see Table 17.1).

Characteristics of Referred Patients

What kinds of seizures and epilepsy are reasonable to consider for referral to a surgical center? Epilepsy is a very heterogeneous disorder, and surgical approaches are necessarily highly targeted. As noted above, medical intractability does not

Table 17.2   Surgical procedures and remediable syndromes

Type of procedure
   Resective surgery
   Hemispherectomy
   Corpus callosotomy
Type of epilepsy
   Symptomatic partial epilepsy caused by a focal disturbance, such as a tumor, vascular
      malformation, gliosis, or sclerotic lesion
   Symptomatic partial epilepsy caused by a widespread hemisphere disturbance, such as
      chronic encephalitis or porencephaly
   Symptomatic generalized epilepsy, such as Lennox-Gastaut syndrome, postencephalitic
      or post-traumatic epilepsy

Table 17.3   Some characteristics of seizures in surgical candidates

1. Impairment of consciousness
2. Injury
3. Stigmatizing ictal behaviors
4. Unpleasant or noxious auras
5. Unpredictability of seizure occurrence
6. Seizures occurring at least once every 1–2 months

equate to surgical candidacy, even though physicians are encouraged to *consider* surgical intervention in every patient with intractable epilepsy. The following paragraphs summarize the kinds of patients who are appropriate for most surgical procedures performed for epilepsy. The procedures are designed to accommodate the different types of processes that cause epilepsy in patients with refractory seizures (Table 17.2). They consist of focal resection or transection for discrete lesions, hemispherectomy when one entire hemisphere is affected, and corpus callosotomy (a disconnection of the two hemispheres to interrupt seizure spread) when a multifocal disturbance makes a resective procedure impossible.

First, how the seizure type influences the need for surgical referral must be considered (Table 17.3). In general, seizures that occur unpredictably and cause impairment of consciousness, injury, or significant disability disturbances are those for which surgery becomes a reasonable choice. Seizures that produce impairment of consciousness cause far more problems than those that do not and typically give rise to significant social, psychological, and medical complications. In contrast, simple partial seizures rarely pose a significant problem; nevertheless, simple partial seizures are rarely profoundly disturbing or even disabling and warrant surgical consideration if medical therapy has failed. For example, simple partial seizures that cause intense vomiting or fear can make life quite unpleasant. Seizures that cause injury, such as tonic-clonic seizures and drop attacks (tonic or atonic seizures), also merit surgical consideration, chiefly because of the dangers inherent in the seizures themselves. The unpredictable timing of most seizures is another troublesome factor. If the patient knew that a seizure would occur on the first Tuesday of each month at 7:20 AM, then accommodations could probably be made for the condition. Not knowing when the next seizure will occur makes epilepsy very hard to handle.

What seizure frequency should be considered a serious problem warranting surgical consideration? No objective answer exists, but most patients who are willing to consider surgery have seizures at least every month or two. As information becomes available about the risks of less frequent seizures, however, this answer might change. After all, one or two seizures per year is sufficient to eliminate driving privileges.

Patients who most commonly undergo surgical intervention for their epilepsy have localized or focal lesions. Indeed, the very beginnings of meaningful surgery for epilepsy was the removal of an offending, localized brain lesion responsible for the seizures. Sir Victor Horsley initiated this therapy in the late nineteenth century and Wilder Penfield commenced the modern era in the late 1920s. It is interesting to note that the EEG was not used to localize a lesion until 1937,[7] when Herbert Jasper teamed with Penfield in Montreal.

Localization is a relative term when referring to epileptogenic lesions, because many people with partial epilepsy have fairly extensive abnormal areas within their brains. Often a large portion of the brain is epileptogenic. The relative disappearance of the term *focal* in favor of the term *localized* reflects not only a semantic change but reflects our more sophisticated understanding of the diverse nature of the extent of epileptogenic lesions.[8] However, when surgical treatment is performed, a fairly discrete lesion can often be removed with subsequent elimination of seizures.

One consideration when thinking about surgery, therefore, is whether a localized lesion is likely to be present. The process begins with the medical history, in which the physician attempts to elicit data from the patient that meet the usual template for partial seizures (i.e., those attacks in which a localized onset can be documented). One begins by searching for the aura, which occasionally offers a clue as to the likely source of seizures. Sometimes the symptoms may not identify the locus of the lesion or may be misleading; attempts to categorize symptoms, such as the "initial stare," for example, remain controversial. Difficulties arise especially when attempting to lateralize a temporal lobe lesion or to distinguish between a temporal and a frontal lesion.[8] Newer techniques, such as magnetic resonance imaging (MRI) and positron emission tomography (PET) are improving our ability to discriminate among these lesions, making the syndrome of frontal lobe epilepsy more approachable.[9] For those patients in whom the diagnosis of frontal lobe epilepsy was correct but who did poorly after frontal lobe surgery, reoperation may be of value.[10]

If the history suggests the presence of localized epilepsy and if appropriate medications have been deemed ineffective, confirmatory laboratory data are required to substantiate the localized nature of the seizures. These evaluations, which include neuroimaging, cognitive testing, and EEG with intensive video monitoring, are all designed to identify an epileptogenic structural lesion. It is now well recognized that scalp EEG recordings, although essential, are at times misleading,[8] and that other tests of brain structure and function must be used before surgery can be offered.

Sometimes the epileptogenic lesion involves much of one hemisphere of the brain, and the bulk of the problem cannot be ascribed to one lobe. Conditions, such as Rasmussen's chronic encephalitis,[11] porencephaly, and dysplastic syndromes, may be associated with widespread hemispheric epileptogenesis. Patients usually have little normal function attributable to that hemisphere and are paretic or plegic in the affected limbs. In that circumstance, the purpose of an evaluation is to determine that the injury is widespread but largely confined to a single hemisphere. If so, a procedure known as hemispherectomy can be performed; this often provides seizure relief with few detrimental consequences.

Other patients have a multifocal brain disturbance affecting both hemispheres. These individuals are usually mentally retarded and suffer from several kinds of seizures, including tonic-clonic seizures and tonic or atonic seizures. The history usually reveals difficulties from an early age and the examination shows bilateral brain dysfunction. The EEG pattern is characterized by bilateral disturbances, and neuroimaging findings may be unremarkable or show bilateral abnormalities (e.g., atrophy, porencephaly, multiple dysplasias). In this circumstance, a partial or complete corpus callosotomy often helps by reducing or eliminating seizures that cause abrupt falls (tonic or atonic) and tonic-clonic seizures. The efficacy of the procedure relates to the degree of cognitive dysfunction, seizure type, and specific EEG findings. This operation is palliative rather than curative and is reserved for seizures that pose risk of injury or disability.

SOCIAL AND MOTIVATIONAL FACTORS

The goal that physicians should establish in treating someone with epilepsy is to help restore as normal a life as possible and limit the adverse medical consequences. The medical repercussions of epilepsy are not obvious to most patients unless they suffer direct bodily injury from a seizure, but the social and psychological consequences are readily apparent. People with epilepsy endure many restrictions that chafe, more so with each passing year, and make life less pleasurable than it could be.

Throughout development, a child with epilepsy requires special arrangements and adjustments that invariably take their toll.[12] Parents, quite justifiably, usually place restrictions on the child's activities and may be overprotective, often leading to abnormal psychological development—particularly in the teen years when gaining independence is a key part of the maturing process. Ordinary childhood joys, such as riding a bicycle, roller skating, and swimming, assume new meanings when a child has epilepsy. The decision to send a child away to camp or college raises different considerations when the child has seizures. Children, like adults, tend to ostracize those who are different, and friendships can be harder to cement and maintain. If seizures are caused by an underlying brain injury and cognitive defects are present, the problems are compounded. In the adolescent years, dating raises even more new issues. Obtaining a driver's license, a rite of passage for most American teenagers, is usually not possible for a teen with active epilepsy, who is then denied one of adolescence's formal certificates of maturity.

An adult with epilepsy may carry some psychosocial baggage from childhood into adulthood if the seizures started early, and new problems develop if the seizures are uncontrolled. Activity restrictions prohibit certain occupations, and, in some people, the seizures are completely disabling.[13] The inability to drive limits where a person with epilepsy can live, how he or she gets to work (if a job can be obtained), what recreational activities can be enjoyed, and how often socialization with others is possible. In general, the level of independence is diminished compared with unaffected adults. Social interactions with others may at times take on a different character. Family responsibilities, such as bathing young children and supervising their outdoor activities, require second thought. Seeing a seizure in a parent may have a profound effect on children and in some way change the relationship between parent and child, particularly as the child ages. Seizures that produce socially stigmatizing behavior, such as inappropriate vocalization, undressing, or incontinence, can lead the patient to restrict activities beyond what is necessary because of embarrassment. Last, unpleasant auras can induce agoraphobia, a not uncommon condition in individuals with epilepsy. These instances are only a few examples of the ways that uncontrolled seizures reduce the quality of life.

Many of these problems can be directly ascribed to seizures themselves. Recent studies suggest that even having a few seizures has an adverse impact on the quality of life and that a seizure frequency of one per month is another significant breakpoint.[14] That is why it is desirable to completely prevent seizures from occurring, and why the term "good control" means *no* seizures, not *occasional* seizures. Consequently, the decision to consider surgery follows naturally from an assessment of the impact of seizures on day-to-day life. The question to pose to a patient with uncontrolled seizures is not whether the patient can live with the seizures, but whether life would be better without the seizures or, failing that, whether life would be better if the seizure frequency were markedly reduced. It is difficult for some patients to pragmatically answer this question because they may have unrealistic expectations, but many are quite insightful. Surgical therapy for refractory epilepsy therefore becomes a rational response to a situation in which uncontrolled seizures lead to loss of control over one's life. Surgery, if successful, enables the patient to reassert control, to have a better quality of life, and to improve employment prospects.[15]

CHOICE OF A SURGICAL CENTER

How is a center for epilepsy surgery chosen? As with other surgical operations, a team experienced in epilepsy surgery is essential. It must know how to properly select patients to optimize results and to operate on the patient safely and minimize complications. Patient selection is not a trivial exercise but requires great skill and experience; high volume leads to lower complication rates and better judgment. Since worldwide the number of surgical procedures performed for the control of epilepsy is still relatively low compared with other types of surgery, the number of desired yearly epilepsy operations per center is not measured in hundreds but rather in dozens. Surgical centers should probably perform at least 25 therapeutic procedures annually to maintain adequate skill levels; higher numbers presumably confer an added advantage. The center should have precise statistics that detail how many operations of each type have been done, the results for each type of operation, and the incidence of complications. These statistics should not be estimates, but should be based on hard data. Results from a center can then be compared with the literature when forming a judgment. Seizure-free rates vary depending on the type of operation, ranging from 70% for temporal lobectomy to 30–50% for extratemporal resections, depending on the cause. The incidence of major, permanent, neurologic complications should be below 1%. Additionally, there is an advantage to centers that perform clinical research with their epilepsy surgery patients; in this way the scientific field advances as patients come to surgery.

RECENT ADVANCES IN SURGICAL THERAPY OF EPILEPSY

Few of the recent advances in surgical therapy for the epilepsies are direct technique-generated studies of new approaches for the surgical operating theater. This is not to say that some new surgical techniques have not been devised, because many have, but most progress in epilepsy surgery lies in improved methods of evaluating patients for surgery. The reason for this is simple; most of the investigative effort in epilepsy surgery has been devoted to the localization of lesions in the partial epilepsies. If the investigative highlights of the last few years are reviewed, the following areas have been the most prominent areas of surgical evaluation: (1) the use of MRI in the localization of the epileptic focus, (2) the continuing refinement of electrocorticography in the localization of the epileptic discharge, (3) the use of the Wada test to localize and predict the outcome of the surgery, and (4) surgical outcomes.

Use of Magnetic Resonance Imaging in the Localization of the Epileptic Focus

The use of MRI has "revolutionized the evaluation of medically intractable epileptic patients who are being considered for epilepsy surgery."[16] Not only can it detect structural lesions, but it has the capability of preoperatively detecting mesial temporal abnormalities, which heretofore has been an impossible task. Some investigators have emphasized the improved outcomes for those patients who have a mass "lesion" or atrophy of a hippocampus, as opposed to those in whom surgical therapy is undertaken in the absence of such a lesion.[17, 18] Although early studies suggested that the ratio of the volumes would yield a reliable predictor of which side was atrophic (and therefore contained the epileptogenic lesion to be removed), recent advances also show that mesial temporal sclerosis can be bilateral and, furthermore, that some patients can have successful surgery in spite of the bilateral nature of the lesions.[19, 20] The MRI criteria continue to advance rapidly, and the impact on surgical evaluation continues. Spencer noted, however, that the MRI scan is "not an independent surrogate for the other functional and electrographic criteria used to diagnose medial temporal epilepsy," but must be evaluated in the context of all the available data from these various sources.[16]

Continuing Refinement of Intracranial Electroencephalography in the Localization of the Epileptic Discharge

The backbone of presurgical diagnosis and localization of lesions to be removed has been EEG and more direct recording modalities, such as intraoperative electrocorticography and chronic intracranial recording. The abnormal focus is defined by the various techniques with a certainty that has ensured the EEG study as the "gold standard" for this process. And new observations continue. In studies of patients with attacks that involve the face, for example, Lehman et al.[21] have successfully used electrocorticography to obtain a more precise excision with fewer additional deficits outside the area designed for removal. The techniques are also applicable to patients with epilepsy and tumors.[22] It should be noted that many patients do not require invasive intracranial EEG recordings in the presurgical evaluation, especially for temporal lobe seizures,[18, 23, 24] although these are used more often for non-temporal seizures.[25] Data obtained noninvasively, such as that from the clinical seizure pattern, interictal and ictal scalp EEG recordings, MRI scan, PET scan, single photon emission computed tomography (SPECT) scan, neuropsychological testing, and the intracarotid amobarbital evaluation, often provide sufficient information to permit surgery without intracranial investigation. In extratemporal epilepsy, clear-cut identification of a lesion on an MRI scan improves the likelihood of a seizure-free outcome.[25]

Role of the Wada Test in Localization and Outcome Prediction

In the pursuit of the locus of onset of the epileptic focus, the first question is whether a locus exists, and then, if it does, can it be defined. The Wada test (also known as the intracarotid amobarbital test) has been routinely used to define the language-dominant hemisphere and to evaluate lateralization of long-term memory, primarily as a measure of the safety of tissue removal in temporal lobectomy. More recent studies of the Wada test, however, strongly suggest that additional, important information can be obtained by proper analysis of the data. Sperling et al.[26] noted that when the memory deficit was lateralized with the Wada test, patients had an increased probability of becoming seizure-free after surgery. Similarly, Loring et al.[27] observed that memory asymmetries were significantly greater in those patients who were seizure free, compared with those whose asymmetry was not as great, and who, on average, had a poorer outcome. Perrine et al.[28] made similar observations in a collaborative effort between two centers. The test has been extended to evaluate memory decline after left temporal lobectomy,[29] and efforts have been made to circumvent some of the deficiencies of the Wada test by using intraoperative thermal inactivation.[30] All of these continuing efforts are aimed at better lateralization and localization of the focus in an attempt to ensure that extirpation is minimal and accurate. Evidence continues to accumulate suggesting that a patient with a well-localized lesion is a much better candidate for successful surgery than if the lesion is poorly localized; this observation is also true in children.[31]

How Good is Surgery?

In addition to all of the technical aspects of surgery and the presurgical evaluation, some investigators are becoming more sophisticated in evaluating surgical outcomes, attempting to put in better perspective the appropriate role of surgery in the management of patients with severe epilepsy. Some investigators[32] suggest that postoperative follow-up should be at least 6 months to be assured of collecting meaningful data, but newer data[33] suggest that, for temporal lobe surgery, at least 2 years of follow-up is needed to reasonably predict a long-term result. Others[34] have analyzed the postoperative EEG recordings and have shown that, in certain patients, the EEG findings predict success or failure; still others use PET findings to make predictions on patient outcome.[35] Using pathologic criteria, Sass et al.[36] observed that the degree of hippocampal neuronal loss was a predictor of the severity of verbal memory loss after dominant temporal lobectomy. On a broader front, others, such as Vickrey et al.,[14] are approaching the issue of health-related quality of life after epilepsy surgery, consistent with the continuing reform of health care delivery in the United States, and are developing a seizure-based surgery outcome system to address this issue specifically.

SUMMARY

Surgery has been proved safe and effective for treating people with intractable seizures. Consequently, patients should be referred for a surgical evaluation as soon as medical intractability is established, provided they have a nonremitting and nonprogressing epilepsy syndrome. There is, indeed, a real disadvantage in continuing to pursue ineffective medical therapy; the risks of developing new complications, such as medical and neurologic morbidity, mortality, and psychosocial impairments, are considerable. The critical task is to recognize when someone has intractable epilepsy. Referral should then be made to an experienced epilepsy center, preferably one that performs many operations yearly, for evaluation for possible surgery. Prospects for attaining a seizure-free outcome after surgery continue to improve, and better methods also continue to be devised for selecting patients for surgery.

REFERENCES

1. Ward AA Jr. Perspectives for Surgical Therapy of Epilepsy. In AA Ward Jr, JK Penry, D Purpura (eds), Epilepsy. New York: Raven, 1983;371.
2. Engel J Jr (ed). Surgical Treatment of the Epilepsies (2nd ed). New York: Raven, 1993.
3. Theodore WH, Porter RJ. Epilepsy: 100 Elementary Principles (3rd ed). London: Saunders, 1995.
4. Dodrill CB. Correlates of generalized tonic-clonic seizures with intellectual, neuropsychological, emotional, and social function in patients with epilepsy. Epilepsia 1986;27:399.
5. Gilman JT, Duchowney M, Jayakar P, Resnick TJ. Medical intractability in children evaluated for epilepsy surgery. Neurology 1994;44:1341.
6. Sperling MR, Liporace JD, French JA, et al. Epilepsy surgery and mortality from epilepsy. Epilepsia 1995;36:140.
7. Flanigin HF, Hermann BP, King DW, et al. The History of Surgical Treatment of Epilepsy in North America Prior to 1975. In H Luders (ed), Epilepsy Surgery. New York: Raven, 1991;19.
8. Porter RJ, Sato S. Candidacy for Resective Surgery of Epilepsy. In H Luders (ed), Epilepsy Surgery. New York: Raven, 1991;105.
9. Laskowitz DT, Sperling MR, French JA, O'Connor MJ. The syndrome of frontal lobe epilepsy: characteristics and surgical management. Neurology 1995;45:780.

10. Salanova V, Quesney LF, Rasmussen T, et al. Reevaluation of surgical failures and the role of reoperation in 39 patients with frontal lobe epilepsy. Epilepsia 1994;35:70.

11. Rasmussen T, Andermann F. Update on the syndrome of "chronic encephalitis" and epilepsy. Cleve Clin J Med 1989;56(Suppl):S181.

12. Rodin E, Rennick P, Dennerll R, Lin Y. Vocational and educational problems of epileptic patients. Epilepsia 1972;13:149.

13. Elwes RD, Marshall J, Beattie A, Newman PK. Epilepsy and employment: a community based survey in an area of high unemployment. J Neurol Neurosurg Psychiatry 1991;54:200.

14. Vickrey BG, Hays RD, Engel J Jr, et al. Outcome assessment for epilepsy surgery: the impact of measuring health-related quality of life. Ann Neurol 1995;37:158.

15. Sperling MR, Saykin AJ, Roberts DF, et al. Occupational outcome after temporal lobectomy for refractory epilepsy. Neurology 1995;45:970.

16. Spencer SS. MRI and epilepsy surgery. Neurology 1995;45:1248.

17. Cascino GD, Trenerry MR, Sharbrough FW, et al. Depth electrode studies in temporal lobe epilepsy: relation to quantitative magnetic resonance imaging and operative outcome. Epilepsia 1995;36:230.

18. Berkovic SF, McIntosh AM, Kalnins RM, et al. Preoperative MRI predicts outcome of temporal lobectomy: an actuarial analysis. Neurology 1995;45:1358.

19. King D, Spencer S, McCarthy G, et al. Bilateral hippocampal atrophy in medial temporal lobe epilepsy. Epilepsia 1995;36:905.

20. Jack CR, Trenerry MR, Cascino GD, et al. Bilaterally symmetric hippocampi and surgical outcome. Neurology 1995;45:1353.

21. Lehman R, Andermann F, Olivier A, et al. Seizures with onset in the sensorimotor face area: clinical patterns and results of surgical treatment in 20 patients. Epilepsia 1994;35:1117.

22. Britton JW, Cascino GD, Sharbrough FW, Kelly PJ. Low-grade glial neoplasms and intractable partial epilepsy: efficacy of surgical treatment. Epilepsia 1994;35:1130.

23. Sperling MR, O'Connor MJ, Saykin AJ, et al. A non-invasive protocol for anterior temporal lobectomy. Neurology 1992;42:416.

24. Thadani VM, Williamson PD, Berger R, et al. Successful epilepsy surgery without intracranial EEG recording: criteria for patient selection. Epilepsia 1995;36:7.

25. Zentner J, Hufnagel A, Ostertun B, et al. Surgical treatment of extratemporal epilepsy: clinical, radiologic, and histopathologic findings in 60 patients. Epilepsia 1996;37:1072.

26. Sperling MR, Saykin AJ, Glosser G, et al. Predictors of outcome after anterior temporal lobectomy: the intracarotid amobarbital test. Neurology 1994;44:2325.

27. Loring DW, Meador KJ, Lee GP, et al. Wada memory performance predicts seizure outcome following anterior temporal lobectomy. Neurology 1994;44:2322.

28. Perrine K, Westerveld M, Kimberlee JS, et al. Wada memory disparities predict seizure laterality and postoperative control. Epilepsia 1995;36:851.

29. Loring DW, Meador KJ, Lee GP, et al. Wada memory asymmetries predict verbal memory decline after anterior temporal lobectomy. Neurology 1995;45:1329.

30. Lee GP, Smith JR, Loring DW, Flanigin HF. Intraoperative thermal inactivation of the hippocampus in an effort to prevent global amnesia after temporal lobectomy. Epilepsia 1995;36:892.

31. Fish DR, Smith SJ, Quesney LF, et al. Surgical treatment of children with medically intractable frontal or temporal lobe epilepsy: results and highlights of 40 years' experience. Epilepsia 1993;34:244.

32. Luders H, Murphy D, Awad I, et al. Quantitative analysis of seizure frequency 1 week and 6, 12, 24 months after surgery of epilepsy. Epilepsia 1994;35:1174.

33. Sperling MR, O'Connor MJ, Saykin AJ, Plummer C. Temporal lobectomy for refractory epilepsy. JAMA 1996;276:470.

34. Patrick S, Berg A, and Spencer SS. EEG and seizure outcome after epilepsy surgery. Epilepsia 1995;36:236.

35. Manno EM, Sperling MR, Ding X, et al. Predictors of outcome after anterior temporal lobectomy: positron emission tomography. Neurology 1994;44:2331.

36. Sass KJ, Westerveld M, Buchanan CP, et al. Degree of hippocampal neuron loss determines severity of verbal memory decrease after left anteromesiotemporal lobectomy. Epilepsia 1994;35:1179.

18
Psychosocial and Behavioral Function in Epilepsy

Orrin Devinsky

The pendulum of medical and lay viewpoints swings slowly. Hippocrates recognized epilepsy as a brain disorder. However, it took more than two millennia for this fact to gain wide acceptance. Overcoming the force of centuries linking epilepsy with evil, curses, violence, and stupidity has been slow and remains incomplete. While we move toward greater understanding and compassion, the trail of discrimination, stigma, and antiquated conceptions remains.

In caring for people with epilepsy, health care professionals must recognize and address the magnitude of the psychosocial burden endured by patients. We must help them understand what having epilepsy means and how they can best lead full and productive lives. This involves more than trying to simply eliminate or reduce the number of seizures and adverse effects of medication and more than achieving a balance between seizure control and side effects. Although seizures and side effects have an impact on psychosocial and behavioral function, they are a small part of the bigger picture that comprises a person's ability to function and thrive (Table 18.1). The health care community must begin to recognize and address this larger realm of where and how patients live their lives.

PSYCHOSOCIAL IMPLICATIONS OF EPILEPSY

The diagnosis of epilepsy has tremendous psychological and social repercussions. The initial reaction to the diagnosis often conjures up horrific images of the attacks and the stereotypes of people afflicted with the disorder. For many, a frightening mental collage emerges—uncertainty about the future, fear of medication effects on the body and mind, when and if the next seizure will strike, progressive mental or physical disability, unwanted disclosure of their secret, loss of driving and other privileges, fear of losing who they are and how they imagined their future. The initial impact of the diagnosis can be minimized by information. Physicians should explore how patients feel about the diagnosis and what aspects

Table 18.1   Psychosocial, cognitive, and behavioral issues in patients with epilepsy

Psychosocial
    Self-esteem
    Independence
    Discrimination: perceived and real
    Stigma of epilepsy
    Need to take medication
    Education
    Employment
    Social activities and restrictions
    Social support
    Physical role limitations
    Driving
    Embarrassment from seizure
Behavioral
    Emotional well-being
    Emotional role limitations
    Depression
    Anxiety
    Paranoia and psychosis
    Fear concerning seizures
    Fear concerning adverse effects of medications
    Level of energy
    Sexual interest
    Sexual function
    Personality disorders
Cognitive
    Speed of mental processing
    Memory
    Language
    Arithmetic skills
    Abstract thought
    Judgment and reasoning

cause them the greatest concern. Pamphlets and books are available to explain the disorder. In some cases, having another epilepsy patient in a similar age and social group to talk to can provide excellent support.

People with epilepsy have higher rates of psychological and psychiatric problems. The disorder typically causes the greatest psychosocial impairment during seizure-free intervals. Medical therapy is often prolonged, drugs often need to be taken several times per day, and side effects can have an impact on a person's daily life; thus, the absence of seizures can lead to questions about the continuing need for medication. People with epilepsy may have limited social, educational, transportation, and employment opportunities. These restrictions may be real or perceived. In either case, they prevent people from even trying to obtain a job or pursue an activity. Parental and societal attitudes often foster low self-esteem and dependence, stigma, discrimination, and restrictions on independence. In considering epilepsy as a chronic burden, we must carefully examine social, psychological, and behavioral problems. These problems are often more disabling than the neurologic and physical disorders, which have been the traditional focus of study.

An individual's response to the psychosocial burden of epilepsy varies depending on his or her premorbid background, including self-esteem and independence, intellect, emotional strength, family and cultural bonds, and knowledge about the disorder. The physician's role in assessing and minimizing the psychosocial problems of epilepsy has rarely received attention. For many patients, however, the psychosocial impact of epilepsy is far greater than its neurologic impact. Physicians must move toward recognizing and handling the cognitive, psychological, psychiatric, and social problems that accompany and often overshadow the traditional neurologic landscape of seizures and medication side effects.

Chronicity and Disability of Epilepsy

Epilepsy is often chronic and disabling. Chronicity leads to a complex reaction over time. Initially, many patients deny the illness through medication noncompliance, failure to follow up with physicians, and continuing lifestyle habits that can provoke seizures, such as excessive alcohol consumption and sleep deprivation. When seizures recur despite the use of antiepileptic drugs (AEDs), many patients become frustrated and angry. Some change physicians or question whether the medication does anything. Others, however, patiently comply as the physician increases the dosage, changes medications or regimens, and systematically attempts to control seizures. Recurrent seizures affect the psyche of patients in various ways and to different degrees. Some acclimate with minimal disruption, continuing their social and occupational lives. For others, the anticipation of or occurrence of seizures prevents them from pursuing their usual activities.

Mild epilepsy, as defined medically, may not be mild when defined by the person with the disorder. A patient may be seizure-free for 1 year; however, the social diagnosis, fear of discrimination, restrictions on lifestyle, and effects of medication often persist. For patients with epilepsy that is difficult to control, the problems imposed on daily life often make living a full and emotionally healthy life quite difficult.

The disability of epilepsy is often overlooked. In the United States, the Americans with Disabilities Act encompasses epilepsy, since it is a neurologic disorder that can substantially limit major life activities. This law protects against discrimination based on disability in employment, activities of state and local governments, public and private transportation, public accommodations, and telecommunications. Similar laws exist in other countries.

Outcome measures for epilepsy patients traditionally include seizure frequency, severity and morbidity (e.g., seizure-related trauma), and systemic and central nervous system side effects of AEDs, such as sedation, nausea, and tremor. Traditional medical factors—seizures and side effects—are viewed quite differently by patients and physicians. "Occasional" or "mild" seizures and "infrequent" and "tolerable" side effects are often considered as "acceptable" by physicians. For patients, the same seizure frequency and adverse effects can be debilitating and are not considered acceptable. In many cases, the patient has difficulty expressing his or her feelings or the physician may not fully understand or attend to complaints. For example, a complaint may not fit the conventional wisdom, such as disabling lethargy or confusion with low therapeutic doses or serum levels of a "cognitively benign" drug. In either case, the physician remains unaware or unimpressed by the magnitude of the problems in the patient's life.

Learning and Education

Children and young adults with epilepsy usually have normal intelligence, although the bell-shaped curve is skewed toward the left, with a higher frequency of mental retardation and cognitive disorders. Short-term memory impairment is very common among children and adults with epilepsy. Academic problems are common in epilepsy groups and can occur even in those with normal intelligence. Whenever academic achievement falls short of expectations, causal factors should be sought. In some cases, expectations are unrealistic. In many more cases, explanations, such as attention or conduct disorders, specific learning disorders, neurologic impairment, frequent seizures, or medications that affect school performance, can be identified. In some cases, problems can be ameliorated with a change in AED dosage, schedule, or type. If parents suspect a problem or the teacher reports an academic or behavioral problem, possible causes should be explored. An educational assessment should be obtained, especially if AED manipulation does not improve school performance. This involves an evaluation of the child's cognitive and emotional status and identification of strengths and weaknesses, after which appropriate referrals for additional support or therapy may be made.

Children with epilepsy have traditionally been excluded from sports, regular classes, and social activities. The current trend, requiring constant reinforcement, is to include children with epilepsy in normal activities with their peers. In the United States and many other countries, the law guarantees a child's right to be educated in a regular classroom environment whenever possible and for as much of the school day as possible. The child should also be included in other social and school-related activities. Parents must serve as the child's advocate to ensure that they are not excluded. Physicians need to "hold the parents' hand," allowing them to comfortably pursue the principle of inclusion. It is often easier for parents to have their child excluded from a class trip or sport activity for fear that a seizure will occur in a potentially dangerous setting. In the vast majority of cases, excluding a child from school trips, sports, camps, or regular classrooms has a more detrimental long-term effect than the risk of a seizure.

Employment

Employment opportunities are limited for many adults with epilepsy, with unemployment and underemployment rates significantly elevated in this population. Despite laws to prevent unfair discrimination, people with epilepsy are often denied jobs or are fired after their disorder is discovered. Employers have discriminated against people with epilepsy largely because of the stigma associated with epilepsy and misconceptions about the social and neurologic aspects of epilepsy. Some employers simply fear the term "epilepsy." In other cases, there are unfounded fears of legal or medical liabilities or assumptions that people with epilepsy will pose more problems and be less productive than others. Employment problems impair self-esteem, limit financial independence, and, in countries such as the United States, affect the ability to obtain health insurance.

Patients often ask their doctors about employment issues. In cases of suspected discrimination with legal ramifications, physicians can offer limited specific advice but can refer patients to local or national epilepsy foundations or associations with experience in handling these matters. Legal advice and intervention are often extremely helpful. In some cases, employers may seek a doctor's opinion in determining if a person can safely perform a job. Physicians should provide their honest opinion, but they have often assumed a conservative position that severely limits employment opportunities. This conservatism is based on two issues: allow no risk to the patient and assume no legal liability. However, patients who are not allowed to work often suffer more persistent and damaging aftereffects than a work-related injury. In most cases, even when a person with epilepsy cannot safely perform a specific job function, the position can often be modified to accommodate the person. For example, persons with uncontrolled complex partial seizures cannot drive a delivery truck and no accommodation will permit them to fulfill this job function. However, this individual could sell shoes, even though the job occasionally requires the person to climb a ladder. The patient may be allowed to climb one or two steps, and can obtain help reaching shoes from other employees when necessary.

Family, Personal, and Social Issues

The social label of epilepsy can often paralyze patients. Children and adults with epilepsy may feel different and become removed from their social group and activities and occasionally from their family. Epilepsy places severe stresses on the family fabric. Epilepsy burdens the patient as well as siblings, parents, and spouses. Siblings often resent the extra attention that the "sick" child receives and resent the additional responsibilities that they must often assume. The emotional and financial impact of epilepsy is felt by the entire family.

People with epilepsy are constantly reminded by society that they are different. For example, children may be required to visit the school nurse for lunchtime medication, teenagers or adults may be restricted from driving or recreational activities, patients may have fears regarding urine tests identifying AEDs when seeking or maintaining employment, and patients may have fears of rejection by peers if a seizure occurs in public or if their disorder is revealed. Epilepsy differs from most other medical and neurologic disorders because of these legal restrictions and requirements. Also, patients may fear dating, sexual relations, marriage, decreased fertility, increased rate of pregnancy complications, birth defects, or the danger of a seizure occurring while holding a baby or giving the baby a bath.

Cognitive and Behavioral Problems

Epilepsy alters behavior during and between seizures. Behavior subsumes an extremely broad range of functions, including primary sensory and motor phenomena; perception, experience, and expression of emotions (e.g., anxiety, depression, anger, happiness); level of energy (e.g., fatigue, vigor) and motivation; understanding of social situations; ability to react to dynamic situations that require rapid responses; and autonomic responses. Cognition (intellectual) functioning is a subset of behavior, including attention, vigilance, speed of intellectual processing, arithmetic and linguistic skills, processing of sensory stimuli, learning, memory, coordination and speed of motor responses, musical appreciation and skills, and visuospatial abilities. Most studies of the cognitive and behavioral aspects of epilepsy and AEDs investigate only a few functional areas. For example, commonly used intelligence tests do not provide information regarding memory and learning and provide limited data regarding attention and vigilance. Furthermore, most cognitive and behavioral studies consist mainly of tests, questionnaires, surveys, and interviews; their relevance for function and success in the real world is limited and often poorly defined.

Most epilepsy patients have normal or even superior intelligence. However, patients with epilepsy often have more cognitive impairment and behavioral problems than individuals in the general population.[1–4] Cognitive impairment and behavioral changes were documented in epilepsy patients before the introduction of bromides and other AEDs.[5, 6] In children and adults with epilepsy, various cognitive problems can occur, including impaired memory, naming, comprehension and fluency, abstract thought and reasoning, judgment of social situations, arithmetic skills, visuospatial skills, and praxis. Neuropsychological testing can identify cognitive disorders and can also reveal areas of relative strength, which may allow for compensatory strategies.

Patients with epilepsy have higher rates of psychiatric disorders, such as depression or anxiety.[7] Other neurobehavioral problems in epilepsy patients include personality disorders, psychosis, mania, and dissociative disorders, including conversion. Anxiety about the occurrence of seizures is common because of lack of control, sudden onset, and possibility of injury or embarrassment.[8, 9] Patients with fear during simple partial seizures may be more prone to certain psychiatric disorders and hospitalization.[10–12] Children with epilepsy have approximately twice the rate of psychiatric disorders as other children. Anxiety and depression are the most frequent behavioral problems in adults with epilepsy.[13] Behavioral and psychiatric disorders need to be recognized. In many cases, counseling or psychotherapy provides valuable support and helps relieve symptoms. In other cases, psychotropic medications are needed. Because behavioral problems are associated with significant morbidity and mortality (e.g., suicide rates among patients with epilepsy are at least five times higher than in the general population),[14] these disorders must receive a higher priority in diagnosis and treatment.[15, 16]

Epilepsy-related factors associated with impaired cognitive or behavioral function include age of onset and duration of epilepsy,[17–21] seizure frequency,[22, 23] history of tonic-clonic seizures,[3, 24] lifetime number of tonic-clonic seizures,[25] and episodes of status epilepticus.[26] These factors suggest that a reduction in seizure frequency, severity, or years of active seizures may improve or prevent deterioration of cognitive or behavioral functioning. Because AEDs control seizures, direct effects of AEDs on cognition and behavior must be evaluated in light of their effects on reducing seizure frequency and severity. The relationship of various etiologic factors can be complex. For example, a social withdrawal syndrome with low rates of employment and marriage may result from a combination of low educational attainment and self-esteem, legislative restrictions, perceived stigma and actual discrimination, and cognitive and behavioral deficits (impaired memory, hyposexuality).[27] Biologic (e.g., cognitive impairment) and medication factors (e.g., depression, lethargy, tremor, weight gain) can further complicate this syndrome.[12, 28]

Physical Issues

Seizures increase the risk of bruises, lacerations, bone fractures and dislocations, burns, and drowning as well as unexplained death.[29–31] Daily medications reduce the seizure threshold but can cause adverse physical effects (e.g., gingival hyperplasia, sedation, nausea, double vision, tremor, hirsutism, osteopenia, and anemia) and mental effects (e.g., memory impairment and psychomotor slowing), some of which are subtle but chronic.[32] Quality of life measures correlate negatively with the systemic or neurologic adverse effects in epilepsy patients.[33]

WHY MEASURE PSYCHOSOCIAL OUTCOME?

Medical attention directed solely at seizure control could have grave consequences, as recognized in the early twentieth century. Gowers[34] and Spratling[35] observed dose-related adverse mental effects of bromides, including general brain depression, impaired memory, irritability, delusions, dribbling, and a tendency toward abuse. Lennox eloquently stated the importance of balancing seizure control and medication effects, for "many physicians in attempting to extinguish seizures only succeed in drowning the finer intellectual processes of their patients."[17]

The cognitive and behavioral problems of epilepsy, noted for centuries, were first systematically studied with neuropsychological testing to define functional brain deficits and the Minnesota Multiphasic Personality Inventory (MMPI) to assess personality issues.[36] Psychiatric rating scales have been used to assess specific problems, such as anxiety or depression, psychosocial inventories have been used to evaluate psychological and social factors (e.g., employment and life activities), and quality-of-life scales have been used to assess the patient's perspective on a broad range of health-related issues.

The first epilepsy-specific psychosocial measure was the Washington Psychosocial Seizure Inventory (WPSI).[37] This 132-item self-report measure consists of eight psychosocial scales (family background; emotional, interpersonal, and vocational adjustment; financial status; adjustment to the diagnosis of seizures and epilepsy; satisfaction with medical management; and overall psychosocial functioning) and three validity scales. The WPSI has been used extensively in evaluating psychological and social functioning among epilepsy patients. The WPSI has also been used to assess outcome after interventions, such as epilepsy surgery or the use of new AEDs.[38]

Several other scales have been developed to assess well-being and social aspects of life in epilepsy patients. The Well-Being Scale[39] examines social and physical functions and includes six subscales: self-esteem, life fulfillment, social difficulty, physical symptoms, worries, and affect-balance. In one study, epilepsy patients had lower well-being scores on all scales than a non-epileptic control group.[39] Lower well-being scores were directly related to seizure frequency and visibility of severe seizures. The Social Effects Scale was developed after extensive patient interviews.[40] Fourteen social aspects of epilepsy were included in the final version, which has been used in the National General Practice Survey of Epilepsy in the United Kingdom.[41]

QUALITY-OF-LIFE MEASURES

The past decade has witnessed the rapid growth of quality of life (QOL) as a vital measure in health care, complementing other traditional measures of medical outcomes. QOL refers to patients' perspective of how they feel and function. In assessing clinical care, QOL measures permit a greater understanding of the role a patient's apparent wellness (or lack thereof) plays in emotional and physical status.[42] The spotlight that QOL has drawn reflects greater recognition than in chronic disorders: The medical symptoms encompass only a fraction of the morbidity and disability. As the population ages and therapies advance, chronic disorders increase in prevalence. QOL outcomes may be the most relevant measure for patients with chronic disorders.

The role of QOL in health care received its most forceful introduction by Karnofsky more than 40 years ago.[43] The zeal to cure or prolong the life of cancer patients needed to be tempered by how the treatment affected the patient's well-being, especially in cases where therapy provided only slight gains in survival. Three additional months in severe pain and no meaningful function does not justify 4 months of unpleasant and time-consuming therapy for cancer. This insight—that the treatment could be worse than the disease (as was recognized in epilepsy by Gowers, Spratling, and Lennox)—is now medical common sense, but was poorly recognized by the academic medical community before Karnovsky introduced scales to assess functional status of cancer patients.

The dramatic rise in QOL assessments in clinical trials, cost-utility analyses, and studies of quality of care reflects the unique nature and value of the data.[44, 45] The patient's perspective provides the "bottom line" of how he or she is doing. The cost of patient bias is far outweighed by the real and direct nature of the measure. Neuropsychological tests and seizure calendars may be less biased and viewed as more quantitative (compared with the qualitative nature of QOL data), but such traditional medical outcome measures (e.g., neuropsychological tests) are of limited relevance to daily life. Also, they are restricted in scope and viewpoint (e.g., seizures affect people in different ways). Medicine myopically focuses on medical outcome, measuring symptoms, signs, and laboratory studies—viewing the disorder from the physician's perspective. Patient histories and reports are used, but their complaints are reformatted. Although the physician's and the patient's perspectives of the patient's QOL might be predicted to be quite similar, such correlations are often poor.[46] QOL recognizes that the patient is the "expert" on his or her own health status.[47]

As patients, payers, health care organizations, and governments demand more effective and cost-efficient care for patients, medicine must find more efficient and rapid methods for evaluating the quality of care than randomized double-blind studies.[48] QOL studies can examine a cross-section of treatment groups and provide rapid assessment of patient outcome. Also, QOL measures can be invaluable in traditional double-blind studies. For example, Croog et al.[49] evaluated different antihypertensive drugs with a QOL battery and helped define optimal therapeutic approaches based on the patient's perspective. This landmark study dramatically changed physicians' prescribing habits and identified major side effects of beta-blockers that were commonly overlooked by physicians—fatigue, depression, and impotence. All of these side effects occur with AEDs.

HEALTH-RELATED QUALITY OF LIFE

The World Health Organization defined health-related quality of life (HRQOL) as a state of complete physical, mental, and social well-being, not merely the absence of disease or infirmity.[50] HRQOL consists of three principal dimensions: physical health (e.g., daily function, general health, seizures, medication side effects, pain, strength, and endurance), mental health (e.g., perception of well-being, self-esteem, perceived stigma, anxiety, depression, and cognition), and social health (e.g., social activities and relationships with family and friends). Economic and environmental factors are encompassed by QOL but are not included in HRQOL assessment. QOL assessments in epilepsy must evaluate seizure frequency and severity, medication side effects, HRQOL, and other social and economic areas, such as employment and driving.

MEASURING HEALTH-RELATED QUALITY OF LIFE IN EPILEPSY

HRQOL issues are most important in chronic disorders associated with problems beyond the experience of the "disease symptoms." Epilepsy is the paradigm of a disorder in which HRQOL issues define the disorder. Seizures are typically infrequent, whereas psychosocial problems and AED therapy and side effects are usually chronic. Psychosocial issues are often the most disabling for epilepsy patients, but physicians receive little or no education about these problems and are often uncomfortable and unskilled in addressing them.

Traditional medical outcome measures (seizures and side effects) as well psychological, psychiatric, and social measures have been the mainstay of quantifying how people with epilepsy "were doing." As HRQOL becomes more important in medical care, research, and health economics and policy, the need for HRQOL measures in epilepsy becomes evident. Such measures must be practical to use, quantify what they purport to measure (validity), and be consistent from one administration to the next (reliability). Generic and specific instruments are available to assess HRQOL.

Generic instruments assess broad functions (e.g., overall feelings of well-being, capacity to perform daily work and social activities, etc.) and can study many disorders. These instruments usually result from extensive development and testing.

They are relatively brief and efficient, and allow comparisons between different groups. However, generic instruments are limited because many questions (e.g., how many blocks can you walk or how severe is the pain) may not be relevant to specific disorders, such as epilepsy. Generic instruments may be insensitive to the most important aspects of specific disorders and therapies.

Specific instruments focus on a certain disorder or population but usually do not permit comparisons between different disorders. In assessing epilepsy, its unique aspects make a specific instrument desirable. QOL assessment in epilepsy is complicated because of the way in which the same symptoms affect different individuals, the diversity of seizure types and manifestations, and epilepsy syndromes. A comprehensive survey of important health-related areas of concern is a difficult task, and the relative importance of each domain might differ considerably between patients.

Several HRQOL in epilepsy scales and instruments have been developed during the past decade and are briefly reviewed here.[33, 51–53]

General Health-Related Quality of Life Assessment in Epilepsy Patients

A well-validated and commonly used generic HRQOL instrument, the RAND 36 Health Survey (also known as the SF-36) was used to assess general HRQOL in 148 epilepsy patients.[54] Data from the epilepsy population were compared with an age-, sex-, and socioeconomically matched healthy population. Epilepsy patients had significantly lower scores in six of eight domains (overall QOL, health perceptions, physical and emotional role limitations, energy/fatigue, and emotional well-being). Patients with seizures occurring within 1 week of the inventory had significantly lower scores than those who were seizure-free for more than 1 year. Patients with systemic and neurologic adverse effects had lower HRQOL scores in five domains than patients without adverse effects.[55]

The RAND 36-item health survey scores from epilepsy surgery patients were compared with those of patients with medical and psychiatric disorders.[56] Patients who were seizure-free after surgery typically had significantly better scores on HRQOL scales than patients with various medical disorders. Patients with persistent postoperative simple partial seizures had similar HRQOL scores as patients with heart disease, diabetes, and hypertension. Patients with persistent postoperative complex partial or tonic-clonic seizures had lower emotional well-being and overall HRQOL scores than other patient groups, except those with depression.[56]

Epilepsy Surgery Inventory-55

The Epilepsy Surgery Inventory-55 (ESI-55) was developed to assess HRQOL outcome after epilepsy surgery.[51] The ESI-55 consists of a generic core and an epilepsy-targeted supplement. The generic core consists of the RAND 36-item health survey[57] with the addition of 19, mostly epilepsy-specific, items. Fifty-four items are comprised by 11 scales assessing HRQOL dimensions. One additional item assesses change in health over the preceding year. Patients undergoing epilepsy surgery represent less than 1% of the epilepsy population, but much of the ESI-55 is relevant for other epilepsy populations. However, some aspects of HRQOL are sparsely covered in the ESI-55, especially those concerning social functioning, for which there was only a two-item scale.

After surgery, patients with persistent seizures had worse HRQOL than those who were completely seizure free on all 11 ESI-55 scales ($p<0.05$). Postoperative auras correlated with poorer HRQOL, thus challenging the traditional classification schema, which places seizure-free patients together with those having persistent auras.[58] The ESI-55 data, collected on a group of more than 100 patients after epilepsy surgery, were subsequently used to provide a methodologic model that is applicable to different diseases. This model enables different aspects of disorder severity to be integrated into a single measure, using HRQOL as the external standard. The study by Vickrey and colleagues has helped provide a more valid method for evaluating outcome based on seizures after surgery.[56]

Liverpool Quality of Life Battery

The Liverpool Quality of Life battery was created to assess the psychosocial outcomes in epilepsy using measures of *physical functioning* (seizure severity, seizure frequency, and activities of daily living), *social functioning* (life fulfillment, stigma, and impact of epilepsy), and *psychological functioning* (affect and balance scale, hospital anxiety and depression scale, self-esteem, and a mastery scale). The battery consists of various scales that have been adapted to study specific clinical settings and questions. Some of these scales were specifically developed to assess the impacts of epilepsy and its treatment; other scales were developed to assess different disorders but were successfully validated in epilepsy.[52, 59, 60] The Liverpool seizure severity scale has been incorporated in this battery and includes seizure variables that can have a significant impact on a patient's QOL but are often overlooked in traditional outcome measures of seizure frequency or severity. These variables include presence and duration of postictal confusion, postictal headache or sleepiness, falling to the ground, and the ability to predict attacks, as well as more traditional features, such as loss of consciousness and incontinence.[61]

Initially used to assess the psychosocial sequelae of AED continuation versus withdrawal,[62] the Liverpool group has applied HRQOL measures to other important epilepsy-related issues, including the impact of a new AED in patients with refractory epilepsy,[63] QOL and quality of services for a community-based population, efficacy of a novel AED in children with epilepsy and learning disabilities, and psychosocial outcomes of immediate versus delayed treatment in single seizures and early epilepsy.[64]

Quality of Life in Epilepsy Instruments

Quality of Life in Epilepsy (QOLIE) test instruments were developed using the ESI-55 as their base, with additional items to better assess social aspects of epilepsy and issues more relevant to a nonsurgical, better-controlled epilepsy

Table 18.2   The QOLIE-89[a] and QOLIE-31[b] scales

Scale	Number of items	
	QOLIE-89	QOLIE-31
Health perceptions	6	—
Seizure worry	5	5
Physical function	10	—
Role limitation, physical	5	—
Role limitation, emotional	5	—
Pain	2	—
Overall quality of life	2	2
Emotional well-being	5	5
Energy/fatigue	4	4
Attention/concentration	9	2
Memory	6	3
Language	5	1
Medication effects	3	3
Social function, work, driving	11	5
Social support	4	—
Social isolation	2	—
Health discouragement	2	—
Sexual function*	1	—
Change in health	1	—
Overall health*	1	1

QOLIE = quality of life in epilepsy.

[a]The QOLIE-89 contains 17 scales with 87 field-tested questions.

[b]The shorter QOLIE-31 includes items from selected scales of the QOLIE-89.

*Two additional items were added after validation studies.

Note: The QOLIE-10 contains one or more questions from each of the seven QOLIE-31 scales. Permission to use the QOLIE-89 and QOLIE-31 and scoring manuals may be obtained by writing to RAND, 1700 Main Street, PO Box 2138, Santa Monica, CA 90407-2138 (Attention: Contracts and Grant Services). Permission to use the QOLIE-10 may be obtained from Professional Postgraduate Services, 400 Plaza Drive, Seacaucus, NJ 07094.

population. As with the ESI-55, the RAND SF-36 serves as a generic core. The general HRQOL core was expanded with a pictorial chart (Dartmouth COOP study) and an overall QOL item (Faces Scale).[33] Eight additional multi-item scales assessed epilepsy-specific areas.[33] The epilepsy-targeted segment was derived from patient interviews, literature review, and expert opinion. An open-ended question encouraged patients to report additional issues affecting their QOL. More than 300 adults with epilepsy of varying severities completed the test inventory. Patients were also evaluated by a proxy (family member or a close friend with whom they had frequent contact). Three instruments were derived from this study: the QOLIE-89 (17 scales, 89 items; validated), the QOLIE-31 (7 scales, 31 items; validated), and the QOLIE-10 screening questionnaire (10 items selected from the 7 scales in the QOLIE-31; nonvalidated) (Table 18.2). Patients also completed a battery of neuropsychological tests and were evaluated for systemic and neurologic effects of medication.

Analysis of the test instrument's 17 multi-item scales suggested four principal factors: epilepsy-targeted, cognitive, mental health, and physical health. Health care use negatively correlated with HRQOL scores, whereas education and employment were positively correlated. The mood factor most strongly correlated with total HRQOL scores. Patients with few or no seizures had significantly better HRQOL scores than those with poorly controlled epilepsy on all four factors.[33] The epilepsy-targeted factor and the seizure worry, health discouragement, and work/driving/social function scales best discriminated between groups with different epilepsy severity.

The QOLIE-89 is a comprehensive instrument designed to assess the outcome of specific interventions (e.g., drug or surgical study). Measures include global QOL issues and areas of specific concern to epilepsy patients (e.g., seizure severity, fear of seizures, loss of control, AED side effects, cognitive and behavioral dysfunction, social limitations, stigma, and driving restrictions). The QOLIE-31 is a shorter instrument providing an overview of a patient's perceptions of his or her disease. It will also be used mainly as a research tool, but it can be used to assess patients in practice. The QOLIE-10 can be completed in less than 5 minutes and the physician can scan the results in seconds to assess the need for further evaluation or intervention.

HEALTH-RELATED QUALITY OF LIFE MEASURES IN EPILEPSY—WHAT IS THEIR ROLE?

The ultimate goal in developing an instrument to measure HRQOL in epilepsy is to change how physicians treating people with epilepsy perceive the disorder and care for their patients. HRQOL scales to assess epilepsy patients have already been accepted into research and are moving into larger numbers of AED trials, surgical trials, and studies on the quality of epilepsy care and services. HRQOL measures can never be used in isolation. They must be incorporated into a more global view of a population and a personal view of an individual.

HRQOL studies in epilepsy may lead to redefinitions of therapy similar to those that occurred in hypertension. Therapeutic studies were largely based on "measurable" outcomes, such as blood pressure, and side effects, such as hypokalemia. However, current trials now recognize that since many drugs effectively lower blood pressure, the important question is how they affect HRQOL. Recent research on newly developed AEDs is beginning to offer new options in caring for epilepsy patients. Since a single AED can control epilepsy in most patients, determining which drug to choose is now often largely based on which one is best tolerated. Such decisions are often made arbitrarily, since side-effect profiles do not clearly differentiate certain AEDs. However, large, double-blind clinical trials of HRQOL may demonstrate that certain drugs are associated with significantly greater or lesser impairment of overall HRQOL or specific HRQOL areas. This information may influence the clinician's decision whether to maintain the patient on the current regimen or try a newer AED that has demonstrated similar efficacy but fewer side effects.

Caution must be exercised in interpreting the results of epilepsy studies using HRQOL measures. The validity of HRQOL instruments is difficult to establish;

there is no gold standard. Many studies have provided validity through correlations with medical outcomes, the very measures from which HRQOL seeks independence. Available instruments have not been studied to assess their sensitivity and validity in different cultural, linguistic, and ethnic groups. Furthermore, study design may be important. For example, consider a study of HRQOL before and after epilepsy surgery. Some patients may undergo preoperative HRQOL testing while in the hospital and undergoing video-electroencephalogram (EEG) monitoring. During this time, AEDs are often withdrawn, and the patient may have had recent seizures, feared an imminent seizure, or experienced AED withdrawal symptoms. Comparison with an inventory obtained 1 year after surgery in an outpatient setting on stable AED doses may reveal more about the test conditions than the effects of surgery.

Data from well-designed HRQOL research studies must be individually applied to patient care. The Veterans Administration Epilepsy Multicenter Cooperative Study I (VAI) revealed that phenobarbital and primidone (Mysoline) have greater adverse effect profiles than carbamazepine and phenytoin.[32] However, some patients tolerate barbiturates and enjoy excellent seizure control. Studies assessing efficacy, tolerability, and HRQOL after specific interventions in large groups do not accurately predict how a patient will respond. We treat patients, not populations.

HEALTH-RELATED QUALITY OF LIFE IN CLINICAL PRACTICE

Studies are in the province of academia. Patients are cared for by physicians, only a small minority of whom are academics. What are the implications of HRQOL in epilepsy for patient care? In addition to HRQOL studies of epilepsy treatments having an impact on care, there is a more direct role of HRQOL— our view of people with epilepsy and our interactions with patients.

Integrating HRQOL issues into routine care of epilepsy patients remains a challenge. The integration must be top-down (physicians in practice) and bottom-up (educating medical students and house officers). We must learn to consider how epilepsy patients perceive overall feelings of well-being, epilepsy, seizures, medications, cognitive functions, emotional well-being, and social and economic functioning—not at the global level of a multicenter study, but at the personal level, during the routine outpatient follow-up visit and on the telephone.

The realities of clinical practice preclude physicians from exploring the full spectrum of QOL issues. However, a middle ground must be sought to improve health care. We can no longer count seizures and grade side effects from the isolated view of a 15-minute office visit. We must view these problems from the vantage point of a life in which these issues are inescapable, in which these issues are but a fraction of those that have an impact on the patient's life. The traditional goal of balancing the impact of seizures and side effects excludes the important psychosocial dimension, in which epilepsy imparts its greatest burden. It is unlikely that even short inventories (e.g., the QOLIE-10) will widely enter clinical practice to screen for HRQOL issues. However, physicians can begin to ask questions, such as, "How have your spirits been lately?" and "Overall, how has your life been going?" Such questions are more important than assessing tandem gait or reflexes at a follow-up visit.

Finally, what does a physician do once a behavioral or psychosocial problem is identified? Just as we have been limited in our ability to recognize these disorders, we have been ill-trained to tackle them. For many patients, the physician's interest and concern and a few words of encouragement will be very helpful. In many cases, the problems are chronic and not easily resolved. Referral to a psychologist, psychiatrist, social worker, support group, or national or local epilepsy foundation can be very helpful. Such referrals are simple and often beneficial.

REFERENCES

1. Barnes MR, Fetterman JL. Mentality of dispensary epileptic patients. Arch Neurol Psychiatry 1938;40:903.
2. MacLeod CM, Dekaban AS, Hunt E. Memory impairment in epileptic patients: selective effects of phenobarbital concentration. Science 1978;202:1102.
3. Smith DB, Craft BR, Collins J, et al. VA Cooperative Study Group 118. Epilepsia 1986;27:760.
4. Perrine K, Congett S. Neurobehavioral problems in epilepsy. In O Devinsky (ed), Epilepsy II: Special Issues. Neurol Clin 1994;12:129.
5. Esquirol E. Mental Maladies. A Treatise on Insanity. Philadelphia: Lea & Blanchard, 1845.
6. Romberg MH. A Manual of the Nervous Diseases of Man. London: Syndenham Society, 1853;202.
7. Devinsky O, Theodore WH. Epilepsy and Behavior. New York: Wiley-Liss, 1991.
8. Mittan RJ, Locke GE. The other half of epilepsy: psychosocial problems. Urban Health 1982;11:38.
9. Nickell PV, Uhde TW. Anxiety Disorders and Epilepsy. In O Devinsky, WH Theodore (eds), Epilepsy and Behavior. New York: Wiley-Liss, 1991;67.
10. Hermann BP, Dikmen S, Schwartz MS, et al. Interictal psychopathology in patients with ictal fear. Neurology 1982;32:7.
11. Hermann BP, Chabria S. Interictal psychopathology in patients with ictal fear: examples of sensory-limbic hyperconnection. Arch Neurol 1981;37:667.
12. Devinsky O. Interictal Behavioral Changes in Epilepsy. In O Devinsky, WH Theodore (eds), Epilepsy and Behavior. New York: Wiley-Liss, 1991;1.
13. Devinsky O, Vazquez B. Behavioral changes associated with epilepsy. Neurol Clin 1993;11:127.
14. Matthews WS, Barabas G. Suicide and epilepsy: a review of the literature. Psychosomatics 1981;22:515.
15. Mendez M. Causative factors for suicide attempts by overdose in epileptics. Arch Neurol 1989;46:1065.
16. Mendez M, Cummings J, Benson DF. Depression in epilepsy. Arch Neurol 1986;43:766.
17. Lennox WG. Brain injury, drugs, and environment as causes of mental decay in epilepsy. Am J Psychiatry 1942;99:174.
18. Serafetinides EA. Aggressiveness in temporal lobe epileptics and its relation to cerebral dysfunction and environmental factors. Epilepsia 1965;6:33.
19. Bourgeois BFD, Prensky AL, Palkes HS, et al. Intelligence in epilepsy: a prospective study in children. Ann Neurol 1983;14:438.
20. Saykin AJ, Gur RC, Sussman NM, et al. Memory deficits before and after temporal lobectomy: effect of laterality and age of onset. Brain Cogn 1989;9:191.
21. Vargha-Khadem F, Isaacs E, Van Der Werf S, et al. Development of intelligence and memory in children with hemiplegic cerebral palsy. Brain 1992;115:315.
22. Gowers WR. Epilepsy and Other Chronic Convulsive Diseases: Their Causes, Symptoms, & Treatment. New York: Wood & Co., 1885.
23. Blakemore CB, Ettlinger G, Falconer MA. Cognitive abilities in relation to frequency of seizures and neuropathology of the temporal lobes. J Neurol Neurosurg Psychiatry 1966;29:268.
24. Matthews CG, Klove H. MMPI performance in major motor, psychomotor, and mixed seizure classifications of known and unknown etiology. Epilepsia, 1968;9:43.

25. Dodrill CB. Correlates of generalized tonic-clonic seizures with intellectual, neuropsychological, emotional, and social function in patients with epilepsy. Epilepsia 1986;27:399.
26. Dodrill CB, Wilensky AJ. Intelletual impairment as an outcome of status epilepticus. Neurology 1990;40:23.
27. Hermann BP, Whitman S. Behavioral and personality correlates of epilepsy: a review, methodological critique, and conceptual model. Psychol Bull 1984;95:451.
28. Robertson MM. The organic contribution to depressive illness in patients with epilepsy. J Epilepsy 1989;2:189.
29. Finneli PF, Cardi JK. Seizures as a cause of fracture. Neurology 1989;39:858.
30. Pear PL. Bilateral posterior fracture dislocation of the shoulder: a case report. N Engl J Med 1970;283:135.
31. Jay GW, Leestma JE. Sudden death in epilepsy: a comprehensive review of the literature and proposed mechanisms. Acta Neurol Scand 1981;82(Suppl):1.
32. Mattson RH, Cramer JA, Collins JF, et al. Comparison of carbamazepine, phenobarbital, phenytoin and primidone in partial and secondarily generalized tonic clonic seizures. N Engl J Med 1985;313:145.
33. Devinsky O, Vickrey BG, Perrine K, et al. Development of an instrument of health-related quality of life for people with epilepsy. Epilepsia 1995;36:1089.
34. Gowers WR. Epilepsy and Other Chronic Convulsive Diseases: Their Causes, Symptoms, & Treatment (2nd ed). New York: Wood & Co., 1901.
35. Spratling WP. Epilepsy and its Treatment. Philadelphia: Saunders, 1904;365.
36. Tartar R. Intellectual and adaptive functioning in epilepsy: a review of 50 years of research. Dis Nerv Syst 1972;33:763.
37. Dodrill CB, Batzel LW, Queisser HR, et al. An objective method for the assessment of psychological and social problems among epileptics. Epilepsia 1980;21:123.
38. Dodrill CB, Arnett JL, Wommerville KW, Sussman NM. Evaluation of the effects of vigabatrin on cognitive abilities and quality of life in epilepsy. Neurology 1993;43:2501.
39. Collings JA. Psychosocial well-being and epilepsy: an empirical study. Epilepsia 1990;31:418.
40. Chaplin JE, Yepez R, Shorvon S, Floyd M. A quantitative approach to measuring the social effects of epilepsy. Neuroepidemiology 1990;9:151.
41. Chaplin JE, Yepez R, Shorvon SD, Floyd M. National General Practice study of epilepsy: the social and psychological effects of a recent diagnosis of epilepsy. BMJ 1992;34;1416.
42. Cramer JA. Quality of life for people with epilepsy. Neurol Clin 1994;12:1.
43. Karnofsky DA, Burchenal JH. The Clinical Evaluation of Chemotherapeutic Agents in Cancer. In CM MacLeod (ed), Evaluation of Chemotherapeutic Agents. New York: Columbia University Press, 1949;191.
44. Spilker B. Quality of Life Assessments in Clinical Trials. New York: Raven, 1990.
45. Guyatt GH, Feeny DH, Patrick DL. Measuring health-related quality of life. Ann Intern Med 1993;118:622.
46. Slevin MB, Plant H, Lynch D, et al. Who should measure quality of life, the doctor or the patient? Br J Cancer 1988;57:109.
47. Devinsky O. Outcome research in neurology: incorporating health-related quality of life. Ann Neurol 1995;39:142.
48. Greenfield S. The state of outcome research: are we on target? N Engl J Med 1989;320:1142.
49. Croog SH, Levine S, Testa M, et al. The effects of antihypertensive therapy on the quality of life. N Engl J Med 1986;314:1657.
50. Constitution of the World Health Organization. In World Health Organization, Handbook of Basic Documents (5th ed). Geneva: Palais des Nations, 1952;3.
51. Vickrey BG, Hays RD, Graber J, et al. A health-related quality of life instrument for patients evaluated for epilepsy surgery. Med Care 1992;30:299.
52. Baker GA, Jacoby A, Smith DF, et al. The development of a novel scale to assess life fulfillment as part of the further refinement of a quality of life model for epilepsy. Epilepsia 1994;35:591.
53. Jacoby A, Baker GA, Smith DF, et al. Measuring the impact of epilepsy: the development of a novel scale. Epilepsy Res 1993;16:83.
54. Wagner AK, Bungay KM, Bromfield EB, Ehrenberg BL. Health-related quality of life of adult persons with epilepsy as compared with health-related quality of life of well persons. Epilepsia 1993;34(Suppl 6):5.
55. Wagner AK, Bungay KM, Bromfield E, Ehrenberg BL. Relationship of health-related quality of life to seizure control and antiepileptic drug side effects. Epilepsia 1994;35(Suppl 8):56.

56. Vickrey BG, Hays RD, Rausch R, et al. Quality of life of epilepsy surgery patients as compared to outpatients with hypertension, diabetes, heart disease, and/or depressive symptoms. Epilepsia 1994;35:597.
57. Ware JE, Sherbourne CD. A 36-item short form health survey (SF-36). I. Conceptual framework and item selection. Med Care 1992;30:473.
58. Vickrey BG, Hays RD, Engel J, et al. Outcome assessment for epilepsy surgery: the impact of measuring health-related quality of life. Ann Neurol 1995;37:158.
59. Baker GA, Smith DF, Dewey M, et al. The initial development of a health-related quality of life model as an outcome measure in epilepsy. Epilepsy Res 1993;16:65.
60. Jacoby A, Baker GA, Smith DF, et al. Measuring the impact of epilepsy: the development of a novel scale. Epilepsy Res 1994;16:83.
61. Smith DF, Baker GA, Jacoby A, Chadwick DW. The contribution of the measurement of seizure severity to quality of life research. Qual Life Res 1995;4:143.
62. Jacoby A, Johnson A, Chadwick DM, on behalf of the Medical Research Council Antiepileptic Drug Withdrawal Group. Psychosocial outcomes of antiepileptic drug discontinuation. Epilepsia 1992;33:1123.
63. Smith DF, Baker GA, Davies G, et al. Outcomes of add-on treatment with lamotrigine in partial epilepsy. Epilepsia 1993;34:312.
64. Devinsky O, Baker G, Cramer JA. Health-related Quality of Life Scales to Assess Epilepsy. In J Engel Jr, TA Pedley (eds), Epilepsy: A Comprehensive Textbook. New York: Raven (in press).

19
Epilepsy Care and the Role of Specialized Epilepsy Centers

Robert J. Gumnit

Treatment of a patient with epilepsy requires a broad range of services from a health care system. Services can be broadly broken down into five categories:

1. Identification of the patient who is suspected of having epilepsy.
2. Diagnostic evaluation.
3. Choice and initiation of treatment.
4. Long-term management of the chronic disease.
5. Re-evaluation and specialized treatment of a patient who has not responded to the initial choice of therapy.

In all societies, the patient initially is seen by whomever provides primary care, usually a physician trained in family or general practice. The primary care physician is expected to possess relatively superficial knowledge of a broad range of medicine. It is very difficult for a primary care physician to be *au courant* with modern diagnostic and treatment knowledge of low-incidence diseases. For example, in the United States, the average primary care physician encounters one new case of epilepsy every 2 years.

In the United States and, to a lesser extent, Great Britain, an ordinary patient with epilepsy may never see a neurologist. In major urban centers, however, even patients with ordinary cases of epilepsy will have at least an initial neurologic consultation. As a result, if we can judge by surveys taken of patients with epilepsy, the majority of patients are unhappy with their plight, in terms of seizure control, vocational adjustment, toxicity, or other aspects of daily living.

As our knowledge of epilepsy increases and the range of treatments becomes broader, it is even more important to make a precise diagnosis of epilepsy type and epilepsy syndrome. This is still the exception rather than the rule.

The response in the United States and, to a lesser extent, in other parts of the world, has been to develop specialized epilepsy centers to which patients whose seizures have not responded to treatment can turn for highly specialized care.

Merely putting the name "Epilepsy Center" on the door to a clinic does not guarantee that a patient with epilepsy will receive the kinds of services that he or she needs. There are many university epilepsy centers that, for all practical purposes, consist of the regular neurology clinic in which patients are seen by the residents, the only difference being that the attending physician has a particular interest in epilepsy. There are other places in the United States where the treatment of epilepsy is looked on as a profit center and in which a grandiose name is given to relatively unsophisticated care. Even worse are those units that call themselves epilepsy centers and provide overly aggressive interventions based on ignorance. The same problems that plagued the 1960s are returning in the 1990s; patients are inappropriately undergoing procedures that produce complications and bad results, giving sophisticated epilepsy treatment a bad name.

Around the world, the term "epilepsy center" means different things. In some countries, an epilepsy center is a residential facility for people with uncontrolled seizures who find a place of refuge from their multiple social and psychological problems. Such centers have largely disappeared from the United States and exist in only a handful of locations in Great Britain. In the United States, the philosophy is to "mainstream" patients with chronic disease. Patients who have difficult epilepsy problems who cannot survive independently in the community often find themselves in residential facilities for the mentally retarded or the emotionally distressed. Usually these placements are appropriate, since to a very large extent most people with epilepsy are unable to live in the community because of emotional or intelligence problems rather than poor seizure control.

Epilepsy centers, in the sense of epilepsy clinics at university hospitals or major medical centers, tend to focus on intermittent interventions. Even patients who are seen over a long period are given very little support other than what they receive during a visit to the clinic, and that support only comes from the physician, perhaps with the assistance of a single nurse clinician.

In the United States, comprehensive epilepsy programs were established following an initiative by the National Institutes of Health (NIH) in the mid-1970s that built on the Public Health Service 314(c) initiatives of the 1960s. These centers were designed to provide a broad range of medical, psychological, psychiatric, social, educational, and surgical care with a commitment made to provide long-term case management. Implicit in this was an organization of community resources and advocacy on behalf of patients. Most of the community activities and advocacy activities were carried out only for as long as NIH funding was available. As NIH funding became more focused on research, especially basic research, the centers have had to struggle to maintain their comprehensive approach. A few have succeeded.

In 1990, the National Association of Epilepsy Centers issued a supplement to *Epilepsia* (volume 31, supplement 1, pp S1–S12) entitled "Recommended Guidelines for Diagnosis and Treatment in Specialized Epilepsy Centers." These recommended guidelines were a typical document of the 1980s. They were heavily process-oriented with very little attention given to outcome studies. Nonetheless, the guidelines did make clear that there were a variety of levels of comprehensiveness and outlined the kinds of expertise and facilities that should be available.

If primary care is provided by a family practitioner, then secondary care is provided by internists, pediatricians, and ordinary neurologists in practice. Tertiary-level medical centers are defined by the guidelines as providing the basic range of medical services needed in an epilepsy referral center. Some of these tertiary centers have competent neuropsychological diagnostic facilities available. Most are encouraged to have psychosocial services.

Fourth level or comprehensive medical and surgical centers were defined as serving as regional or national referral facilities providing services to a catchment area of millions of people. The centers provide the more complex form of intensive neurodiagnostic monitoring (video-electroencephalographic [EEG] monitoring, computerized ambulatory EEG) and other diagnostic procedures. They are expected to have extensive neuropsychological and psychosocial services. Many of them also provide fourth-level surgical services carrying out complete surgical evaluations and having the ability to perform a broad range of surgical procedures for epilepsy.

In the United States, the manner in which health care services are carried out is undergoing rapid change. There is great variability from locale to locale. Nonetheless, there is still a consensus that the following services should be provided: (1) diagnosis; (2) antiepileptic drug selection and long-term treatment; (3) psychological evaluation and treatment (especially for psychogenic seizure cases); and (4) surgical intervention.

A. Diagnostic services
    1. Electrodiagnostic
        a. Twenty-four–hour video-EEG monitoring with surface and sphenoidal electrodes with supervision by an EEG technologist or epilepsy staff nurse supported when appropriate by a monitoring technician or automated seizure and interictal activity detection computers
        b. Invasive 24-hour recording with subdural electrodes, depth electrodes, or epidural electrodes
        c. Intercarotid amobarbital or Wada testing
        d. Functional cortical mapping
        e. Electrocorticography
    2. Imaging
        a. Modern high-resolution magnetic resonance imaging (MRI)
        b. Computed axial tomography (CT)
        c. Cerebral angiography
        d. Possibly single photon emission computed tomographic (SPECT) scanning
        e. Possibly positron emission tomographic (PET) scanning
B. Medical treatment
    1. Pharmacologic expertise
        a. Epileptologist (neurologist) with special expertise in antiepileptic medications
        b. Individualized pharmacokinetic analysis
        c. Individualized pharmaceutical treatment plans for the patient
        d. Twenty-four–hour antiepileptic drug level service
        e. Quality-assured antiepileptic drug levels
C. Psychological evaluation
    1. Neuropsychological/psychosocial services
        a. Comprehensive psychogenic inpatient treatment
        b. Interventive/supportive inpatient and outpatient psychological and social services

      c. Comprehensive neuropsychological test battery for evaluation and localization of cerebral dysfunction as well as complete assessment of characterologic and psychopathologic issues

      d. Supervision of the neuropsychological testing component of the intra-carotid amobarbital test

      e. School services for children

D. Surgical treatment

    1. Epilepsy surgery. If epilepsy surgery is performed, it is expected that the center will be prepared to provide a full range of epilepsy surgical services. This includes:

      a. Emergency neurosurgery

      b. Complication management

      c. Open biopsy

      d. Stereotactic biopsy

      e. Excision of lesions

      f. Intracranial electrodes and cortical resection

      g. Corpus callosotomy

      h. Cortical resections, including hemispherectomy

      i. Clinical experience of greater than 25 cases per year

    2. Rehabilitation; inpatient and outpatient. The center should have available for its patients:

      a. Physical therapy

      b. Occupational therapy

      c. Speech therapy

      d. Vocational education

    3. Consultative expertise

      a. Psychiatry

      b. Other medical specialties

      c. Other surgical specialties

The guidelines recommend that neurologists be board certified in neurology with special training in invasive, intensive, neurodiagnostic monitoring per the American Clinical Neurophysiology Society guidelines, that the neurosurgeon be board certified with special interest and experience in epilepsy surgery, that other staff members be similarly trained, and that at least one physician be certified by the American Board of Clinical Neurophysiology.

Implicit in the guidelines is the concept of a team focused on the needs of the epilepsy program and not distracted by multiple hospital responsibilities. As hospitals attempt to reduce personnel costs to meet the changes in the health care system, existing teams are being threatened or dissolved. It is necessary to meet the spirit and not just the words of the guidelines.

Index

Note: Page numbers followed by f indicate figures; page numbers followed by t indicate tables.